D1238275

Bullets and Bandages

Bullets and Bandages

The Aid Stations and Field Hospitals at Gettysburg

James Gindlesperger

BLAIR

Copyright © 2020 by James Gindlesperger
All rights reserved

Printed in South Korea
Cover design by Callie Riek

Blair is an imprint of Carolina Wren Press.

The mission of Blair/Carolina Wren Press is to seek out, nurture, and promote literary work by new and underrepresented writers.

We gratefully acknowledge the ongoing support of general operations by the Durham Arts Council's United Arts Fund.

All rights reserved. No part of this publication may be reproduced, stored in a retrieval system, or transmitted in any form or by any means, electronic, mechanical, photocopying, recording, or otherwise without the prior permission of the copyright owner.

ISBN: 978-1-94-946742-0

Library of Congress Cataloging-in-Publication Data

Names: Gindlesperger, James, 1941– author.
Title: Bullets and bandages : the aid stations and field hospitals at Gettysburg / James Gindlesperger.
Other titles: Aid stations and field hospitals at Gettysburg
Description: Durham, NC : Blair, an imprint of Carolina Wren Press, [2021] | Includes bibliographical references and index. | Summary: "At Gettysburg, PA, during three days of July 1863, 160,000 men fought one of the most fierce and storied battles of the US Civil War. Nearly one in three of those men ended up a casualty of that battle, and when the two armies departed a few days later, 21,000 wounded remained. This book is the story of how those soldiers were cared for in a town of 2,500 people. Historian and author of several other guides to Gettysburg, James Gindlesperger provides a context for the medical and organizational constraints of the era and then provides details about the aid stations and field hospitals created in the aftermath of the battle. Filled with historical and contemporary photos, as well as stories about the soldiers and their healers, this book is a detailed guide for visitors to the site as well as others interested in American Civil War history"— Provided by publisher.
Identifiers: LCCN 2020014747 (print) | LCCN 2020014748 (ebook) | ISBN 9781949467420 (hardcover) | ISBN 9781949467437 (epub)
Subjects: LCSH: Gettysburg, Battle of, Gettysburg, Pa., 1863. | Military hospitals—Pennsylvania—Gettysburg—History—19th century. | United States—History—Civil War, 1861–1865—Hospitals. | United States—History—Civil War, 1861–1865—Medical care. | Gettysburg (Pa.)—History—19th century.
Classification: LCC E475.53 .G53 2020 (print) | LCC E475.53 (ebook) | DDC 973.7/349—dc23
LC record available at https://lccn.loc.gov/2020014747
LC ebook record available at https://lccn.loc.gov/2020014748

To Suzanne, my beautiful wife, travel companion, research partner, and best friend.

This book would never have been written without your realization

that the wounded and those who treated them had rarely received

the recognition they deserved.

And to Greg Coco,

who pioneered the study of Gettysburg field hospitals

Probably at no other place on this continent was there ever congregated
such a vast amount of human suffering.

Union Second Corps surgeon Justin Dwinell

Contents

Chapter 9   Baltimore Pike, East of US 15   199

Chapter 10   York Road/Hanover Road Area   223

Chapter 11   Old Harrisburg Road/ Hunterstown Road Area   241

Preface

THERE ARE THOUSANDS OF BOOKS ABOUT THE Battle of Gettysburg, and hundreds of new titles are written every year. The topics address every phase of the fighting, with many focusing on some particular detail of the battle, others studying troop movements or individual regiments, some looking at strategies and tactics, and still others broadening their investigation to the entire three days of the battle, or even to include the entire Gettysburg Campaign.

In our more than a quarter century of visiting Gettysburg and studying the battle, at some point my wife, Suzanne, pointed out that, among those thousands of works, there are only a handful dedicated to the aid stations and field hospitals that arose during and after the battle.

This realization haunted both of us, although we rarely talked about it. Eventually, though, while walking the battlefield in the vicinity of the McPherson barn one autumn day, the discussion took root: the wonderment of the carnage that had taken place in such a serene and beautiful location, the contrast between the horrors of those three days in July 1863 and the serenity of our surroundings, and finally, a bit of wonder that few people had taken the time to delve into the sufferings of those who had actually taken part in that epic battle, or those who did all they could to relieve those sufferings.

Then it struck us. Suzanne pointed out that we were just as guilty as anyone for not looking deeper into the pain of those who had seen and experienced the misery firsthand. We had several published books to our credit—why had we not done anything? Why were we wondering why someone else had not taken on the task? And the idea for this book was born.

We spend a lot of time in bookstores, and we learned that there were two books on field hospitals: *A Vast Sea of Misery* and *A Strange and Blighted Land*, written in the mid-1990s by a man we knew, Greg Coco. A licensed battlefield guide, Greg had reviewed one or two of our earlier books and, although we did not know him well, we knew him well enough to know we liked him. Unfortunately, he had passed away just a few years earlier, so we could not talk to him about his work. However, we were inspired to embark on our own project when we read the last sentence of Greg's introduction to *A Vast Sea of Misery*: "It is my anticipation that *A Vast Sea of Misery* will serve as only the forerunner of a more complex and elaborate work by some other writer in a not-too-distant day."

We accepted Greg's challenge, recognizing that there is still much to learn about this little-discussed topic. Along the way, Suzanne realized that writing this book would be difficult for her in light of the fact that it would take significant time away from some of her other projects. We both agreed that she would help with some of the research, particularly any that we could do on-site in Gettysburg, and I would take on the task of the actual writing. And so our roles evolved.

I have to admit that I felt some pangs of guilt, as if I had taken over her idea for the book. She assured me that this was not the case; that she actually felt some relief from the (self-induced) time pressure that came with the writing, and that she enjoyed the research part of the project more anyway. She insisted that she not be identified as coauthor, since she would do none of the writing. This is why, as you may have noticed, I dedicated the book in part to her. (Greg Coco is the other person to whom the book is dedicated, for all his early work.) Suzanne came up with the original idea. She helped with the research. She helped seek out some of the hard-to-find (and long-gone) hospital sites that are such an important part of the story. The least I could do was give her the credit she deserved.

The question of what actually constituted a hospital came next. Was it only the official hospitals established by the armies? Was it every house that provided even basic first aid to a passing soldier? For the purposes of this work, we arbitrarily decided on four criteria. The first was obvious: Was it officially established by a corps, division, or regiment as a hospital or aid station? The second criterion was the presence of multiple wounded. Third, if a doctor or surgeon was present, we considered it a hospital or aid station. Finally, we chose to include sites that may have only treated one wounded soldier if that soldier was of significant importance or presented an interesting story.

Many soldiers were treated in private homes that kept no specific records. Those homes are not included in this work. One such home is the John Hennig house at 45 W. High Street (39°49.717' N, 77°13.948' W). We only learned of the possibility that this family treated the wounded when we came across the obituary for Philip Hennig, which noted that Philip's parents, John and Susan Hennig, had cared for an unspecified number of wounded in their home during the battle. Unfortunately, no supporting documentation can be found for this claim. There were undoubtedly more homes like this.

Having chosen which sites to include as aid stations or hospitals, we then divided the battlefield and its surroundings into specific areas based roughly on geography. Each of these areas constitutes a chapter, headed by a map of that area. Numbers on the maps represent specific locations in that geographical area that we consider either an aid station or a hospital. In addition to showing its location on the map, we also include an address, if one exists, plus GPS coordinates to further aid the reader in locating the site. In some cases, current site owners asked that we not divulge their exact location, and we have honored those requests, listing the site's information without any address, map location, or GPS coordinates. This raises the obvious warning that most of these locations are privately owned, and we ask readers to respect that privacy. We found that most of these property owners are proud of their property and are more than willing to allow visitors to take photos or ask questions, as long as it is done with courtesy.

Using Greg Coco's wish that someone expand on what he had started as inspiration, we would issue the same invitation to others who wish to expand the research even further. Build on what we have learned. Grow the story. We owe it to those whose sufferings have been forgotten, and to those unsung heroes who opened their homes and farms to ease the pain of strangers.

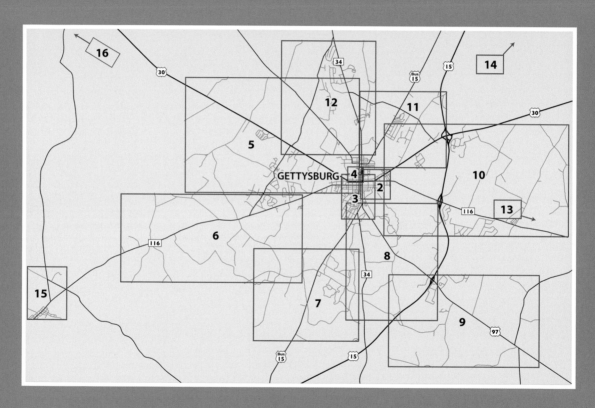

Gettysburg area map showing the areas discussed, with corresponding chapter numbers. (Map by Bill Nelson)

Prologue

On April 12, 1861, Confederate soldiers fired on Fort Sumter in South Carolina, launching what would become known in the North as the Civil War. The South referred to it by numerous names, including the War for Southern Independence, the War between the States, and others. No matter the name, the fighting would rage until April 9, 1865, when General Robert E. Lee surrendered his Army of Northern Virginia at Appomattox. Some smaller skirmishes continued after the surrender, but the Appomattox surrender ended any chance of success for the South and is generally recognized as the end of the war.

With an extra day for the leap year in 1864, those four years constituted 1,459 days. July 1–3, 1863, made up a minute portion of them, slightly more than 0.2 percent, to be exact. Yet on those three days the future of the nation hung in a precarious balance. During them, the Battle of Gettysburg saw approximately 160,000 combatants struggle to gain supremacy, with roughly one of every three becoming a casualty. Of these casualties, 7,058 were fatalities (3,155 Union, 3,903 Confederate). Another 33,264 had been wounded (14,529 Union, 18,735 Confederate) and 10,790 were missing (5,365 Union, 5,425 Confederate).[1] Of the wounded, some 21,000 would remain behind when the armies left town. Those 21,000 would have to be cared for. Neither army was equipped to treat casualties of such a magnitude. It would fall on the people of Gettysburg and the surrounding area to lend assistance, despite their own hardships.

In 1863 Gettysburg had a population of approximately 2,400. The 21,000 wounded represented a burden of nearly 9 wounded for every man, woman, and child in town. Because not all wounded were treated within the confines of the town itself, the ratio was obviously somewhat lower, but still significant, and the message was clear: it was going to be overwhelming.

Furthermore, it was not only the wounded whom the citizens had to accommodate. It was not long before thousands of outsiders arrived in town, compounding the hardship. Most of those outsiders came with good intentions. Many came as badly needed volunteers to assist the wounded. Others came to search for loved ones, not knowing what they would find. Would they be looking for a wounded son or husband, or would they be accompanying their loved one's remains back home?

Unfortunately, many of those who came had less altruistic motives. There were the inevitable curiosity seekers who appear after every disaster, even today. Local citizens tolerated this group of visitors, even if they preferred that they leave. Others, however, came to make a profit from the battle, most notably the grave robbers, looters, and those who charged inflated fees for their services, such as the itinerant coffin makers and embalmers, or the wagon owners who charged exorbitant fees to transport the wounded. In one blatant example, a local farmer was said to charge fifty cents for each wounded soldier he transported to the nearest field hospital. To maximize his profit, he made each man sit up, no matter how serious the wounds. This enabled the farmer to squeeze more passengers into his wagon. It was said that he could carry as many as eight wounded soldiers per trip in this manner.[2]

Whatever their purpose, those from outside the area all required shelter and food. Local citizen Sarah Broadhead wrote in her diary on July 13 that the town was being "overrun and eaten out by two large armies" and that there were ten thousand to twelve thousand visitors.[3] Her thoughts were echoed by Private William A. Rupp of the Twenty-Sixth Pennsylvania Infantry, who noted that, while on picket duty, he personally observed "hundreds of people from all parts of the country going to and coming from the Battle field [sic] at Gettysburg."[4]

But it was the wounded who raised the most concern. Very early it became apparent that divisional and regimental aid stations and field hospitals were not going to be able to treat them all. With so many needing treatment, the wounded began to take refuge anywhere they could find shelter, including private homes. Hundreds of houses, shops, and farms became refuges for the wounded. It was not long before virtually every church and public building was serving as a hospital, as well as several homes. Sergeant Wilfred McDonald of Company H, 118th Pennsylvania Infantry, noted in his diary, "Every house, woods, and barn is a hospital, and they are all full."[5]

The bullets had stopped. Their butchery was over. The task of caring for their victims was about to begin.

Bullets and Bandages

Chapter 1

Treatment of the Wounded

Early Medicine

Compared with today's standards for battlefield medicine, or even basic general medicine, medical knowledge and treatment during the Civil War was tragically crude. Hospitals were virtually unheard of, doctors received only minimal training, and physicians had no understanding of the causes of infection or effective medications to treat it.

It was the "heroic" era of medicine, an era characterized by the belief that diseases, especially those accompanied by fever, were caused by a collection of poisons in the body. The theory followed that the patient could be treated by removing those poisons, with the most popular removal methods being bleeding, cupping, sweating, skin blistering, and inducing vomiting. Surprisingly, even chest wounds were treated by inducing additional bleeding.[1] Conversely, it is not surprising that survival rates for these treatment methods were low.

Gradually these methods gave way to less harsh treatments that turned away from bleeding and the use of chemicals that we know today to be poisonous themselves, such as mercury. One of those updated theories relied on botanical treatment, using herbs. Another used homeopathy, relying on small doses of drugs that would cause symptoms in healthy people. A third was referred to as eclectic medicine, borrowing something from various types of practice (conventional, botanical, and homeopathic).[2]

There were about forty medical schools across the country by 1845, with an average faculty size of five to seven instructors. The number of medical schools increased slightly to about sixty by the time the Civil War broke out. The instructors were paid from the proceeds of attendance tickets sold to students who attended the lectures. Instruction consisted of two terms of six months each, with first-term classes in anatomy, chemistry, pharmacology, surgery, and diseases of women and children. These classes give mute testimony to the fact that there was still no knowledge of germ theory or antiseptic practices. The second term repeated the same classes and labs in the belief that students learned best by repetition. Following completion of this curriculum, students then usually apprenticed with a practicing physician.

Medical Organization of the Armies

When the Civil War broke out, the Confederate army emulated the organization that had already been established in the North. Each had a surgeon general with the rank of colonel who was in charge of all field and general hospitals. The surgeon general for the Union at the beginning of the war was Thomas Lawson. Unfortunately, Lawson died on May 15, 1861, with the war still in its infancy, and Clement Finley, a veteran of the Black Hawk War, succeeded Lawson. A rapid succession of surgeons general would follow. The South had only one surgeon general, Samuel Preston Moore, throughout the entire war. Before the war, Moore had served in the Medical Department of the US Army, and he structured the Medical Department of the Confederate Army after the North's system.

Reporting to the surgeon general were medical officers, including surgeons, assistant surgeons, and acting assistant surgeons. The acting assistant surgeons were usually private physicians serving as contractors. The Union army had thirty surgeons, given the rank of major, and eighty-four assistant surgeons with the rank of first lieutenant. The Confederate army had even fewer of each.

By the time general hospitals were established, the number of surgeons had increased, and each general hospital had a surgeon in charge, with assistant or acting assistant surgeons responsible for the individual wards.

Each regiment was assigned one surgeon and one or two assistant surgeons. They, in turn, supervised stewards, individual soldiers who were responsible for obtaining supplies, preparing food, and dispensing drugs. Nurses were used during times of battle, or for soldiers who fell ill or were injured. Those nurses usually were assigned from the ranks of the regiment or from the Nursing Corps. Both men and women served as nurses, although many questioned the propriety of using women in hospitals. As the war progressed, volunteers were utilized to supplement the nursing staffs, particularly when large battles required an abnormally high number of nurses.

With more soldiers dying from disease than from wounds, the Union army established a medical inspection staff in April 1862 that reported to the surgeon general. This unit continued to operate after the war concluded. The roles of the medical inspectors included monitoring sanitation conditions and the spread of disease in camps, hospitals, and prisons; providing recommendations for food and medical supplies; analyzing surgical procedures; and ensuring the validity of medical records. Deaths from illness were recorded and tracked, and the cleanliness and orderliness of kitchens, sleeping quarters, and toilet facilities were closely monitored. Even though it was not fully understood, a connection between cleanliness and disease had been established, and the inspectors were instructed to monitor drainage, water supply, and sewage in both camps and hospitals. At Gettysburg the inspectors included Surgeon Edward P. Vollum (US Regulars), Surgeon John M. Cuyler (Third Corps), Surgeon G. K. Johnston (First Michigan Cavalry), and Surgeon John H. Taylor (Army of the Potomac).[3] Cuyler was so diligent about his duty that when his scalpel slipped and he cut his finger while operating on a gangrenous wound at Gettysburg, he immediately had his own finger amputated to avoid contaminating his patients.[4]

The Letterman Plan

For the first year of the war, treatment of the wounded was haphazard at best. It was generally up to the wounded to find their way to an aid station or hospital. Those who could not walk often lay on the battlefield for several days. Many did not survive.

That changed for the Union army in June 1862 when Jonathan Letterman was named medical director. An 1849 graduate of Jefferson Medical College in Philadelphia, Letterman introduced many significant innovations that immediately improved conditions for the wounded. Taking over a department that was in disarray, Letterman created a system that utilized three areas of treatment. In the first, field dressing stations were established on or immediately adjacent to the battlefield. Here, the wounded received basic treatment. No operations were performed at these primary sites. The doctor there simply stabilized and dressed the wound, provided whiskey to prevent shock, or administered morphine for pain, if it was available. The physician then sent the less seriously wounded back to the battle. Concurrently, other attendants gathered the more seriously injured to an ambulance collecting point for removal by wheeled conveyances to the second, more serious level of treatment: the divisional field hospitals.

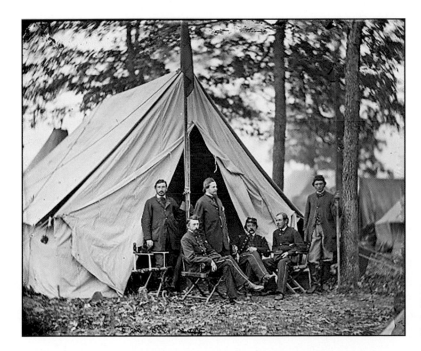

Letterman (seated on the left) and his staff. (Courtesy of Library of Congress, Reproduction Number LC-DIG-cwpb-03769)

This second level of Letterman's system required each division of the army to set up field hospitals in the rear of each unit before battle, away from the fighting but close enough for ambulances to reach quickly. The more seriously wounded were transferred from the dressing station to these field hospitals for further treatment. Three surgeons and three medical officers were assigned to each divisional hospital. These facilities, usually a home or barn not far from the battlefield but more protected than a dressing station, provided emergency surgery and amputations. Finally, those needing long-term treatment were sent from the field hospitals to larger facilities located some distance from the battlefield.

Letterman's plan also established a three-tiered organized triage plan. Priority was given to those whose wounds were deemed serious but survivable. Those with lesser wounds were only treated after the serious wounds had been addressed. The lowest priority was given to those who had suffered wounds so serious that their chances of survival were considered unlikely. Head, chest, or abdominal wounds were generally considered to be mortal, and the wounded were made comfortable and left alone to either recover or die.

While this resulted in better treatment for those in the first two categories, it relied on the judgment of the attending physicians, many of whom had never seen a gunshot wound before. Occasionally, it arbitrarily doomed some who might otherwise survive with treatment, or caused needless pain for those incorrectly triaged. One of the latter was Private John Chase of the Fifth Maine Battery, who was wounded an unimaginable forty-eight times when a case shot prematurely exploded as he was loading it into a cannon. Chase's right arm was shattered and his left eye blown out. He was taken to the farm of Isaac Lightner and given a cursory triage. Not expected to survive, he was placed outside the barn with no protection from the elements. Still alive after three days, he was given minimal treatment and moved inside the barn, where he lay for several more days in agony before being moved inside the house, where he stayed for another week, still not expected to survive. He was eventually relocated to the Lutheran Seminary, where he finally received more advanced treatment. He survived his wounds and was awarded the Medal of Honor in 1888 for his heroism at Chancellorsville just two months before he was wounded at Gettysburg.[5]

To address the problem of keeping the wounded lying on the battlefield until a battle was over, Letterman also established an ambulance corps for the first time. Before Letterman's plan was introduced, musicians and convalescents were often pressed into service as stretcher bearers and ambulance drivers, under command of the Quartermaster Department. Letterman took that responsibility away from the Quartermaster Department and instituted trained attendants. He also assigned one four-horse ambulance and two two-horse ambulances to each regiment, with three privates assigned to specific duties for each ambulance. Brigade officers were assigned to oversee the ambulance service, and brigades were assigned their own medicine and supply wagons.

Divisional ambulance trains were organized with forty to fifty ambulances and ten to fifteen supply wagons per train. Each ambulance had four stretchers and hand litters, plus a supply of bandages, lint, astringents, chloroform, whiskey, brandy, condensed milk, and concentrated beef soup. These supplies were to be used in an emergency only.

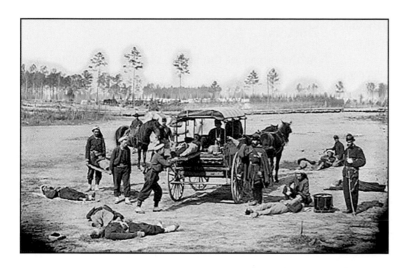

Zouave ambulance crew demonstrating removal of wounded. (Courtesy of Library of Congress, Reproduction Number LC-DIG-cwpb-03950)

Those assigned to the Ambulance Corps had the responsibility of removing the wounded from the battlefield as quickly as possible, no longer waiting until the battle was over, as had been the practice. This undoubtedly saved many lives, but proved to be dangerous duty for the men of the corps. Enemy troops fired indiscriminately at anyone in the line of fire, combatants and noncombatants alike. At Gettysburg one officer and four privates were killed and seventeen wounded while in the discharge of their ambulance duties. A number of horses were killed and wounded, and some ambulances damaged.[6]

Letterman's system also provided for blacksmiths to maintain the ambulances, or to assist as stretcher bearers as needed. The old two-wheel ambulances, called "gut busters" by the soldiers, were replaced by smoother, four-wheel types. Despite this, at Gettysburg and other large battles, the system became overwhelmed and both sides often had to resort to farm wagons when regular ambulances broke down.

Notwithstanding the efficiency of Letterman's plan, its effectiveness was hampered when orders were given to send all wagon trains except for ambulances and those carrying ammunition to the rear, between Union Mills and Westminster, Maryland. While Letterman still had his ambulances, many of his supplies were carried in wagon trains separate from the ambulances. Their removal to the rear deprived the Union army of the means of treating the wounded as quickly as it otherwise would have. The exception to this was the Twelfth Corps, which had its own medical wagons and ambulances and chose to ignore the order. This allowed it to provide faster treatment to its wounded.[7]

When the armies left Gettysburg, the Union army left six ambulances and four wagons from each corps to convey the wounded from their hospitals to the railroad depot for transportation to the outlying hospitals in Baltimore, Philadelphia, York, and Harrisburg. Because the Cavalry Corps had several ambulances captured at or near Hanover a few days before the fighting at Gettysburg, that corps only kept four ambulances behind.

Letterman also established organized plans for establishing better communication between surgical field hospitals and ordered that surgeons be selected based on their qualifications and abilities, rather than by rank. He also assigned specific personnel the tasks of organizing food tents, various supplies, and administrative duties, and all medical personnel had particular assignments on the day of battle. Even before the battle began, surgeons, assistant surgeons, hospital personnel, ambulance drivers, litter bearers, nurses, teamsters, and other attendants knew their posts and duties. That efficiency was credited with reducing the number of fatalities at Gettysburg.

Doctors

At the outset of the battle, some 650 surgeons were available to the Union army. When the armies left, however, that number decreased rapidly. Fearing another battle could be imminent, the Union took 544 of those doctors along, leaving only 106 Union surgeons and an unknown, but small, number of Confederate doctors to treat the 14,000 Union and 7,200 Confederate wounded. Of the Confederate wounded, 5,400 were too badly wounded to take part in the retreat. The remaining 1,800 were prisoners of war, many of whom had been wounded when they were captured and also required treatment, albeit at a lesser level.

Along with the doctors who were taken away after the battle, hundreds of attending nurses and stewards,

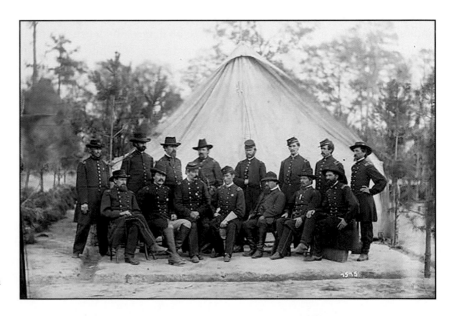

Second Division surgeons. (Courtesy of Library of Congress, Reproduction Number LC-DIG-cwpb-04060)

plus three thousand ambulance personnel, also left with the army, which was then pursuing Lee's scattered and retreating forces. This further depleted the number of medical personnel available for treating the wounded.

To alleviate the shortage, Surgeon General William Hammond sent twenty extra physicians. These were augmented by some seventy-five to one hundred civilian volunteer doctors. Among the doctors who served at Gettysburg but who were not shown in the records as having been assigned to a specific hospital were Surgeon George L. Cook (volunteer), civilian surgeon John Dickson, civilian volunteer surgeon Joseph Dickson, civilian volunteer surgeon Thomas J. Gallaher, Dr. Thomas W. Shaw (civilian volunteer), Dr. A. W. Arewald, a Dr. Brown, a Dr. Davenport (from Michigan), a Dr. Gorton (from Michigan), a Dr. Gunn (from Michigan), a Dr. Kin (from New York), a Dr. Ladd, Dr. S. Weir Mitchell, a Dr. Quackenbush (from New York, who may have been representing the Surgeon General's Office), a Dr. Stonedale, and a Dr. Ellerslie Wallace.

The civilian doctors may or may not have been of much help. Justin Dwinell of the Second Corps had between seventeen and thirty doctors available to him at various times between July 4 and August 8 when the Second Corps hospital closed, many of them civilians. Dwinell spoke for many army doctors when he bluntly assessed the civilian doctors, saying that they only showed up for the free breakfast, watched the army doctors for a while, then disappeared. He noted that they did not like dressing wounds and seemed only to be interested in "taking off limbs."

Dwinell did not limit his criticism to the civilian doctors. He had a similar opinion of the hundreds of able-bodied skulkers who invaded these hospital areas under the guise of helping but who only "consume the food and occupy the shelter provided for the wounded."[8]

One of the more colorful volunteer doctors at Gettysburg was Mary Walker. Walker tried to become an army surgeon when the Civil War broke out but was refused because of her gender. Uninterested in becoming a nurse, she volunteered first at a temporary

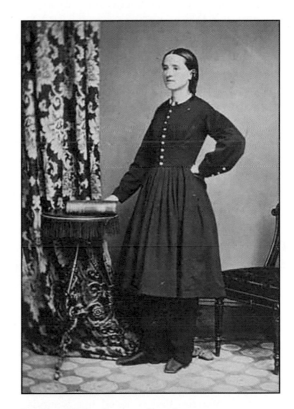

Dr. Mary Walker became the only woman to be awarded a Medal of Honor. (Courtesy of Library of Congress, Reproduction Number LC-DIG-ppmsca-19911)

hospital in Washington, then at various field hospitals. Along the way, she began wearing a calf-length skirt over men's trousers, and a military jacket. Her attire was often finished off with a low silk hat. She would become a prisoner of war in 1864, released later in a prisoner exchange.

As a way of recognizing her service, President Andrew Johnson presented her with the Medal of Honor in January 1866, making her the only woman to receive the award. In 1916 Congress revised the Medal of Honor standards to include only actual combat with an enemy, and a year later 912 Medals of Honor were rescinded, including Walker's. Ever the contrarian, when the army's judge advocate general ruled that the army did not have authorization to require that the medals be returned, Walker opted to keep hers and wore it for the rest of her life as a show of pride and defiance. In 1977 her Medal of Honor award was restored.

Surgeons operated virtually around the clock with little rest. The stress took a toll on them all. Surgeon Cyrus Bacon, who served at the Jacob Weikert farm with the Union's Fifth Corps, noted that of the eleven surgeons on duty there at different periods, eight were taken ill, including Bacon himself, who was seized with an inflammatory diarrhea. At one point Bacon was so exhausted that he fell asleep across the operating table.[9]

Treatments became personal. At Pennsylvania College, Dr. L. P. Warren of Pettigrew's North Carolina Brigade was able to save the life of his own eighteen-year-old brother, Lieutenant John C. Warren. The younger Warren had suffered five wounds and had been thought to be beyond help.[10]

While every effort was made to set up field hospitals in relatively secure areas, they were still in a war zone, and thirteen medical staff were wounded at Gettysburg. One, Assistant Surgeon W. S. Moore of the Sixty-First Ohio Infantry, suffered a thigh wound while serving at an aid station near the Catherine Guinn home on Cemetery Hill and died of his wounds on July 6.

Nurses

As in every war, the unsung heroes were the nurses, both professional and those who were pressed into service, often involuntarily, by the presence of wounded men in their homes. In addition to treating the wounded, changing bandages, and feeding those

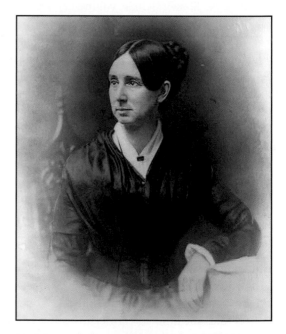

Dorothea Dix. (Courtesy of Library of Congress, Reproduction Number LC-USZ62-9797)

who could not feed themselves, nurses wrote letters home and sat with dying soldiers to provide comfort. The stories of their work at Gettysburg are legion.

When it became apparent that the war was not going to be over in a matter of months, as officials on both sides had originally thought, sixty-one-year-old Dorothea Dix proposed that women perform the nursing duties previously performed by men. Her thinking was that this would free up more men to do the actual fighting. After several months of fighting, accompanied by more and more wounded needing treatment, Union secretary of war Simon Cameron agreed and authorized Dix to organize a female nursing corps, with Dix as its head.

The US Bureau of Nursing that she organized labored under draconian rules, all established by Dix. Applicants had to be plain looking, could only dress in brown or black, and had to be available day or night. Further, no hoop skirts, curls, bows, or jewelry were permitted, and applicants under the age of thirty were not considered, no matter how impressive their credentials. A strict Unitarian, Dix decreed that only Protestants would be considered, a rule that caused friction between her and some of the non-Protestant organizations that came to Gettysburg to help. Dix quickly gained a reputation as one who was difficult to work with, garnering such unflattering nicknames as "Dragon Dix" and the "Dictator in a Petticoat."[11]

Almost immediately, outside organizations began arriving to assist in treating the wounded. Among the first to appear were the Sisters of Charity from nearby Emmitsburg, Maryland, under the direction of Father James Francis Burlando. Traveling on roads made nearly impassable by heavy rains, eight Sisters of Charity arrived the day after the battle concluded.

Father Burlando noted, "We were compelled to drive cautiously to avoid passing over the dead. Our terrified horses drew back or darted forward reeling from one side to the other. The further we advanced the more harrowing the scene; we could not restrain our tears."[12]

The priest's observations were not exaggerated. Carrying food, bandages, sponges, and clothing, the small group made their way around puddles red with blood and countless pieces of weaponry and other military accoutrements that had been discarded. The short trip from Emmitsburg was made longer by the number of wounded that they encountered. Reasoning that they were coming to Gettysburg to assist the wounded, they began providing aid to those they encountered along the way, long before they reached the battlefield. After providing basic assistance, the sisters transported the wounded to locations where farm wagons were gathered to convey them to field hospitals.

The dead, both human and animal, littered the approach to Gettysburg. Already beginning to decompose in the summer heat, the stench forced Father Burlando and the Sisters of Charity to cover their noses to avoid becoming physically ill. Eventually, there were so many bodies that the horses balked and reared, refusing to go any farther until led by hand. Sentinels stood guard over the bodies as they were being prepared for burial. Others could be seen digging graves.

Just outside town, Burlando and his group encountered pickets, still edgy from the three days of fighting. Thinking that they may have been Confederate sympathizers, the pickets leveled their weapons at them. Burlando waved a white handkerchief, which was ignored because the pickets had been given orders not to recognize any flag of truce. Only when the eight sisters got out of their wagons so the pickets could see them better was the tension relieved. Hearing of their mission, the pickets provided an escort to allow them to pass through later checkpoints.

Once in town, Father Burlando dispersed his charges in teams of two, with two going to each of St. Francis Xavier Roman Catholic Church, the Methodist Episcopal Church on East Middle Street (now the Grand Army of the Republic Hall), and the Pennsylvania College. The remaining two returned to Emmitsburg to prepare others to come the next day. Altogether, some forty representatives of the Sisters of Charity ultimately served in Gettysburg hospitals.

Also arriving were the US Sanitary Commission (USSC) and the US Christian Commission. The USSC was a private relief agency created by federal legislation shortly after the war began, to provide help and comfort to sick and wounded soldiers. This forerunner of the American Red Cross worked with the Army Medical Department to improve sanitation and provide well-ventilated hospitals. The USSC did nursing and general hospital work, directed battlefield aid, and collected medicines, food, clothing, and personal items, distributing supplies to both sides. It set up a storehouse about a mile north of White Church, on Baltimore Pike, and eventually moved into Fahnestock's store in town. When the army began sending the lesser wounded to hospitals in cities such as Baltimore and Philadelphia, the USSC established a place for the wounded to wait, providing additional aid until the wounded could board the trains.

While the USSC focused on the physical benefits to be derived from good sanitation, cleanliness, and fresh food, the US Christian Commission focused more on spiritual and emotional benefits, while also

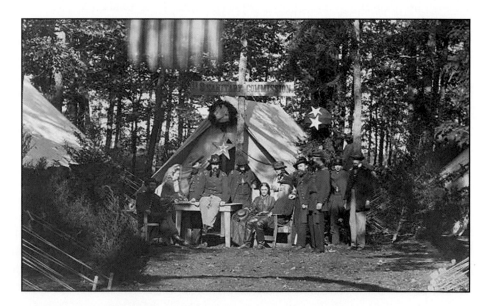

Headquarters of the US Sanitary Commission at Camp Letterman. (Courtesy of Library of Congress, Reproduction Number LC-DIG-ppmsca-33752)

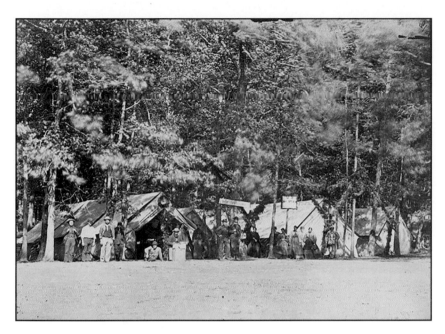

The US Christian Commission at Camp Letterman. (Courtesy of Library of Congress, Reproduction Number LC-DIG-ppmsca-33638)

providing assistance to the wounded. Based in Philadelphia and supported by the YMCA, the commission set up its headquarters in the Stoever-Schick Building in town, with an annex across the street in what was then the Apollo Hall. From there it passed out bibles, stationery, and food, while providing medical and spiritual guidance to soldiers. Over the next several weeks, the commission set up stations in each corps hospital except the Sixth.

Sarah Broadhead, a local civilian who served as a nurse in both her own home and at the Lutheran Seminary, praised both organizations, writing in her diary on July 9, 1863, "The merciful work of the Sanitary and Christian Commissions, aided by private contributions, was to be seen at every hospital."[13]

Other organizations that assisted the wounded at Gettysburg included the Women's Central Association of Relief, the Soldiers' Aid Society of Northern Ohio, the New England Women's Auxiliary Association, the Northwestern Sanitary Commission, the General Aid Society for the Army, the Michigan Soldiers' Aid Society, the Wisconsin Soldiers' Aid Society, the Department of the South, the St. Louis Ladies' Union Aid Society, the Patriot Daughters of Lancaster, Ladies' Aid Society of Philadelphia, the Hospital Corps of Adams Express Company, the Fireman's Associations of Baltimore, the Soldiers' Relief Society of Philadelphia, the New York Soldiers' Relief Agency, the Germantown Field Hospital Association, the Indiana Soldiers' Relief Agency, the Soldiers' Aid

Association of Philadelphia, and the Benevolent Society of East Thompson, Massachusetts.

Hundreds of private citizens also assisted, some in their own homes, others in one of the scores of hospitals that were created. Many carved out reputations that are still talked about. One of those was a ninety-eight-pound nurse at Pennsylvania College. Born in Maryland, Euphemia Goldsborough, or Miss Effie, as she was known to the wounded in her care, made no attempt to hide her allegiance to the South. When the Confederate wounded were being moved to other facilities, they gave her a book of letters and signatures of one hundred of her patients as a show of appreciation for her work. One soldier hand-carved a wooden ring for her with the name Effie on its face.[14]

Cornelia Hancock, of the Second Corps, Third Division Union Hospital, evoked the same type of admiration from those in her charge. As their stay at the division hospital neared its end, the men pooled their money and gave her a twenty-dollar silver medallion with the inscription on one side, "Miss Cornelia Hancock, presented by the wounded soldiers 3rd Division, 2nd Army Corps." The other side said, "Testimonial of regard for ministrations of mercy to the wounded soldiers at Gettysburg, Pa.—July 1863."[15] Hancock had been turned down for admission to the Bureau of Nursing by Dorothea Dix. She was only twenty-three years old.

Helen Gilson was yet another nurse turned down by Dix. Young (twenty-eight years old) and attractive, the independent nurse from Massachusetts distinguished herself at the Schwartz farm by her compassion. She was singled out by many of the men, as well as both the Christian Commission and the Sanitary Commission in their formal reports, for the respect the wounded accorded her. She tended to their wounds, fed them, sang to them to calm their fears, read to them, wrote letters for them, sat with many dying men until they drew their last breath, and calmed arguments. On occasion she even assisted with amputations and conducted religious services. She also took it upon herself to forward personal effects of the dead to their families. She did the same at Fredericksburg, Antietam, the Peninsula Campaign, Chancellorsville, Morris Island, Brandy Station, the Wilderness, Spotsylvania, Cold Harbor, Petersburg, and other lesser battles.[16]

One of the nurses at the Jacob Weikert farm was Mary "French Mary" Tepe. Considered a bit eccentric, Tepe wore a uniform that consisted of a blue Zouave

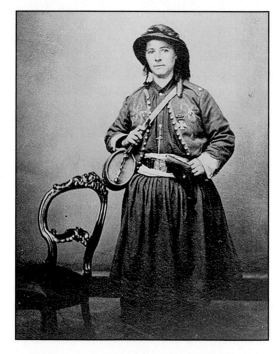

Mary Tepe, a.k.a. French Mary. (Courtesy of National Archives, Local Identifier 79-T-2148)

jacket, a short skirt trimmed with red braid that reached to just below the knees, and red trousers over a pair of boots. The ensemble was completed by a turned-down sailor hat. Over her shoulder she carried a small keg containing contraband whiskey, which she sold to the soldiers, commanding a price of five dollars a pint. Although the soldiers protested the price, she must have had plenty of customers, and she was said to have earned a tidy sum. Recognizing that soldiers also enjoyed cigars, hams, and tobacco, she added those to her inventory. With Annie Etheridge, Tepe had been awarded the Kearny Cross of Honor for her bravery at Chancellorsville. The two women were the only ones among the three hundred awardees that day. In true French Mary fashion, she refused to accept it.[17]

The task of providing spiritual comfort to the dying, as well as assisting as needed in nursing the wounded, came under the purview of the chaplains. Dozens of Union chaplains filled that need, and each infantry division of the Confederate army was ordered to leave behind one chaplain as well. Anderson's Division chose to leave two behind. Confederate chaplains who stayed back during the retreat included Crawford H. Toy of the Fifty-Third Georgia (McLaws's Division), Peter Tinsley of the Thirty-Eighth Virginia (Pickett's Division), George E. Beitler of the Third Arkansas (Hood's Division), John L. Pettigrew of the Thirty-First Georgia (Early's Division), Harvey Gilmore of the Twenty-First Virginia (Johnson's Division), Joseph W. Murphy of the Thirty-Second North Carolina (Rodes's Division), John M. Stokes of the Third Georgia and J. Osgood A. Cook of the Second Georgia Battalion (Anderson's Division), and William Burton Owen of the Eleventh Mississippi (Heth's Division). Presumably Pender's Division also kept one chaplain

back, but his name is not recorded. It could reasonably be assumed that, much like the doctors, chaplains would rarely be exposed to enemy fire, but as many as twenty-five chaplains died from their wounds during the war, although none died at Gettysburg.

Sallie Myers, a private citizen who said she got sick at the sight of blood yet went to St. Francis Xavier Catholic Church to do her part, may have summed up the feelings of those who served as nurses when she said, "The sight of blood never again affected me and I was among the wounded and dying men day and night. . . . I shall always be thankful that I was permitted to minister to the wants and soothe the last hours of some of the brave men who lay suffering and dying for the dear old flag."[18]

Hospitals

Wounded men knew to look for the nearest aid station for their initial treatment. The sheer number of wounded often made this impractical, however, and many either made their own way or were carried by comrades directly to a field hospital, which was designated by a red or yellow flag. Others, desperate for help, stopped at the first farm or house they encountered, forcing many homes to become unwilling aid stations. Dozens of private homes thus became small hospitals where citizens nursed the wounded.

The sites for field hospitals were left up to the medical staff, who looked for places somewhat distant from the actual fighting while still accessible by ambulance. Often this had to be nothing more than an old barn or a small grove of trees.

Arriving at a field hospital did not mean a soldier's problems were over. Understaffing and overcrowding meant that an individual may not receive rapid care, or even so much as a blanket. Set up quickly under less than ideal conditions, field hospitals were often disorganized and underequipped. Operations and amputations were carried out in near-primitive conditions, with little or no concern for those wounded who lay in the immediate area. A constant cacophony of groaning, crying men begging for help or calling for their mother assaulted the senses of those unable to avoid the din. The sights were no less offensive, as attested to by H. S. Peltz, who wrote in the *Gettysburg Compiler* several years after the war. Time had not diminished the impact, as Peltz recalled, "I noticed with horror, as I assisted the dressing of a bleeding wound, that the blood of the patient (on the floor) above filtered through the cracks . . . and dripped upon the sufferers below."[19]

Wounded soldiers lay on the bare ground in the open, with no shelter from the weather or the thousands of biting blowflies that seemed to appear out of nowhere. Regarding this, Nurse Jane Boswell Moore wrote of the Union's Second Corps hospital, "Scarcely had one man out of a thousand anything more than the ground, covered with an old blanket or oil cloth, to lay on, and hundreds had undergone amputation since the battle. Miserable little shelter-tents alone protected them from the rain, whilst numbers of the poor wretched Rebels had not even these, but were exposed through all the heavy rain of Tuesday night, with scarcely covering enough to keep warm in dry weather."[20]

Lack of sanitation, although already mentioned, cannot be overemphasized. Most of the hospitals outside town lacked clean water. Rain began on July 4 and continued almost daily. Runoff carried the detritus of the battlefield: human waste from thousands of soldiers, the blood of the wounded that had pooled and then soaked into the ground, and the products of decomposition of human remains hastily buried in shallow, inadequate graves.

More than seventy thousand horses and mules had arrived with the two armies, producing several hundred gallons of urine and nearly two thousand tons of manure.[21] Runoff carried all this material through camps where wounded and dying men lay on the bare ground, ending up in creeks that were used for drinking water and for what passed as scrubbing and cleaning water.

The air surrounding these hospitals was similarly foul, not only from the camps themselves but also from the surrounding area. In addition to the odor of corpses decomposing in the summer heat, the remains of some five thousand horses that had also been killed added to the unpleasantness, a smell that changed to the odor of burning horseflesh when the unfortunate animals were dragged into piles and burned. Overall, the air in Gettysburg and its surrounds became so sickening that many citizens carried bottles of pennyroyal and peppermint to apply under their nostrils to block out the stench.

Confederate hospitals were more spread out than the Union's because so many were established as the Southerners retreated. Logistically, this compounded an already difficult situation for the Southern army. The wounded now had to be cared for while the army was on the move, and obtaining supplies became even more challenging. Many of the wounded Confederates were in no condition to be moved, leaving the responsibility for their treatment to a Union army already struggling under the load of treating its own, or the put-upon citizens of Gettysburg.

Hospitals in town were subject to being hit by artillery, as they were the first established while the fighting was at its peak. Union artillery fire badly wounded an attendant for Dr. James L. Farley, taking off his thumb. The rear of the Washington House Hotel was also struck, blowing out an entire wall and showering patients with dust and debris.

The phrase "every house a hospital" was often used to describe the conditions in the aftermath of the battle. Although this is an exaggeration, the point is well taken that the hospital system as it had been planned quickly became overwhelmed, leading to untold suffering and needless deaths.

Treatment

Wounds at Gettysburg were a microcosm of all battlefield wounds. Most were caused by projectiles from rifles or muskets, called minié balls. These lead bullets were heavy (.45 and .69 caliber) and traveled relatively slowly, tearing tissue and organs when they struck a body. Bones hit by a minié ball were usually so shattered that they could not be saved. As a result, the shattered limb was typically amputated.

After bullet wounds, injuries from shell fragments caused the second most common type of battle injury. The last wound category, saber blows and bayonets, caused relatively few wounds compared with bullets and shell fragments.

When a soldier was wounded, his first line of care was at a field dressing station. There, a bandage or lint dressing was applied, and whiskey was given for shock and morphine for pain. The injured man was then either returned to battle or transported to a field hospital.

At the field hospital, usually a barn or tent but sometimes just an open field, the wounded were triaged. Wounds to the chest or abdomen usually were considered mortal and treatment consisted of keeping the unfortunate victims as comfortable as possible (usually with opium) until they died.

For those needing surgery, laudanum would often be given before the operation. When laudanum was not available, brandy became an acceptable substitute. The injured was then placed on a makeshift table, the bleeding was controlled, and the wound was probed, usually with the surgeon's fingers, to remove any foreign objects, including bullet fragments, bits of clothing, or pieces of splintered bone. With no knowledge of sepsis, surgeons rarely washed their hands during extremely busy times, and instruments were rinsed with bloody water. Sponges and cloths were reused. There was little attempt at sanitation as we know it today. Feces, urine, vomit, amputated limbs, and removed internal organs all littered the operating floor.

Anesthesia, which was used in 95 percent of Civil War surgeries, would then be administered. Despite the romantic notion of having the patient bite down on a bullet, it actually was a rare occurrence. Chloroform was the preferred anesthetic, although ether was also used. Smaller dosages of chloroform were needed, as opposed to ether, and it had a much more rapid effect. It was also more stable than ether and could safely be used around open flame.

The chloroform was administered by placing the anesthetic on a sponge at the top of a cone and placing the open end of the cone over the patient's nose and mouth. It was administered gradually to avoid shock. Once the patient was unconscious, the cone was removed. The average time needed for the administration of chloroform was nine minutes.

Ether, on the other hand, took an average of seventeen minutes to work. When it was used, the preferred method of administration was to use a folded towel or bell-shaped sponge that was large enough to cover the nose and mouth. This was then soaked with the anesthetic.

Only a low dose of anesthetic was used during the Civil War, just enough to make the patient insensitive to pain. In some cases, men did not lose consciousness despite the anesthesia. Witnesses reported patients thrashing wildly and shrieking in pain throughout the operation. Adding to the chaos were soldiers begging to be taken next, to relieve their suffering. At the same time, many of those requiring amputation protested vehemently, all adding to the stress of the surgeons.

Three of every four surgeries required amputation, leading to the unfair characterization of surgeons as butchers. As previously noted, the minié ball did such devastating damage that saving a limb, particularly under battlefield hospital conditions and time constraints, was virtually impossible.

A typical amputation began as soon as the patient was anesthetized. The surgeon would wipe any blood off his scalpel that remained from the previous patient, then proceed with little or no additional sterilization. He deftly cut flesh and tissue above and below the wound, cutting to the bone and leaving a small semi-circular-shaped flap of skin, which would be used to close the wound after the procedure was completed. A bone saw was then used to cut through the bone, with the severed limb tossed onto a nearby pile from previous amputations. Amputated limbs would only

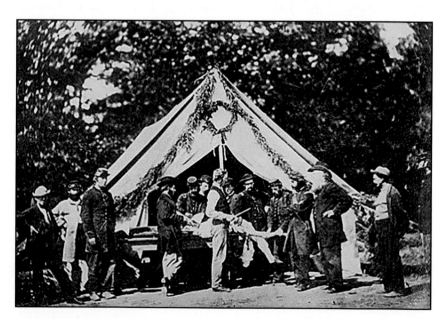

An amputation being performed at Camp Letterman. (Courtesy of National Archives, Local Identifier 79-T-2265)

be removed when the pile grew so large that it became a hindrance.

With the limb successfully removed, arteries were then tied off with cotton thread. If thread was not available, horsehair would be used. Those whose arteries were tied off with horsehair saw faster recovery than those with cotton thread, although there was no recognition of this phenomenon at the time. It would be some time before it became apparent that boiling the stiff horsehair to make it supple enough for use had the added benefit of sterilization.

Sharp edges of remaining bone would then be scraped to make them smoother, although many surgeons skipped this step. The flap of skin that had been left when the surgeon cut through the muscle and tissue was then folded over the open stump and sewed shut, leaving a small opening for drainage. The entire stump was then covered with a piece of cloth, which in turn was coated with a form of gelatin made from fish bladders, called isinglass. This dried to a rugged but flexible cover to keep the wound relatively dry and clean. Unfortunately, the cloth used was often just a dirty rag that may have been used earlier.

The patient was then removed from the table and placed wherever space could be found, often in a filthy barnyard. Many amputees who survived said that their wounds never healed completely, necessitating periodic draining for the rest of their lives. It is no surprise that a wounded soldier was as likely to die of infection as he was to die of his actual wounds.

While amputating a limb seems like a long and laborious process, a good surgeon could perform an amputation in about twelve minutes from start to finish, and as many as seventy thousand to eighty thousand amputations took place over the course of the war.

The mortality rate for amputations depended a great deal on what part of the body was amputated. The lowest rate of mortality was for amputated fingers, with only 3 percent of those victims not surviving. Amputated toes resulted in a mortality of 6 percent. Those who lost an arm saw mortality rates of 14 percent if the amputation was below the elbow, 24 percent if it involved the upper arm. One of every three who had their lower leg amputated did not survive, a number that jumped to 54 percent if the leg was amputated at midthigh and 58 percent if the knee joint was the site. The highest mortality rate was 83 percent, for those who had their amputation at the hip.[22]

When all the amputations had been completed, the surgeon could now turn his attention to those with lesser injuries. Many of those who had been triaged to this category did not receive treatment for several days if there were many with more serious wounds, which was nearly always the case. Nurse Cornelia Hancock wrote that five days after the battle ended, "there [were] hundreds of brave fellows who ha[d] not had their wounds dressed since the battle."[23]

These patients also had their wounds probed to remove any foreign objects. For smaller wounds, treatment methods varied from surgeon to surgeon. Many used "home remedies" with surprisingly good results. Other wounds were treated with the application of a dressing. Smaller wounds usually received a dressing of flaxseed or bread poultice. Large wounds were covered with cotton dipped in cold water. If bandages were not available, cornhusks were used.

Some wounds were left unbandaged to promote drainage of "laudable pus," which was believed to be beneficial. Many doctors thought pus had to form to aid the healing process, not knowing that pus was indicative of infection. Considering the state of medical knowledge at the time of the Civil War, it is not surprising that many of the wounded let their wounds heal on their own, rather than have them treated at a field hospital.

Both sides used similar medicines, but the North had better infrastructure to deliver those medicines to its field hospitals, despite the decision at the beginning of the battle to relegate the supply wagons to the rear. Letterman alluded to this problem several times during and after the battle. In his official report he wrote, "I may here instance the hospital of the Twelfth Corps, in which the transportation was not reduced nor the wagons sent to the rear at Gettysburg. Surgeon [John] McNulty, medical director of that corps, reports that '. . . it is with extreme satisfaction that I can assure you that it enabled me to remove the wounded from the field, shelter, feed them, and dress their wounds within six hours after the battle ended, and to have every capital operation performed within twenty-four hours after the injury was received.'"[24]

While Letterman's complaints had some merit, the Confederates had their own problems, including the logistics of moving supplies in an unfamiliar and unfriendly area. There were very few sources for medical instruments in the South, and the blockade made it even worse, as many surgeons on both sides got their instruments from Europe. Instruments on ships destined for Northern ports got through, but those hoping to reach Southern ports were only successful if they were able to run the blockade.

Both sides had labs capable of producing medicines, but once again Lee's army often encountered problems that hampered production or delivery. An example of this was noted by a druggist in Alabama, who reported that he could manufacture high-quality medicinal alcohol but could not get glass bottles to ship it.[25]

These issues, along with the huge number of wounded, overwhelmed the system at Gettysburg. Further, the success or failure of wound treatment was complicated by the generally poor physical condition of most Civil War soldiers. Recruits were supposed to have a physical examination, but these were usually very superficial. Many entered their service with chronic diseases. Others acquired illnesses in camps, having never been exposed to disease. This was especially true of Southern soldiers, most of whom had grown up on farms with little interaction with large groups of people outside their own families.

Unsanitary camp conditions added to the misery. Poor diets saw many on both sides come down with scurvy, caused by vitamin deficiencies created by the lack of fresh vegetables. Typhoid, dysentery, and chronic diarrhea, magnified by contaminated water supplies and generally poor sanitation, were prevalent. Long, difficult marches, often in severe weather conditions, further wore down the troops, lowering their resistance and making it more difficult to recover from even the slightest injury. The result was that diseases were far more responsible for Civil War deaths than wounds, with nearly two of every three deaths coming from disease.[26]

Burials

Considering that many of the dead lay for several days in the heat of July, it is immediately apparent that burial of the dead was a task that was beyond distasteful. Expediency dictated that the dead be buried where they were found, where feasible. Most of the Union dead were buried by their own regiments, particularly those in the Eleventh and Twelfth Corps.

During the day and night of July 4, Union soldiers who were not assigned burial duty went out into the fields looking for fallen comrades. The first burial parties were sent out at dusk that same day and the men were instructed to stay out until midnight, burying Union and Confederate soldiers alike wherever they had fallen. An unnamed New Jersey soldier graphically described what he saw:

Burial Parties were sent out, and those who could get away from their commands went out to view the scene of carnage, and surely it was a scene never to be forgotten. Upon the open fields, like sheaves bound by the reaper, in crevices of the rocks, behind fences, trees and buildings; in thickets, where they had crept for safety only to die in agony; by stream or wall or hedge, wherever the battle had raged or their waking steps could carry them, lay the dead. Some with faces bloated and blackened beyond recognition, lay with glassy eyes staring up at the blazing summer sun; others, with faces downward and clenched hands filled with grass or earth, which told of the agony of the last moments. Here a headless trunk, there a severed limb; in all the grotesque positions that unbearable pain and intense suffering contorts the human form, they lay. Upon the faces of some death had frozen a smile; some showed the trembling shadow of fear, while upon others was indelibly set the grim stamp of determination. All around was the wreck the battle-storm leaves in its wake—broken caissons, dismounted guns, small arms bent and twisted by the storm or dropped and scattered by disabled hands; dead and bloated horses, torn and ragged equipment, and all the sorrowful wreck that the waves of battle leave at their ebb; and over all, hugging the earth like a fog, poisoning every breath, the pestilential stench of decaying humanity.[27]

Despite the admonition to bury Confederate soldiers as well as their own, some Union burial details chose to take care of their own first. Only after all their comrades had been buried did the grim task of burying the enemy dead begin. Some burial details also took shortcuts by throwing bodies, or body parts that had been amputated or shot off, into wells. This was only discovered when those using the well water complained of getting sick.

Southern prisoners of war were also used to bury their dead until the prisoners were moved to Northern prisons. Mass graves were utilized, with the Confederate dead buried in trenches, often 150 or more in a single mass grave. Confederates who died in the field were usually unidentified when they were buried. Those who died in hospitals usually, but not always, had marked graves. Even the dead who were identified often became unknowns as farmers plowed over graves in the years following the war.

Robert P. Nevin of the Christian Commission described the typical burial of dead Confederate soldiers: "Hour by hour they die off, are carried to the trenches, a foot or two deep, in which they are to lie. They are laid side by side conveniently to those trenches and remain there in continually increasing groups until the parties whose duty it is come around

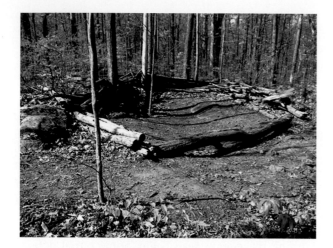

An unknown Confederate grave can be visited on Culp's Hill, a short distance behind the Second Maryland Battalion (Confederate States of America) monument. The logs are no longer there.

to tend to their interment. It is awful, it is terrible, it is horrible beyond expression."[28]

With most of the dead interred in temporary graves across the battlefield, the unenviable task of disinterring Federal dead for reburial in the new national cemetery began in late summer. Bids were solicited from civilian contractors, with F. W. Biesecker receiving the contract for $1.59 for each body disinterred. In turn, Biesecker hired Samuel Weaver to serve as the overseer of the exhumations. Weaver was not inexperienced at the task, also working closely with Dr. John W. C. O'Neal in the identification of Confederate remains and the salvaging of personal effects from Confederate bodies for shipment to their families in the South.

One of those who assisted Weaver was Basil Biggs, a local veterinarian, whose job was to place the bodies into coffins and transport them to the cemetery for reburial. Biggs had a two-horse team and was able to haul nine coffins on each load, while those who had only a one-horse team could only haul six.

The Confederates, for the most part, remained where they were originally buried until about 1871, when 385 sets of remains were shipped to Raleigh, Savannah, and Charleston by Rufus Weaver, son of Samuel Weaver. Rufus Weaver was the demonstrator of anatomy at Hahnemann Medical College in Philadelphia, and he had taken on the task of returning Confederate remains after his father died.

The next summer, the Ladies' Memorial Association of Richmond hired Rufus Weaver to disinter their sons and husbands on a larger scale and ship them home for burial in Southern soil. The negotiated price was $3.25 per body.

Under this contract he shipped 3,320 sets of remains to the South. The bulk of these went to Richmond, with 2,935 bodies shipped in numbered boxes, where they were interred in trenches in Hollywood Cemetery. Records of where each box was buried were either lost or never kept, and the locations of specific bodies have been lost to history.

Weaver's bill came to $9,536, indicating that he may have given a slight discount to individual families. Whatever the final agreement, he only received $2,800 because the memorial association defaulted on the agreement when it did not receive the full anticipated compensation for burials and acquisition of new ground.

Families requesting the return of their loved ones had the option of having the bodies embalmed, a service not widely practiced before the war. The work was done by embalming surgeons who often followed the armies, knowing there would be a need for their services at some point.

Embalming was not regulated in 1863, leading to wide variations in costs. It was inevitable that fraud would become a problem. Private Justus Silliman of the Seventeenth Connecticut wrote, "Gettysburg has been an extensive coffin mart and embalmer's harvest field. . . . These coffin makers made an enormous profit."[29]

At the beginning of the war, embalming cost about one hundred dollars. By war's end, the cost had dropped to about fifty dollars for officers and twenty-five dollars for enlisted men. The average price for embalming at Gettysburg was twenty dollars, with an additional fee of fifteen dollars to cover the cost of a coffin. Transportation costs were additional and averaged about thirty dollars. Gravedigger fees at both ends of the journey added still more.[30]

Dr. Richard Burr of the Seventy-Second Pennsylvania Infantry was one of the most notorious embalmers for price gouging and questionable business practices. There were so many complaints lodged against him that the Union army established a formal licensing system and set uniform fees. The widespread fraud, even after the licensing requirements were established, was so brazen that eventually licensed undertakers took over the duty.

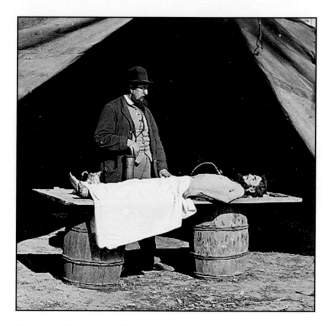

Dr. Richard Burr embalming a dead soldier. (Courtesy of Library of Congress, Reproduction Number LC-DIG-cwpb-01887)

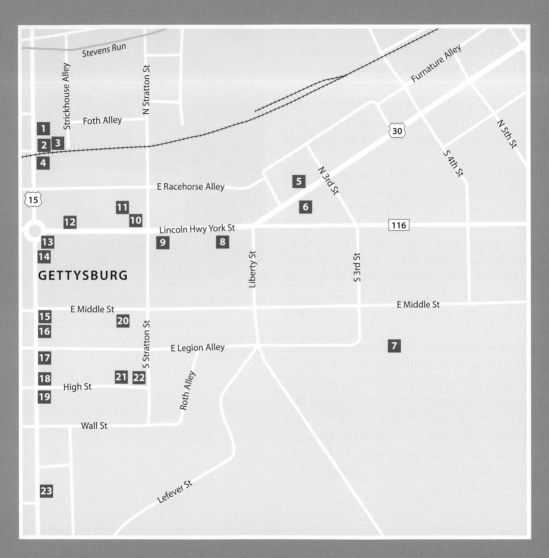

Chapter 2 sites: in town, east of square. (Map by Bill Nelson)

1. McCurdy-Diehl Warehouse Site, Carlisle Street, 39°49.948' N, 77°13.856' W

This warehouse, co-owned by Robert McCurdy and Jeremiah Diehl, sat immediately north of the Sheads and Buehler warehouse on Carlisle Street. The wood frame structure was only opened a short time before the battle, a strategic move by McCurdy, who was said to have profited greatly from the venture. McCurdy was president of the Gettysburg Railroad Company and saw the advantage of having a warehouse beside the railroad station.

Louis B. Brainard, assistant surgeon for the Seventh Wisconsin, was in charge. McCurdy-Diehl initially treated the wounded of the Union First Corps but found itself under control of the Confederates later in the first day of fighting. Thus, wounded from both sides were treated here.

In McCurdy's damage claim, he said the building was in complete possession of the Confederate army and suffered heavy damage. He claimed $391.89 for lost groceries, three barrels of shad, mackerel, molasses, tobacco, and various sundries. McCurdy also said that he lost some wagon harnesses and other

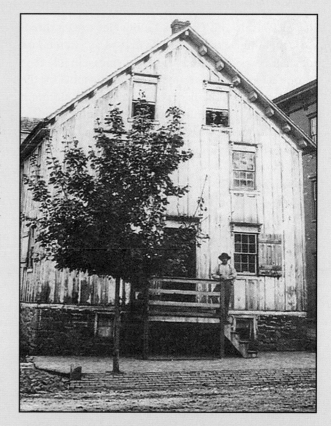

The McCurdy-Diehl Warehouse became a Union hospital early on July 1 but changed hands later in the day. (From a wayside marker on the McCurdy-Diehl Warehouse site)

equipment, as well as grain and grocery sacks. He eventually received full reimbursement.[1]

The McCurdy-Diehl warehouse was torn down in the 1960s in conjunction with the razing of the neighboring Sheads and Buehler warehouse.

2. Sheads and Buehler Warehouse Site, Carlisle Street, 39°49.933' N, 77°13.860' W

Robert Sheads and Charles H. Buehler used a three-story building on this site, build in 1858, as a warehouse for their coal, stove, and lumber business. In July 1863 it took on a new role: temporary field hospital for the wounded. Situated adjacent to the railroad station, it provided shelter for those awaiting transport by rail to outlying hospitals. There is also evidence that the First Brigade, First Division, First Corps used the building as its hospital. Lieutenant William H. Myers of the Seventy-Sixth New York Infantry was in charge of the hospital.

The building housed the Porter Guards, also known as the Tenth New York Cavalry, in the first months of the war. The second floor was used for amputations during the battle, allowing the removed limbs to be tossed out the windows. There, they gathered in the hot sun until they were shoveled into carts and removed for burial in long trenches. Residents of nearby homes complained that the odor got so intrusive that they were unable to open their windows for weeks.

The building was one of the last to close as a hospital. By July 18, 1863, only three hospitals remained open in town, including the Sheads and Buehler warehouse. The other two were the High Street School and the Lutheran Seminary. All others had had their

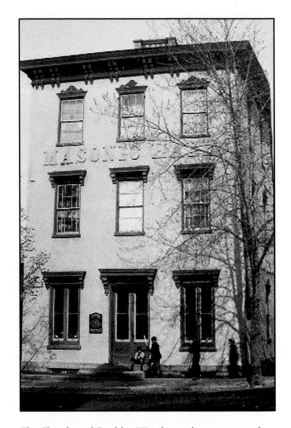

The Sheads and Buehler Warehouse became one of the last hospitals in town to close. (From a wayside marker on the Sheads and Buehler Warehouse site)

occupants moved to the Camp Letterman General Hospital on York Pike.

When the warehouse finally saw its last wounded soldier depart, Sheads and Buehler returned the building to its prior use as a warehouse. By the 1880s it had become the location for the local Masonic hall.

In the 1960s the building, by then known as the M. A. Hartley Building, was purchased by the Gulf

Oil Corporation. Gulf offered to donate the structure to anyone willing to move it back about sixty feet so the company could construct a gas station. The move was determined to be too costly, and there were no takers for the offer. After all attempts to find someone to move it, Gulf decided to raze it, relegating the building to memory.[2]

3. Adams Express Site, Carlisle Street, 39°49.933' N, 77°13.860' W

In the early to mid-1800s, packages were delivered by stage coach or Pony Express. The development of the transcontinental telegraph system put the Pony Express out of business, and the growth of the nation's railroad system provided a faster and more efficient delivery system than the use of stage coaches. As a result, four package delivery agencies took over most of those duties: Adams Express, Wells Fargo, American Express Company, and Southern Express Company. Adams Express hauled freight of all types, including mail, into and out of nearly every American city with a railroad depot.

As the nation learned of the battle that had taken place at Gettysburg, the company's superintendent in Baltimore, S. M. Shoemaker, saw a need that the company could fill. Shoemaker proposed to Secretary of War Edwin Stanton that the Adams Express set up a hospital corps of its own in Gettysburg, offering to send men and supplies to the war-torn town. When Stanton approved Shoemaker's plan, the company's Gettysburg office quickly converted from a delivery service to a field hospital and ambulance service. Wagons were sent to bring in the wounded from the field, and supplies were transported to other aid sta-

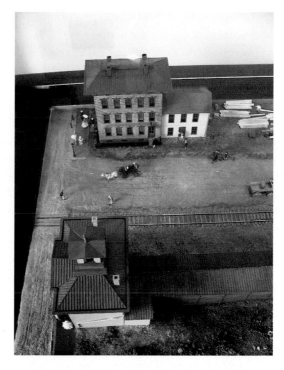

Model display at the railroad station. The Sheads and Buehler Warehouse is at the top. The small, white frame addition to the rear of the warehouse is likely the Adams Express Office.

tions and hospitals. When the railroad system around Gettysburg was restored, the company transported the remains of those killed.

The Gettysburg agent for Adams Express was Charles Buehler, who operated the office near the railroad station. The exact location for the office is not known with certainty, but considering Buehler's position with Adams Express and noting further that there was a small frame building attached to the rear of the Sheads and Buehler warehouse, it is likely that this building housed the Adams Express office, which became a hospital during the battle.

The company established its headquarters a block away, in Michael Spangler's store on the northwest corner of the town square (39°49.874′ N, 77°13.874′ W). A local representative, Harry Eiglehart, was appointed and J. H. Beach of the Twenty-Fourth Michigan became surgeon in charge. Surgeon Abner Hard (Eighth Illinois Cavalry), Surgeon D. C. Ayres (Seventh Wisconsin), Surgeon Jacob Ebersole (Nineteenth Indiana Infantry), Dr. Alexander Collar (Twenty-Fourth Michigan), Dr. George W. Towar (Twenty-Fourth Michigan), and Dr. John C. Hall (Sixth Wisconsin) split their time between this facility and the nearby railroad station. The Twenty-Fourth Michigan's chaplain, William C. Way, floated between several hospitals in the area of the railroad station, including the Adams Express facility.

On July 24 Felix Blanchard of the Twenty-Fourth Michigan wrote to a Mrs. Worthy that many of the wounded at the Adams Express office had missing limbs. He also noted that the smell was so terrible that it was responsible for about one of every three deaths, and that about one person was dying every day at this location.[3] On August 6, Blanchard wrote again, this time to his mother. In this letter he mentioned that Eli Blanchard, presumably a relative, and Webb Wood were both safe and working as nurses at the Adams Express office hospital.[4]

After Confederate troops overran the town, Confederate general Jubal Early sent a message to Union surgeon Ayres, asking whether he might want some whiskey for his patients. "Does a duck like to swim?" Ayres responded. The patients got their whiskey.[5]

By August 7, about thirty wounded remained at this site.

4. Gettysburg Railroad Depot, 35 Carlisle Street, 39°49.922′ N, 77°13.861′ W

In 1851, local citizens Robert McCurdy, Josiah Benner, and Henry Myers created the Gettysburg Railroad Company, receiving their official charter the following year. The first passenger train arrived in the town in September 1857. The next year, George McClellan, owner of the McClellan House (on the site of today's Gettysburg Hotel), donated property to the company for the purpose of constructing a passenger station, freight station, and engine house.

The passenger station contained two waiting rooms for passengers. One was for men, the other for women. Access to these waiting rooms was through one of the two doors on the building's front, which are still there. Women entered their waiting room through the door on the left (north) side of the building, with the men's waiting room accessed by the door on the right (south) side of the depot.

By December 1858 the project was completed sufficiently to provide service, although the ticket office and passenger portion of the station would not be completed until May 1859 at a final cost of $2,070. During that period, the Washington House Hotel (where the Lincoln Diner now sits across the street) served as the ticket office.

Rail service moved into and out of Gettysburg uninterrupted until June 26, 1863, when Confederate general Jubal Early destroyed the railroad bridge over Rock Creek, burning several freight cars at the same time and rendering the track impassable.

When Union general John Buford's First Cavalry Division arrived in Gettysburg on June 30, 1863, he had with him several men who were ill. Buford's medical

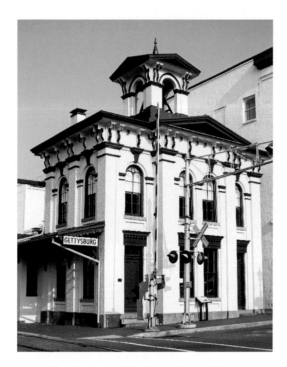

The railroad station still looks much as it did in 1863.

officer requested accommodations for them. With the railroad station out of service until the bridge over Rock Creek could be replaced and the track restored, the station was deemed suitable for Buford's men and twenty beds were set up, making it unofficially the first field hospital at Gettysburg. Surgeon Abner Hard of the Eighth Illinois Cavalry attended to the sick. The next day, with the battle escalating and facilities needed to treat the wounded, the building and passenger platform were pressed into service for treatment of the wounded. Buford's sick men were transferred to the Presbyterian Church on Baltimore Street. They, along with their doctors, were destined to become

prisoners of war within a few hours of their arrival at the church.

The Nineteenth Indiana's surgeon Jacob Ebersole and four unnamed surgeons from the Iron Brigade operated the hospital in the railroad station and several surrounding buildings for the First Corps. Nurses known to have been in attendance included Sue Elizabeth Stoever, Harriet Ann Harper (who headed the Union Relief Society), Susan Hall, Sarah Montford, Mary Montford, and Jennie Wills. Sarah Montford and her twelve-year-old daughter, Mary, traveled each day from their home on York Street to do what they could to help the wounded, only to discover that Sarah's husband and Mary's father was one of their patients. Struck by a shell, he was mortally wounded.

While rail service was suspended for weeks, the station was actively accommodating the wounded's needs. Those whose wounds were less severe used the building's cupola as an observation platform, and ten to fifteen were said to have watched the entirety of Pickett's Charge from that vantage point.

On July 10, train service was finally restored, but only for transporting the wounded and receiving badly needed incoming supplies. By then, some four thousand wounded had already been taken by ambulances to temporary terminals in Westminster and Littlestown, from where they were sent to hospitals in Baltimore and Harrisburg. The reopening of the Gettysburg railroad depot allowed for faster and more efficient transport of the wounded.

With train service resumed, the US Sanitary Commission set up a large tent across the tracks from the rear platform to help facilitate the transfer of wounded men. Trains were scheduled to leave at nine o'clock in the morning and three o'clock in the afternoon daily, and long lines of ambulances soon arrived, filled with wounded soldiers who waited for hours to board. Volunteer Georgeanna Woolsey recalled, "Twice a day the trains left . . . and twice a day we fed all the wounded who arrived for them."[6] Those who could not get on either of the two trains were forced to return the next day and try again.

On November 18, 1863, President Abraham Lincoln arrived at the railroad depot when he came to dedicate the new national cemetery. Alighting from the train, he was greeted by the somber sight of coffins stacked around the railroad platform as part of the reburial operation.

5. Elizabeth Culp House, 240 York Street, 39°49.892' N, 77°13.544' W

Elizabeth Culp, eighty-four years old at the time of the battle, lived with her fifty-seven-year-old daughter, Susan Smyser, owner of this house on York Street. Smyser was listed in the 1860 census as being unable to read or write.[7]

Culp, who was known to neighbors as Aunt Polly, and Smyser were said to have treated several wounded here. Aunt Polly was the widow of Peter Culp, who had died in 1841. When Peter died, Aunt Polly sold the family farm to her son Henry. The Henry Culp farm became famous in its own right during the battle as a hospital for the Confederate army.

On July 3, as the East Cavalry Field fighting wound down, the Confederates brought a wounded Michigan soldier named Smith to the Jacob Rinehart farm on the edge of the battlefield along Hoffman Road. There, he was given basic treatment for his injuries by Rebecca Rinehart and her daughter, Sarah King, and moved to

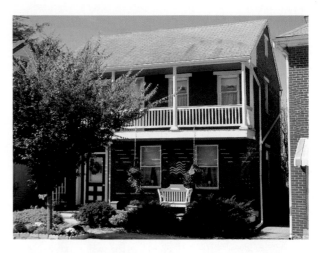

The Elizabeth Culp House.

the nearby Isaac Miller farm. After additional treatment there, he was moved into town, where Aunt Polly cared for him, along with several other wounded men, until he was well enough to return to Michigan. The connection between the Rineharts, the Millers, and Aunt Polly has not been established.

Aunt Polly died in 1867 and is buried in Evergreen Cemetery in Gettysburg.

6. Jacob Hollinger House Site, 225 York Street, 39°49.871' N, 77°13.568' W

Jacob Hollinger; his wife, Sarah (age forty); daughters Liberty (sixteen), Julia (fifteen), Annie (nine), and Bertie (seven); and their son, Gussie (five), lived on this triangular parcel of land formed by the junction of York and Hanover Streets. The 1863 brick farmhouse fronted on York Street, while the barn and sheds were on the Hanover Street side. The buildings

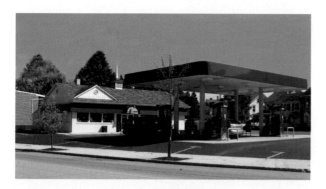

What was once the home of Jacob Hollinger and his family is now a convenience store and service station.

were torn down in the early 1900s for the construction of a school. Several years later, the school was torn down to make room for the convenience store and gas station that currently sits on the historic plot.

On the first day of fighting, two wounded Union officers asked whether they could take refuge in the Hollingers' cellar. One had a wound of the neck; the other was shot in the wrist. Both appeared to be in great pain. Once in the cellar, they found that Liberty's mother, Sarah, had fainted from the excitement. The two wounded officers brought her a rocking chair and then realized that they were in danger of being captured. Despite their injuries, they left and did not return.

The Confederates filled the town, taking possession of nearby houses that had been abandoned. Some made biscuits in a house across the street and called to Liberty's younger sister Julia, asking for butter for their biscuits. She saucily answered, "If you are hungry you can eat them as they are." Liberty reported that they laughed and went back into the house.

Jacob owned a warehouse that sat adjacent to the railroad tracks about a block from the railroad station.

When several Southern soldiers demanded the keys to the warehouse, he refused. Undaunted, the rebels said they would get in anyway. True to their word, the Confederates forced the locks of the warehouse and took what they wanted. What they didn't need, they destroyed by opening the spigots of the molasses barrels and allowing the contents to run over the floor. They also scattered the supply of salt and sugar on the floor and surrounding shelves of goods.

The family stayed in the cellar most of the time during the three days of battle. Liberty wrote that a few bullets struck the cellar doors, and occasionally the brick walls of the house, but they never felt they were in danger, except for her father, Jacob, who was shot at several times by Union sharpshooters stationed in Henry Culp's wheat field. It happened each time Jacob left the cellar to feed the chickens or to milk the cow. Finally, he confronted them about it, only to be told by an officer, "Take off that gray suit; they think you are a Johnny Reb." Liberty noted that her father quickly put on a black suit and had no further trouble.

Several wounded were treated at the Hollinger house, including at least four from the Sixth Wisconsin. One of them had brought with him a captured Second Mississippi flag. Another of those treated was a young man named Paul, whose right arm had been amputated at the shoulder. Liberty was assigned the task of dressing the wound each morning and evening. In great pain, the young man had to be administered an anodyne, or painkiller, so he could sleep, and the family became quite attached to him. His father came and took him home, and the Hollinger family was distraught later when they learned that the youth had died of his wound.

With so many outsiders coming to Gettysburg to assist, many families, including the Hollingers, took some into their home and provided them with a place to stay. Four such women arrived from Baltimore and were introduced by John A. Swope, a neighbor. The four would spend the day in the field and at Confederate hospitals. The Hollingers soon learned that they were purchasing civilian clothes, to be used to aid Confederate prisoners to escape. Upon hearing of their ruse, Jacob Hollinger insisted that he would not tolerate any Confederate sympathizers in his home and that they must leave. Liberty wrote that the four ladies "left our home very reluctantly and we could not help wondering whether they found another place they liked."[8]

Conditions on the battlefield were such that residents found body parts for several weeks after the battle. On one particular day, young Annie Hollinger was walking over the field and found a hand, which she brought home. It had dried to parchment so that it looked as though it was covered with a kid glove. There was nothing repulsive about the relic, and the family remarked about the smallness of the fingers. They guessed that it must have belonged to a very young soldier or a Southerner who had never worked with his hands.[9] Stories such as this were common in the days and weeks following the battle.

7. Henry Culp Farm, Middle Street, 39°49.748' N, 77°13.441' W

Henry Culp (age fifty-four), Anna (forty-four), Rufus E. (twenty), Livina A. (eighteen), Calvin B. (fifteen), Mary C. (thirteen), Sarah (ten), and Edward (three) lived on this farm during the battle. Also in the home were Peter Johns (twenty-four), described

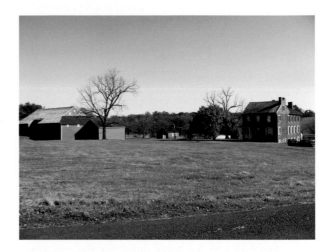

The Henry Culp farm became a hospital for Ewell's Corps.

as a hireling, and Elizabeth Snyder (twenty-one), a domestic worker.[10]

The two-story house with attic and basement was built in 1840 and the interior is largely unchanged. A two-story bank barn was constructed ten years later. The farm also contained a smokehouse, springhouse, wagon shed, carriage house, and woodhouse.[11] The family stayed in the cellar throughout the fighting and later filed a damage claim for more than $1,000.

During the battle, the Culp farm buildings were within and behind the battle lines of a portion of Confederate lieutenant-general Richard Ewell's Confederate Corps. The buildings came under fire from Union small arms and artillery firing on July 2–4 but, despite the heavy fighting, they sustained relatively little damage. Because of its location near a large concentration of Confederate troops, the farm served as a Confederate field hospital for Ewell's Second Corps, General Jubal Early's Division, and the grounds surrounding the buildings and within the orchard became a vast temporary Confederate cemetery. The farm proper contained at least thirty-three burials, plus two more on the south side of the house. Many more were buried in the area around the farm but are categorized as Culp's Hill burials.[12]

Of those treated at the Culp farm, thirty-four-year-old Colonel Isaac Avery of the Sixth North Carolina Infantry is the best known. Avery was shot in the neck and shoulders on July 2 as he led an attack up Cemetery Hill. As he lay in Culp's barn, he wrote his famous note to his friend Major Samuel Tate. Using his left hand because his right side had been paralyzed by his wound, Avery wrote, "Tell my father I died with my face to the enemy."[13]

Avery died on July 3 and his body was taken along on the retreat with the intention of giving it to his family. When his men arrived at Williamsport, the Potomac River was determined to be too high for safe crossing. Avery was buried in a temporary grave under a pine tree by the men who were with him when he fell. Eventually his body was removed and reburied in the Washington Confederate Cemetery section of Rose Hill Cemetery in Hagerstown, Maryland.

The Culp family is a good example of the brother-versus-brother aspect of the war. Wesley Culp, a relative of Henry, was working in Virginia when the war broke out and he enlisted in the famous Stonewall Brigade. Wesley's brother William and cousin David fought in the Eighty-Seventh Pennsylvania Volunteer Infantry. Wesley got a pass to visit his sister the night of July 2 and was killed the next day.

William Reese and John Geddings Hardy, both of the Sixth North Carolina Infantry, served as physicians on the Culp farm. The farm also served as an ambulance depot for Early's Division.

8. Jeremiah Culp Carpenter Shop, 141 York Street, 39°49.852' N, 77°13.661' W

Cabinetmaker Jeremiah Culp (age forty-one) and his wife, Rebecca (forty), lived with their seven children, John F. (seventeen), M. Luther (fifteen), M. Welle (thirteen), Sarah E. (eleven), Reuben H. (eight), George M. (six), and Ella V. (four), at this York Street home.[14] Liberty Hollinger noted that a carpenter shop near her home, believed to be the one Jeremiah operated at the rear of his residence, served as an operating room during the battle. The carpenter's bench was pressed into service as an operating table, and a pile of arms and legs quickly accumulated outside under the window.[15]

It is not known where the Culps spent their time during the battle. It is possible that they went to Daniel and Mary Paxton Culp's home on Baltimore Street. Daniel and Mary were Jeremiah's uncle and aunt, and

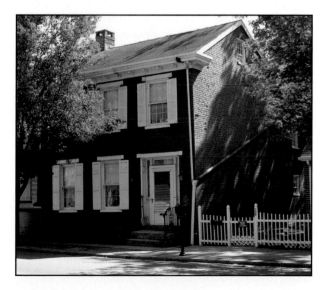

Jeremiah Culp's home and carpenter shop.

Daniel also operated a carpenter shop at his home. It is known that Jeremiah was there at some point during the battle, because he and Daniel worked together at Daniel's shop to build a coffin for Confederate brigadier-general William Barksdale. The coffin was left behind when the Confederates retreated and was eventually used for the burial of Jennie Wade, the only civilian killed during the battle.

Daniel and Mary's teenaged son James was killed shortly after the battle when an artillery shell exploded in his hands as he worked to open it.

9. St. James Lutheran Church, 109 York Street, 39°49.850' N, 77°13.730' W

In 1789 a group of German Lutherans formed the church that would become St. James. Built in 1847–1848, the original church had a cupola that was used as an observation post during the battle. Torn down in 1911, it was replaced by a new structure, which suffered extensive damage in 1928 and 1969 from fires. The 1969 fire was ruled arson, and the church had to be rebuilt again. In 1997 a twelve-thousand-square-foot addition was constructed.

Rev. Abraham Essick, pastor during the battle, recorded that the church was used for five weeks as a hospital, with the wounded filling every area of the church. A young Union drummer boy is said to have died in the vestibule, and wounded from both sides left scribbled messages in the hymn books, with the word *mother* appearing twenty times on consecutive pages of one particular hymnal.

The pastor said that he went to the steeple several times to observe the fighting, not realizing the danger at the time. It was only when the steeple was taken

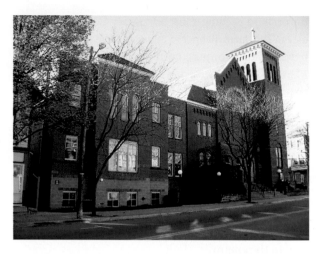

The St. James Lutheran Church was a hospital for five weeks.

down that it was found to have been riddled with bullets. Essick also noted that Jennie Wade was confirmed here on April 20, 1862.

The Civil War was not the only national crisis in which this church served the community. In World War I the church opened its social rooms to the soldiers serving at Camp Colt, a tank training facility located on the ground covered by Pickett's Charge, and during the 1918 flu epidemic the church became a free place of refuge for families of the men at Camp Colt.

10. George Swope House, 60 York Street, 39°49.861' N, 77°13.740' W

This home was built in 1836 when George Swope tore down the original two-story log cabin that had been built in 1793 by James Gettys, the founder of Gettysburg. Shown in the 1860 census as the wealthiest man in Gettysburg, Swope had combined real estate and

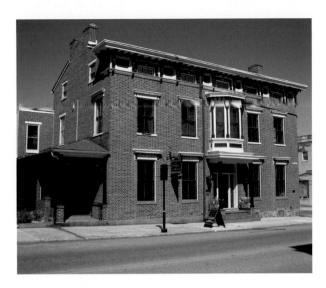

The George Swope House.

personal estate listed at $86,000; his wife, Margaret, was shown as having an estate worth $14,000.[16]

At the time of the battle, George was serving as the president and director of the Bank of Gettysburg, as well as president and director of the Gettysburg Railroad Company, the Gettysburg Water Company, the Adams County Mutual Fire Insurance Company, and the Gettysburg and Petersburg Turnpike Company. The sixty-two-year-old Swope lived here with his wife, Margaret (sixty), and daughter Lena (sixteen). Also in the home were Jane Copeland (forty-three, shown on the census as Help) and A. J. Cover (a thirty-one-year-old attorney).[17] Some sources say the Swopes also had a son named John, but he was not shown to be in the home at the time of the battle.

The Swope house is believed to have been used to handle the overflow of wounded from St. James

Lutheran Church, which sits across the street. William Pohlman, a twenty-two-year-old lieutenant from the Fifty-Ninth New York, was wounded on July 3 in the defense of Cemetery Ridge during Pickett's Charge. He had been treated in an unnamed field hospital until July 11, when he was moved to the Swopes' house, where it was thought he would be more comfortable. His health improved daily until July 20, when he suffered an unexpected secondary hemorrhage. He died the next day, his last words being, "Cease firing!"

11. Peter Stallsmith House Site, 52 York Street, 39°49.891' N, 77°13.752' W

This building sits on what was the front lawn of the Peter Stallsmith house in 1863. The original Stallsmith house sat behind the existing building. Peter himself had died a year before the battle at the age of forty-seven, but his widow, Ann (age forty-two); daughter Sarah (twenty-one); daughter Mary (fourteen); and son Harry (eight) all still lived in the home.[18] The Stallsmiths had three additional children who had died not long before the war. Anna Margaret (nine) and Elisabeth Catherine (eight) had died within three weeks of each other in 1855. Emma Grace died within a week of her birth in April 1861. There is no doubt that Ann Stallsmith had known sorrow, so having badly wounded soldiers in her home might have been less daunting to her than to others in Gettysburg.

The Stallsmiths also owned a farm just off Fairfield Road and west of Willoughby Run but did not live there. It was not far from the George Arnold farm and was occupied by tenant farmer William Keefauver.

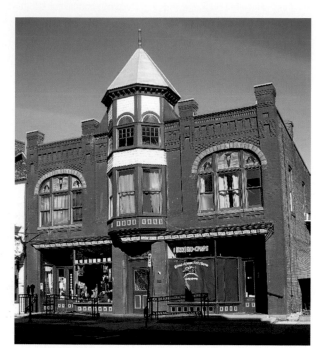

The Peter Stallsmith House sat to the rear of the lot where this building now stands.

An 1887 newspaper article confirmed that it was the house in town that was the hospital, rather than the farm. That article noted that several officers were treated at the Stallsmith house, including Captain Henry C. Parsons of the First Vermont Cavalry, who was wounded on July 3 in Farnsworth's Charge. Parsons was first taken to the Adams County Courthouse, then moved to Stallsmith's home.[19] He survived his wounds and moved to Virginia, where he became president of two railroads. He was also a wealthy landowner, and his possessions included the property on which the famous Natural Bridge is located.[20]

12. T. Duncan Carson House Site, 6 York Street, 39°49.859' N, 77°13.817' W

T. Duncan Carson began his career with the Bank of Gettysburg in March 1857 when he was elected a teller at the annual salary of $800. He was promoted to assistant cashier in November 1857 with a $200 annual raise, and when cashier John B. McPherson died in January 1858, Carson assumed the top position in the bank. At the time, the bank was housed in McPherson's home on York Street, where it remained until 1882. Carson remained at the helm of the bank throughout the war, resigning in 1867 to take a position with the Fidelity Insurance Trust and Safe Deposit Company in Philadelphia.[21]

The bank itself, built in 1814, sat on the site now occupied by the Grand Ballroom of the Gettysburg

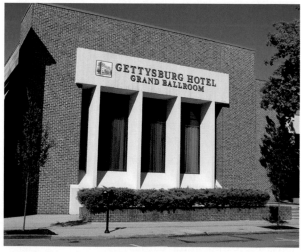

The Gettysburg Hotel's Grand Ballroom sits where the Bank of Gettysburg, with T. Duncan Carson's home, sat in 1863.

Hotel. The thirty-year-old Carson lived either in the bank itself or in the structure adjacent to it. Living with him were his wife, Mary (thirty), and son Robert D. (five). The Carsons also provided housing for their twenty-two-year-old domestic worker, Ann Rollman.[22]

Late in June 1863, when fighting appeared imminent, Carson suspended operations at the bank and removed all the bank's assets, taking them to York. From there they were shipped to Philadelphia for safekeeping. The bank remained closed until late in July.

When fighting broke out, the family took shelter in the bank's vault. Accompanying them were fifteen additional people, plus two dogs and a cat. Among the group were the family of Dr. Robert Horner, which proved to be fortuitous when the wounded began arriving.

At least three wounded were brought here, one of whom would succumb to his wounds. One of the three was Mary Carson's brother, Lieutenant Charles O. Hunt, of the Fifth Maine Battery. Horner removed a bullet and cared for Hunt until July 12, when he was able to go to his own home.

Lieutenant Charles Fuller, of the Sixty-First New York Infantry, was treated here for wounds to his leg and shoulder suffered in the Wheatfield on July 2. His leg had been removed at an unnamed field hospital, where the surgeon had somehow missed a second bullet that was discovered a few days later in the remaining stump of his leg. He also had a three-inch piece of humerus bone removed from his shoulder.

Fuller said that other wounded men around him were groaning in pain as he lay in the Wheatfield.

Not knowing the extent of his wounds, he wondered whether they were slight enough to allow him to groan like the others were groaning. He wrote, "I determined to try it, and drew in a good breath, and let out a full grown man groan. I was satisfied with the result and then kept quiet."[23]

While Horner and Carson's wife and mother tended to the wounded in their home, Carson assisted at another hospital during the battle. He would become one of the civilian casualties, sustaining a slight wound of the arm from a stray bullet.

The house sustained some damage, with several bullet holes noted on the inside walls. An artillery shell entered one of the windows but failed to detonate. Carson's action in taking the bank's funds away for safekeeping was widely praised by the bank's customers, none of whom lost any of their money.

13. David Wills House, 8 Lincoln Square, 39°49.852' N, 77°13.837' W

As far back as the late 1700s, a small stone house stood here, the home and shop of Samuel Keplinger, a local watch- and clockmaker. In 1807 Keplinger sold the property to Alexander Cobean. It was Cobean who built what is now known as the Wills house, sometime around 1814. Unfortunately, Cobean died bankrupt in 1823 and his property was taken over by the Bank of Gettysburg. In 1859 David Wills purchased the structure for his home and law office.

Wills was thirty-two years old at the time of the battle. His wife, Catherine Jane, was two years younger. The couple had three children, all under the age of six. Catherine Jane was eight months pregnant with a fourth child during the battle. Eventually the

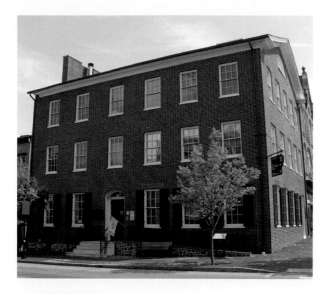

The David Wills House.

couple would have seven children. Also in the home during the battle were David's father, James, and the family domestic worker, Catherine Rollman.[24] Despite her pregnancy, Mrs. Wills made the daily trek to the McPherson farm to help with the wounded there.

Wills was a prominent attorney who frequently sparred for power with another local attorney, David McConaughy. A graduate of Pennsylvania College, Wills was active in community affairs and his home was destined to become one of the most famous houses in Gettysburg.

Wills wanted a soldier's cemetery to be created on Cemetery Hill where artillery had fought, and he submitted his idea to Pennsylvania governor Andrew Curtin. He had already negotiated the purchase of 3.5 acres from Peter Raffensperger and 4.5 acres from Edward Menchey at the cost of $200 per acre if Curtin

agreed. Wills proposed that burials be conducted at $3.50 to $4.00 each.[25] Meanwhile, a similar proposal on behalf of Evergreen Cemetery was submitted to the governor by David McConaughy. The relationship between Wills and McConaughy was not improved when Curtin selected the plan submitted by Wills, with the cemetery to be constructed adjacent to the town's Evergreen Cemetery.

Among the wounded treated here was Union general Winfield Scott Hancock. Colonel Henry Morrow of the Twenty-Fourth Michigan, who had been shot in the head, was also brought to the Wills house on July 1 but was soon captured and marched to the rear as a prisoner of war. Left behind when Lee's army retreated, Morrow made it a point to return to thank the Wills family for his treatment.

It was Wills who invited President Abraham Lincoln to attend the dedication of the new national cemetery and make a "few appropriate remarks."[26] Those remarks would make up what is arguably the most famous speech in American history.

On the night of November 18, 1863, Lincoln spent the night as a guest of David Wills, where he finalized his Gettysburg Address. In addition to Lincoln, featured speaker Edward Everett and thirty-six others were dinner guests.

After the war, merchant Henry Carr filed a damage claim for items he said he had stored in Wills's basement storeroom. He said that his losses included dry goods, clothing (both men's and women's), spices, silverware, gunpowder, soap, fishing tackle, books, musical instruments, drugs and medicines, jewelry, whiskey, wine, cider, a Union flag, carriages, and numerous other items. Carr claimed that the Confederates had broken into his store with an ax to gain access to his items. Many other local merchants, however, cast doubt on his claim, testifying that his business was too small to require such a large inventory, and that he never had as much as his claim indicated.

David Wills died on October 27, 1894, while working in his office.

14. Robert G. Harper House Site, 9 Lincoln Square, 39°50.840' N, 77°13.842' W

The same year Adams County was formed, Robert G. Harper's father, Robert Sr., founded the Gettysburg *Centinel* [*sic*] newspaper. When the elder Harper died in 1817, Robert G. took over the paper and continued to operate it for the next fifty years. Then, the newspaper combined with the *Star* to form the *Star and Sentinel*.[27]

As editor of a prominent local newspaper, Harper became quite influential in Gettysburg, and was a force in the Masonic movement in the early 1800s. With no Masonic lodge existing in town, Harper filed a petition to form the Gettysburg Good Samaritan Lodge No. 200 of the Free Masons in 1824. The lodge became chartered the next year. Within three years, the lodge had thirty-seven members, but soon withdrawals and suspensions cut into membership, and the lodge dissolved in December 1832.

Until 1860 there was no new lodge in Gettysburg. Then, Harper and two other local citizens, Joel B. Danner and John Geiselman, worked to establish Good Samaritan Lodge No. 336. The new lodge grew steadily throughout the Civil War.

By the summer of 1863, Harper was sixty-three years old and shared the house that sat on this site with several family members, a cook, a nurse, and three apprentice printers.[28] The two-story brick building was Harper's residence. The office for the *Centinel* was immediately adjacent on the same lot. When Lincoln came to town for the dedication of the new cemetery, Secretary of State William Seward was a part of the group that accompanied the president. Seward stayed at the Harper residence and met with Lincoln there for more than an hour the night before the dedication.

During the battle, several members of the Twenty-Fourth Michigan Infantry were treated in

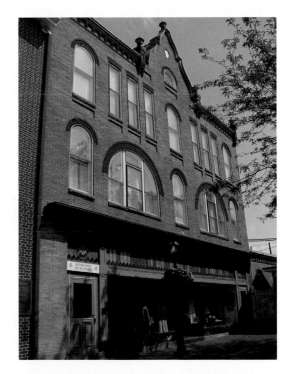

Robert Harper's house (replaced by this building, a Masonic Lodge) became a hospital for the Twenty-Fourth Michigan.

Harper's home, including Lieutenant Colonel Mark Flanagan. Flanagan, a former sheriff in Wayne County, Michigan, had been badly wounded on July 1 in the fighting on McPherson's Ridge. His wound was so severe that he had to have his leg amputated.

After the battle, the remains of a Confederate officer were found near the Codori farm buildings on Emmitsburg Road. In the process of burying the body on the south side of the Codori barn, papers were found on his person that showed him to be a Mason. Harper's Masonic lodge, Good Samaritan No. 336, heard of the dead Confederate officer and the location of the grave and came to help. Several of the men, including Harper, cared for the grave on the farm by enclosing it with a fence, putting up a headstone, and trimming the grass for their fallen brother. Some years later, the lodge was instrumental in having the remains of the officer returned to his family in the South.

Both Harper's home and the *Sentinel* office were demolished before 1900 and replaced with the existing building, which is now the home of Good Samaritan Lodge No. 336, Free and Accepted Masons, the lodge that Harper was instrumental in establishing.

15. John Cannon House, 100 Baltimore Street, 39°49.778' N, 77°13.860' W

In 1863 John Cannon, his wife, and his thirteen-year-old son were living as tenants in a home on this site. The deed for the property shows that it was jointly owned by Drs. Robert Horner, Charles Horner, and local merchant David Kendlehart. Cannon, a marble cutter, operated a marble-cutting

yard with James Adair in the rear in which Confederate general Jubal Early may have established his headquarters on July 2.

Not much is known about the property's use as a hospital, but a letter written by Chaplain William C. Way of the Twenty-Fourth Michigan notes that at least two men from his regiment, Privates Thomas Ballou and Alfred Willis, were treated here.[29] Willis's wounds were slight enough that he also served as a nurse at Cannon's, implying that there may have been additional wounded here. Way

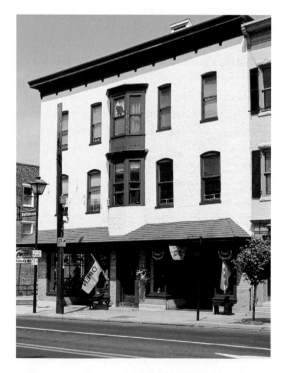

John Cannon's house took in at least two wounded men from the Twenty-Fourth Michigan.

moved from hospital to hospital in the area of the town square and became familiar with the buildings used as hospitals, especially those treating the men of his regiment.

16. David Buehler House, 112 Baltimore Street, 39°49.763' N, 77°13.859' W

Attorney David Buehler lived in this house with his wife, Fannie, and their six children, who ranged from infancy to twelve years of age. Before he became an attorney, David had edited the *Centinel* newspaper for a dozen years. He was now the town's postmaster, and when they first heard in late June that Confederates were approaching Gettysburg, he and Fannie thought it was just another false alarm. They had heard the rumors before. In fact, two weeks earlier, the rumors sounded so certain that their African American servant Elizabeth Brien had fled to avoid possible capture by the rebels. The Buehlers would never see Brien again, although Fannie said she had heard that the woman had gone to Philadelphia.

This time they ignored the warning until David looked outside and saw Confederates coming down Baltimore Street. Taking a satchel packed with valuable government property and a valise of clothes, he left on the run, making it to Hanover and then to Fannie's family's home in New Jersey. Fannie remained in town and spent the battle in her home with her children, the family dog, Bruno, and several wounded soldiers.

When the battle was over, Fannie was astounded to see dead soldiers and their belongings lying on the streets as far as she could see. Exhausted men took refuge on her porch, unable to go any farther. Those who

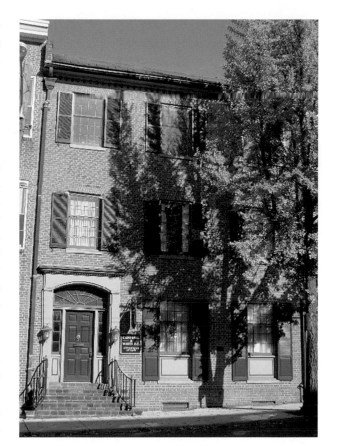

Fannie Buehler was accused of hiding wounded Union soldiers in her home. No action was taken against her or the wounded men.

were wounded were brought into the house for treatment. Taken at first to the basement, the wounded eventually were brought upstairs and placed on the dining-room floor. Neighbors came to help, and Fannie set up food on the front porch, free for anyone who needed it.[30]

At least six and possibly as many as a dozen wounded were treated here. Many were officers, including Colonel John C. Callis of the Seventh Wisconsin, seriously wounded by a buckshot that struck him in the right side of his chest, broke a rib, and came to rest in his right lung during the retreat from McPherson's to Seminary Ridge on July 1. He lay on the battlefield until the afternoon of July 2, when he was carried to the office of Gettysburg physician John W. C. O'Neal on Baltimore Street, then sheltered in one of the private homes nearby. Hearing of his injury, the colonel's wife immediately traveled from Wisconsin to Gettysburg and, finding him in less than satisfactory conditions, had him moved to the third floor of the Buehler home. Here, she nursed her injured husband until released to journey home that September.[31]

Fannie wrote that Confederate lieutenant colonel Harry Gilmore, provost marshal, came to her house and accused her of concealing Union soldiers. Fannie said she was not concealing anyone, but that there were Union wounded in her home and they were lying all over the first floor. She said Gilmore was welcome to come in and see them himself, which he did. Gilmore said he would write up parole papers for all of them but he never returned with the paroles. No action was taken against Fannie.[32] One of the wounded men later swore in an affidavit that Fannie's neighbor and editor of the *Gettysburg Compiler*, Henry Stahle, had told the Confederates of their whereabouts.[33]

17. Henry J. Stahle House Site, 126 Baltimore Street, 39°49.746' N, 77°13.859' W

Henry Stahle was the outspoken editor of the *Gettysburg Compiler*, the local Democratic newspaper in

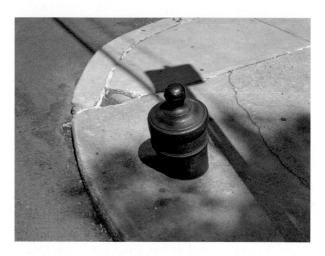

This cannon, named Penelope, was fired when a Democrat won an election. After it exploded in 1855, it was partially buried in the sidewalk, where it remains.

town. Although he was loyal to the Union, he was also an unabashed critic of Abraham Lincoln, which did not endear him to some of the local citizenry. Stahle was noted for firing a cannon, which he had named Penelope, after every Democratic election victory. In 1855 Penelope's tube burst after an overexuberant assistant loaded her with too much powder. Penelope can still be seen today, buried in the sidewalk outside the site of the old *Compiler* office.

One of twelve children, Stahle was thirty-nine years old at the time of the battle and married to Louisa B. (age thirty-six). The couple had four children: Thomas J. (sixteen), Mary L. (fourteen), Hattie M. (eight), and Annie D. (five). Also in the home were M. E. Dull (twenty-six), a journeyman printer, and Marie Noel (eighteen), a domestic worker.[34]

On the first day of the battle, Lieutenant Colonel William Dudley of the Nineteenth Indiana was

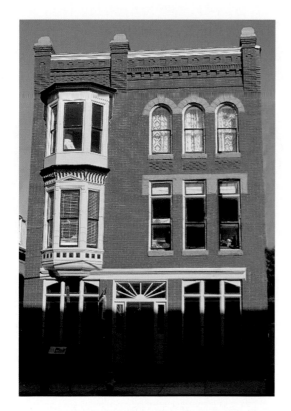

The site of the Henry Stahle home and the *Gettysburg Compiler* office.

geon available, a Confederate doctor, to come look at the wounded officer. Hoping to save Dudley's leg, the surgeon removed 187 pieces of shattered bone. While the gesture was noble, it proved unsuccessful and the leg was ultimately amputated. A story associated with the case claims that the amputated leg was buried in a wooden box, and almost immediately Dudley began complaining that he could feel pain in the toes of his missing limb. When the leg was disinterred it was discovered that the toes had been pushed into the box so the leg would fit. Once the toes were rearranged and the leg reburied, Dudley was said to have had no further pain.[35]

When one of Stahle's political opponents, David McConaughy, learned that Stahle had summoned a Confederate surgeon to treat a Union officer, he complained to Union provost marshal Marsena R. Patrick that Stahle had disclosed the location of a hidden Union soldier. Stahle was arrested and sent to Fort McHenry, where he took the Oath of Allegiance and was paroled and released on July 19. After returning to Gettysburg, he was arrested a second time and returned to Fort McHenry. Released a few days later, no further action was taken against him, although many in town insisted that he had turned in others, in addition to Dudley. That suspicion was supported when a wounded man being treated at David Buehler's home later swore in an affidavit that Stahle had told the Confederates of their whereabouts.

Dudley had given his spurs and sword to Mrs. Stahle for safekeeping. The spurs had been given to him by a Confederate officer named Cussons when Dudley had captured him at the Second Battle of Bull Run (Manassas). Years later, on a return visit to Gettysburg, Dudley met with a *Compiler* employee. A conversation

severely wounded in the leg during the fighting in Herbst Woods, where the regiment's monument now stands. He was brought to Stahle's home by four soldiers who told Mrs. Stahle that they had a dead man with them. They left Dudley with Mrs. Stahle and quickly departed to avoid capture. Dudley was brought inside, where the Stahles realized that, although badly wounded, he was still alive.

While a neighbor cleaned Dudley's leg, Stahle went to the courthouse, where he summoned the only sur-

between the two led to the realization that Cussons was now head of a Virginia company that had been supplying calendars to the *Compiler* for the past four years.

The old *Compiler* building was located here at 126 Baltimore Street. The site of Stahle's adjoining house is the northern end of what is now the county library property. Both buildings were razed in 1912 to make room for the construction of the US Post Office building, which became the library building in 1992.

Stahle died in 1892 and is buried in Evergreen Cemetery.

18. Drs. O'Neal, Taylor, and Cress Office Site, 140 Baltimore Street, 39°49.720' N, 77°13.855' W

The Adams County Library now sits on the site of the former offices of Drs. John William Crapster O'Neal, William Taylor, and James Cress. Little is known of Taylor and Cress, but O'Neal was a prominent figure in not only treating the wounded but also identifying and recording burial locations of Confederate remains for later retrieval by their families.

O'Neal was born in Fairfax, Virginia, in 1821 and attended Pennsylvania College in Gettysburg. Following graduation, he received his medical degree from the University of Maryland in 1844 and opened a practice in Baltimore. He married Ellen Wirt, and the couple had five children by the time of the battle, with a sixth born five years later. One son, Walter, followed in his father's footsteps and also became a doctor after the war.

O'Neal had assisted in treating the wounded at Antietam and had been persuaded to move to Gettysburg by local politicians who promised him that he could treat local prison inmates and residents of the

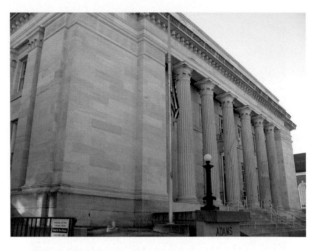

The offices of Drs. O'Neal, Taylor, and Cress sat on the site now occupied by the Adams County Library.

almshouse. With that enticement, he brought his family to Gettysburg just a few months before the battle. He rented an office in the Wills Building on the town square for a short time, then opened his office in space leased from Professor Charles Krauth at this location.

As he had moved from Virginia, local citizens suspected him of being a Confederate sympathizer, a sentiment that was only partially dispelled when men from Confederate brigadier-general James Pettigrew's brigade took him captive late in June. He was taken to Cashtown and questioned before his release a day later.

O'Neal, Taylor, and Cress treated an unknown number of wounded here, in addition to assisting in various homes, churches, and other public buildings throughout the town. Dr. Robert Hubbard of the Seventeenth Connecticut also treated wounded here, so it is likely that at least a few from that regiment were brought here. Colonel John C. Callis of the Seventh

Wisconsin was initially treated here before being moved to David Buehler's house a short distance away.

When President James Garfield was shot in 1881, Callis's friend Lieutenant Colonel William Dudley (see the previous section) was serving as commissioner of pensions in Washington. Dudley rushed to the White House, where he realized that Garfield's wound was remarkably similar to the wound Callis had received at Gettysburg, and that Callis's life had been saved. A telegram was dispatched to Callis, who sent information back about the treatment of his wound. The president's physicians used that information in an unsuccessful attempt to save the president.[36]

During the battle, O'Neal treated wounded soldiers from both sides. As he made his rounds throughout the community, he would record in his journal the locations of Confederate graves. He would also include the individual's name and regiment if that information was available to him. He performed this service to make it easier for the loved ones of dead Confederates to find their bodies. Between O'Neal and another local citizen, Samuel Weaver, who was doing the same thing, as many as 1,200 Confederate dead were able to be returned to their families.

O'Neal became a battlefield guide after the war and died in 1913 at the age of ninety-two. He is buried in Mt. Olivet Cemetery in his wife's hometown of Hanover, Pennsylvania.

19. Presbyterian Church, 208 Baltimore Street, 39°49.708′ N, 77°13.859′ W

The first Presbyterian church built in Gettysburg was erected in 1813 at the corner of North Washington and Railroad Streets. At that location it served the local

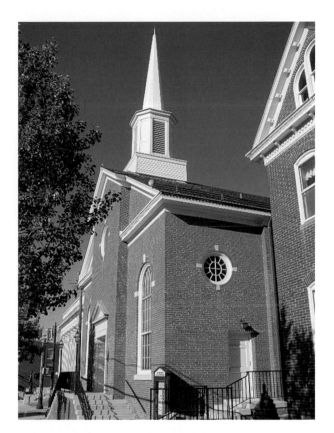

The Presbyterian Church sits on the site of the church that served as a hospital for the Cavalry Corps.

congregation until 1842, when it moved to the present location. During and immediately following the Battle of Gettysburg in July 1863, the church, along with many other public buildings in town, was converted into a temporary hospital. It would be many weeks before the church resumed normal activities. Local citizen Sarah Broadhead lamented the shortage of church services: "We have had no Sundays. The churches have all been converted into hospitals."[37]

This hospital, primarily established to serve the Cavalry Corps, as well as the Third Division, First Corps, was used for several weeks. The pews were covered with boards and straw, and blankets were placed on top to make the wounded as comfortable as possible. Patients brought here from the railroad station on July 1, as well as attending Union physicians and nurses, were captured when the Confederates overran the town later that day.

It is not known with certainty how many wounded were treated here, but all the Cavalry Corps hospitals together treated some three hundred injured troopers.

While most people took refuge inside their homes during the battle, Agnes Barr, a member of the church who lived three doors from it, would have none of that. Along with her sisters, Barr provided food for the nurses and doctors at the church hospital. Although she lived less than 150 feet from the church, traversing the short distance proved to be a daunting task. She described dodging bullets to get to the church to help with the wounded: "We ladies went the back way through the yards to help the wounded. Their shrieks and groans were heartrending."[38]

Three plaques are mounted on the outside wall of the church. The first two identify the church as having hosted two presidents. On November 19, 1863, four months after the battle, President Abraham Lincoln came to town to take part in the dedication of the Gettysburg National Cemetery. Late in the afternoon, following the delivery of his famous Gettysburg Address, Lincoln attended a patriotic meeting in this church with local citizen John Burns, who had fought on McPherson Ridge as a civilian. The pew where Lincoln and Burns sat is marked with a bronze plaque. The second plaque notes that President Dwight D.

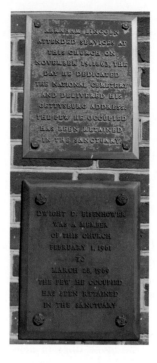

Plaques recognizing the attendance of Presidents Lincoln and Eisenhower at the church.

Eisenhower was a member of the church from 1961 to 1969. His pew is also marked, and the Eisenhower Lounge, containing prints of paintings and memorabilia of the late president, is named in his honor.

The third plaque, on the outside wall, identifies the church as the Cavalry Corps Hospital. The inscription on the plaque reads,

Army of the Potomac
Medical Department
Field Hospitals
Cavalry Corps

The hospitals of the First Division Cavalry Corps
were located in this church and other nearby

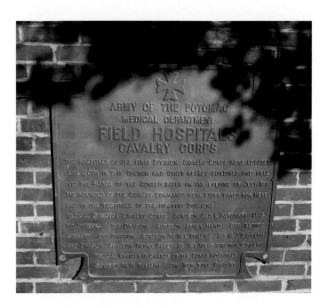

Plaque identifying the church as a Cavalry Corps hospital.

buildings and fell into the hands of the
Confederates on the evening of July 1st.
The wounded of the Cavalry Commands were later
cared for here and in the Hospitals of
the Infantry Division.

Medical Director Cavalry Corps, Surgeon Geo. L.
Pancoast, U.S. Volunteers
1st Division, Surgeon Abner Hard, 8th Illinois Cavalry
2nd Division, Surgeon Henry Capeheart, 1st West
Virginia Cavalry
Medical Officer in charge of the Corps Hospitals,
Surgeon W. H. Rulison, 9th New York Cavalry

Other doctors who assisted here included Eugene
F. Sanger (US Volunteers), Assistant Surgeon Hiram
D. Vosburg (Eighth New York Cavalry), a Dr. Patterson
(regiment unknown), Assistant Surgeon P. O'Meara
Edson (First Vermont Cavalry, medical officer in
charge of the corps hospital), Surgeon E. W. H. Beck
(Union, no unit), Dr. John Runkle (a local citizen who
lived on Baltimore Street), and a Dr. Gates (regiment
unknown). Rev. H. G. Finney was serving as pastor at
the time of the battle.

The 1863 church building was completely dismantled and replaced with the current structure in 1963.
The only original portions of the structure reused
were the wooden ceiling beams. All of the pews except
the Lincoln pew were replaced.

20. Methodist Episcopal Church (GAR Hall), 53 E. Middle Street, 39°49.781' N, 77°13.770' W

Built in 1822, this building was the first permanent
house of worship in Gettysburg for Methodists. In
1863, during and after the Battle of Gettysburg, most
public and church buildings were used as hospitals to
care for the wounded and dying, and the Methodist
Episcopal Church took on a new role.

Only a few wounded were treated here, and no
deaths were reported to have occurred among those
who were brought to the church. In the true spirit
of ecumenicity, the Catholic Sisters of Charity from
Emmitsburg, Maryland, had several of their order
at the Methodist church to administer aid to the
wounded. This small hospital remained in operation
until mid-August 1863. Few records remain concern-
ing those who were treated here.

By 1871 the congregation had grown to the point
where they needed a larger building. With completion
of a new building, the old church, including the graveyard, was put up for sale. It would take nine years to

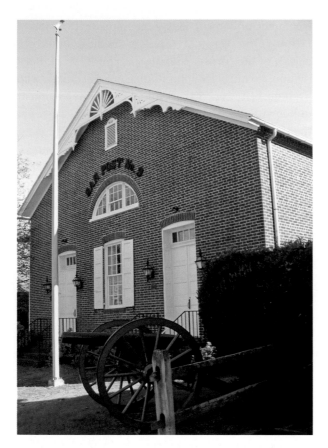

The Methodist Episcopal Church became a small hospital until the middle of August 1863.

find a buyer: a local branch of the Grand Army of the Republic (GAR). The GAR was a national organization of Union veterans of the war, and the local branch had been organized just a few years after the war ended. This would be their first permanent home in Gettysburg. They named their post the Corporal Johnston H. Skelly Post No. 9 of the GAR, after a local

veteran who had been mortally wounded at the Battle of Winchester on June 13, 1863. The purchase price of their new home was $600.

A few years after moving into their new facility, the local post had seen such a surge in membership that an addition was constructed on the rear of the building. This addition is said to have covered as many as two dozen graves.

During the summer of 1918, a deadly flu epidemic struck especially hard at Camp Colt, a US Army tank training facility established on the fields of Pickett's Charge. Commanded by a young Captain Dwight D. Eisenhower, many of those at the camp succumbed to the effects of the flu. The GAR Hall became the holding point for the coffins used to convey the remains.

For many years the GAR remained a powerful veterans' organization, lobbying on behalf of veterans for benefits and serving as a source of patriotic information for all Americans, but especially those of school age. Gradually, however, the number of surviving veterans decreased to the point where it was no longer economically feasible to try to maintain the building. In 1930 the few remaining members voted to turn the building over to an offshoot of the original organization, the Sons of Union Veterans. In 1988 the Historic Preservation Society of Gettysburg–Adams County purchased the property and began restoration efforts.

The Methodist Cemetery, the oldest burial ground in Gettysburg, is located behind the building. Although most of those interred were eventually relocated to Evergreen Cemetery, it still holds the remains of some forty-five local residents.

Today the facility is used as a meeting hall for the local community.

21. High Street (Common) School, 40 East High Street, 39°50.718' N, 77°13.783' W

Gettysburg's elementary school system was begun in 1834 to provide children with free education. Classes were segregated by gender and race and were conducted in several buildings around town, often in the home of a teacher. In 1857, the High Street, or Common, School was constructed as Gettysburg's first consolidated public school building. Both genders were taught here, although races remained separated.

On July 1, during the chaotic Union retreat from Oak Ridge, this hospital was established for the Union Cavalry Corps, as well as the First and Eleventh Corps. It would soon house Union and Confederate casualties on separate floors, with an estimated forty Union men on the first floor and about thirty Confederates on the second. Being a hospital did not spare the building from the dangers of the fighting. Several doctors reported that the school was struck several times by bullets over the first two days of fighting.

Gettysburg physician Theodore Tate, who had been in the Third Pennsylvania Cavalry only a month, was placed in charge of the Confederate wounded. Surgeon William W. Weidman of the Second Pennsylvania Cavalry also treated wounded Confederates on the second floor. Assistant Surgeon P. O'Meara Edson (First Vermont Cavalry), Assistant Surgeon George L. Potter (Fifth US Cavalry), Surgeon Ethanan W. Rowe (Confederate, unknown unit), and Surgeon E. W. H. Beck (Union, unknown unit) were also known to have been here, and Dr. Abraham Stout (153rd Pennsylvania Volunteers) would soon relocate to the school from the nearby Reformed church. The Ladies of the Confederate Aristocracy of Baltimore were among the nurses.

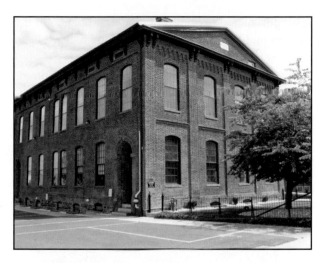

The High Street, or Common, School.

The exterior of the building looks nearly identical to its 1863 appearance except that the original bell cupola has been removed. The bell is now on display in Alumni Park at Baltimore and Lefever Streets. On July 1 a Union soldier became cut off from the rest of the Union army as he retreated through town. Taking refuge in the bell cupola, he remained hidden for three days with only a few drops of water from his canteen and no food the entire time.[39]

The school was one of the last three public buildings serving as hospitals to close (the Sheads and Buehler warehouse and the seminary were the other two).

22. Trinity German Reformed Church, 60 E. High Street, 39°49.718' N, 77°13.738' W

Now named the Trinity United Church of Christ, the congregation of this church formed as far back as 1790, and the original German Reformed Church was constructed here in 1814. The first portion of the present building was erected in 1851 and had just been refurbished at the time of the battle.

On July 1, Dr. Abraham Stout of the 153rd Pennsylvania Infantry was captured. One of his captors suggested he open a hospital. Stout did so at this church and it was filled, mostly with Union men, within thirty minutes. A red banner was hung from the cupola to signify that the church was now a hospital, where men from both sides took refuge.

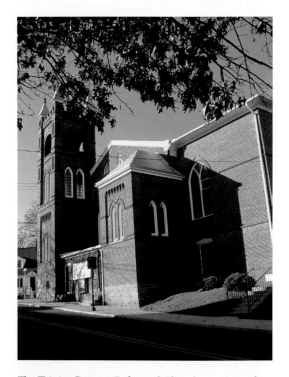

The Trinity German Reformed Church. A captured Union doctor opened a hospital here on the suggestion of his captors.

The lecture room was used for surgeries for several days, and the newly painted walls became blood-spattered. The new pews became soaked with blood, and surgeons had to bore holes in the floor to allow blood to drain out. Private Reuben Ruch of the 153rd Pennsylvania Infantry minced no words in describing the scene, calling it a slaughterhouse. He went on to say that he saw all he wanted to see when he observed the surgeons covered in blood, compelling him to go to an upper floor where he found an empty pew to lie down in. As soon as he could safely leave, Ruch made his way to the George Spangler farm, where the Eleventh Corps hospital was located.[40]

The hospital eventually became so crowded that many of the wounded were moved to the Common School. The church graveyard served as the second resting site for Jennie Wade, the only civilian killed in the battle. Initially buried outside her sister's home, she was later moved to the church cemetery and ultimately to Evergreen Cemetery, where she rests today.

23. Samuel Witherow House, 302 Baltimore Street, 39°49.613' N, 77°13.853' W

Samuel Witherow, fifty-four years old at the time of the battle, worked as an auctioneer and lived here with his daughters, Mary R. (twenty-two) and Sarah H. (a.k.a. Sally, twenty), and son Charles W. (eleven). Anna McGinley (sixty-six) was also listed in the 1860 census as being in the house, but her exact role is uncertain. She is believed to be the actual owner of the house and the sister of Witherow's deceased wife, Jane Eliza McGinley Witherow, who had died in 1857 at age forty-nine.[41]

The two Witherow sisters did double duty as nurses. In addition to helping with the wounded in their own home, both also assisted at the John Edward Plank farm.

One of those treated at the Witherow house was Lieutenant James Purman of the 140th Pennsylvania Volunteer Infantry. He had been wounded on the second day of fighting, receiving a severe leg wound. On October 30, 1896, Purman would be awarded the Medal of Honor for his heroism. His citation reads, "Voluntarily assisted a wounded comrade to a place of apparent safety while the enemy were in close proximity; he received the fire of the enemy and a wound which resulted in the amputation of his left leg."[42]

Purman obviously did not forget his hosts in Gettysburg. He returned after the war and married Mary. She wrote, "Like most families in Gettysburg, we took in wounded soldiers during the battle. I cared for Lt. James Purman of the 140th Pennsylvania in our home. Purman's injury was so severe that it required the amputation of his left leg. Later, I married this courageous soldier, creating a touching story of love against the backdrop of war."[43]

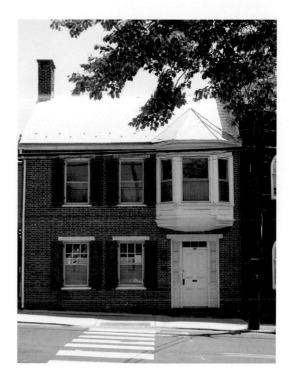

The Samuel Witherow House.

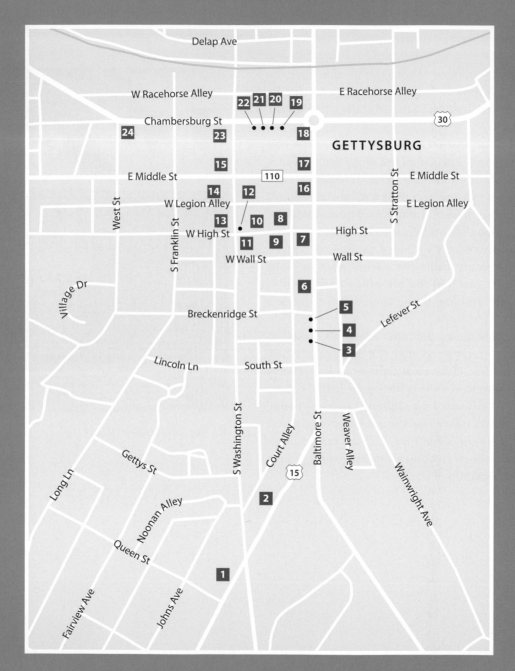

Chapter 3 sites: in town, southwest of square. (Map by Bill Nelson)

1. George George House, 237 Steinwehr Avenue, 39°49.257' N, 77°14.011' W

Although it may be difficult to visualize in today's landscape, the George George house actually sat on an open seven-acre plot of ground in 1863. George was a tenant in the house, which was owned by Captain John Myers, who also owned the house on Baltimore Street that would become the National Orphans Homestead. The house is believed to have been built before 1800 and, in addition to the sixty-three-year-old George, was occupied by George's wife, Susannah (age forty-three), and their six children, Jacob (fourteen), Sarah (twelve), Louisa (nine), John (six), Philo (four), and Samuel (thirty-one). Both George and his eldest son, Samuel, were day laborers.[1]

Assistant Surgeon Murdock McGregor of the Thirty-Third Massachusetts documented the house as a hospital, although it does not appear that it treated a large number of wounded. McGregor noted that all the sheets, quilts, pillows, and provisions were used for the injured. He then went on to say that George estimated his loss as about $100, indicating that his note may have been meant to serve as a receipt and

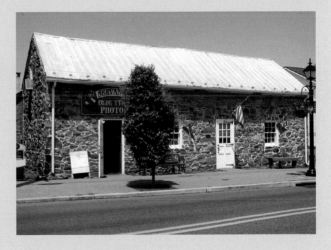

The George House received the body of General John Reynolds after he was killed in Herbst Woods.

documentation that the house had served as a hospital, in the event that George ever needed to prove it to authorities.[2]

The George house has become famous as the house where the body of Union general John Reynolds was brought on July 1 after having been killed in Herbst Woods. He was brought to George's by his staff to allow them time to locate a suitable coffin in which to transport him to his home in Lancaster, Pennsylvania, for burial.

2. Dobbin House, 89 Steinwehr Avenue, 39°49.365' N, 77°13.967' W

Using two of the slaves he held, Presbyterian minister Alexander Dobbin built this house on three hundred acres in 1776, making it one of the oldest buildings in Gettysburg. A one-and-a-half-story springhouse at the southern end of house was built at the same time. In the early 1800s the springhouse was raised to two stories and incorporated into the main house. This can be identified by the recessed balcony on the second floor of the front of house. The house is documented as being used as a hospital during the battle.[3] Neither the number of wounded treated here nor the names of the attending physicians were recorded.

Born in Ireland, Dobbin operated the first classical school west of the Susquehanna for young men in his home. A combined theological seminary and liberal arts college, it operated from 1788 to 1799. When Dobbin first settled in the area, Adams County was part of York County. He was one of the community leaders who worked to establish Adams County in 1800 and one of two appointed commissioners to choose Gettysburg as the county seat.

Dobbin's first wife was Isabella Gamble, with whom he had ten children. After Isabella died on August 19, 1800, at age forty-nine, Dobbin married Mary Irvin Agnew, the widow of Daniel Agnew, with whom she had had nine children. Alexander and Mary Irvin Dobbin had no children from their marriage.

Dobbin died in 1809 and the house changed hands several times over the next few years. It became a

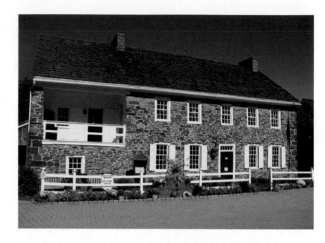

The Dobbin House served as a hospital, a stop on the Underground Railroad, a theological seminary, and a liberal arts college.

stop on the Underground Railroad, and by the time the war came to Gettysburg, the house was no longer in the Dobbin family. During the battle, twenty-nine-year-old Alvira Ziegler and her five children, Anna (thirteen), John (ten), Elizabeth (nine), Alice (six), and Rufus (four), lived here. Her husband, John, was away with the Union army and was not at Gettysburg.[4]

On July 2, Confederate sharpshooters used the barn as a stronghold to shoot at Union soldiers on Cemetery Hill, and the house itself was struck at least four times by artillery shells.

3. Henry Garlach House, 323 Baltimore Street, 39°49.574' N, 77°13.862' W

Forty-five-year-old Henry Garlach, his wife, Catherine B. (forty-one); and their four children, Anna L. (seventeen), George E. (fourteen), William (eleven), and

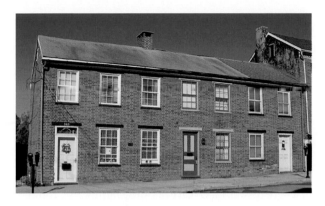

Henry Garlach's house is best known for its role in hiding Union general Alexander Schimmelfennig.

Catherine (a.k.a. Katie, age four), lived in the south end of this Baltimore Street house, with the rest of the building used as Henry's cabinetmaking and coffin shop.[5] Henry made many of the coffins used to send dead soldiers home, and he found that he had more business than he could handle after the battle.

Henry had gone to the crest of Culp's Hill to observe the fighting. Arrested as a possible spy, he was detained for several days and did not get home until the fighting was over. Katie had also left on the first day with some neighbors, for her safety. It fell on Catherine B. and Anna to care for the family throughout the battle, as well as the wounded who made their way to the house. Anna also went to the Presbyterian Church on July 4 to help with the wounded there.

Seeking refuge in her cellar, Catherine found that a foot of rainwater had accumulated there. Undaunted, she and her son William used wood from Henry's shop to build a platform above the water level. Once that was done, Catherine invited several of her neighbors into her home, where they would be safer. This proved

to be a prudent move, as the Garlach home and several others in the area were all struck several times by bullets. By the evening of July 1 there were eleven neighbors in the Garlach house. Everyone slept on the floor, fearing stray bullets could enter windows and strike them if they slept on the beds. They spent most of their time in the kitchen, preparing their meals after dark and going to the basement any time there was firing. They got their water at night from a well in the yard, with Confederate soldiers often helping to draw the water and carrying it to the house.

At one point a Confederate soldier attempted to take advantage of the uneasy acquaintance he had made with Catherine. She described the incident: "(A rebel soldier) tried to come into my house to use it as a sharpshooter position but I grabbed him and told him that he couldn't come in because the house was full of women and children. Luckily he saw I was serious and left."[6]

The Garlach home would become the scene of one of the more unusual incidents of the battle when Union general Alexander Schimmelfennig had to hide in the backyard for three days. Schimmelfennig was a veteran of the Prussian army and had come to the United States in 1853. He had been hand-picked by Lincoln for promotion from colonel to general, a strategy employed by Lincoln to get support from the German American community for the war effort. Schimmelfennig was serving as brigade commander in the Eleventh Corps during the battle.

The first day of fighting found Schimmelfennig retreating on his horse on Washington Street. Unfamiliar with the town, he turned down a dead-end alley as the rebels pursued. When his horse was shot, the general jumped over a fence into Garlach's yard but quickly saw that rebels on Baltimore Street were cutting off his escape. An old watercourse that had been converted into a sewer ran through the yard and had been covered with a wooden culvert. Schimmelfennig ducked into the culvert, where he remained until dark. He then came out and hid in Garlach's woodshed, behind two barrels containing swill for the hogs. This part of the story has led to some accounts saying he stayed in the pen with Garlach's hogs, but that has been proved to simply be an overdramatization to embellish the story.

When Catherine came out to feed the hogs, he called to her. "Oh, the fright he gave me when I saw him," she exclaimed later.[7] She brought him some food and water the next day but feared she would be seen, so the general hid there until the morning of July 4 with no more food or water.

On the night of July 3, Confederate soldiers asked Catherine for wood from Henry's shop so they could make a coffin for General William Barksdale. Catherine directed them to the yard, telling them it was too dangerous to make a light in the shop but that they could use any wood they found. They complied with her request but had to retreat in the morning before the coffin was finished.

Daniel Culp, who owned the woodworking shop near the courthouse, claimed that the Confederates brought the wood to his shop to make the coffin as the retreat began. It is likely that Culp and his nephew, Jeremiah Culp, worked on the coffin but discontinued the effort when the Confederates left. It is known that the coffin eventually was finished by Charles Comfort, who also lived nearby. However, when it was done, the coffin was eventually used to bury Jennie Wade, the lone civilian killed at Gettysburg.

The exact number of wounded treated at Garlach's is unknown, but there was at least one amputee cared for in the home. Lieutenant Charles W. Roberts, adjutant of the Seventeenth Maine Infantry, had been badly wounded on July 2 in fighting against the Eighth Georgia Infantry in the Wheatfield. Lieutenant Colonel Charles B. Merrill cut a strap from his sword belt and used it as a tourniquet on Roberts's leg, saving his life. Unfortunately, the leg had to be amputated at the division hospital. Roberts was moved to Garlach's on July 6, where he was taken care of by the family and Thomas Dennett, a nurse from the Seventeenth Maine. Roberts remained at Garlach's home for about five weeks until his father was able to come and take him home.

4. George Shriver House, 309 Baltimore Street, 39°49.593' N, 77°13.862' W

George and Henrietta "Hettie" Shriver were twenty-three years old and had been married for five years when they paid $290 for a plot of land on Baltimore Street in 1860. They immediately built this house and moved in, making a home for themselves and their daughters Sarah (a.k.a. Sadie) and Mary (a.k.a. Mollie). A son, Jacob, had died in infancy. At the same time that he built his home, George built a saloon in the cellar and a two-lane, ten-pin bowling alley in a building just behind the house.

In September 1861, George mustered into Company C of Cole's Maryland Cavalry and was not present during the Gettysburg fighting. The company was made up of sixty-eight Gettysburg residents and was known as the Keystone Rangers. Shortly after George left with his regiment, the Tenth New York Cavalry moved into Gettysburg and occupied the town from

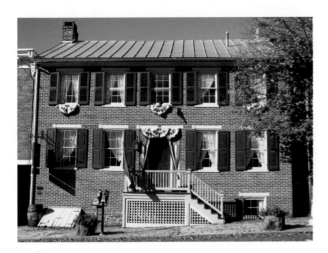

When George Shriver's family fled for safety, Confederates quickly moved into the house and established a hospital.

Christmas Eve 1861 until March 7, 1862, many of them staying in the saloon and bowling alley.

When the battle started, Henrietta took her daughters to the home of her neighbor James Pierce. Pierce was concerned for his daughter Tillie's safety and convinced Hettie, her daughters, and Tillie to leave. Hettie's father, Jacob Weikert, owned a farm three miles from town that Hettie believed would provide them with a safe place to sit out the battle. They immediately began the trek to Weikert's farm on foot. When they arrived, she learned that the farm was not as far from the fighting as she had hoped, and it had become a field hospital for the Union's Second, Third, and Fifth Corps. She immediately was pressed into service nursing the wounded.

Hettie and her daughters returned home on July 7 to find that nothing in their house was left. Her new home had been occupied by Confederate soldiers, and all the food, clothing, and blankets were gone. Two rebel sharpshooters had been killed in an upstairs garret. The Confederates had also used the house as a hospital, and medical supplies were scattered around the house.

Decades later, forensic detectives from the Niagara Falls Police Department received permission to test stains found in the attic. Using luminol, a chemical used to detect trace amounts of blood at crime scenes, the forensic team confirmed that the stains were from human blood. They also found a bottle of Civil War–era medicine and a jar of salve that had been hidden under some floorboards.[8]

George was able to obtain a furlough to come home for Christmas 1863. On December 29, he left home for the last time. He would be captured near Winchester, Virginia, by Mosby's Raiders and sent to Andersonville Prison, where he died of scorbutus (scurvy) on August 25, 1864.

On July 19, 1866, Henrietta Shriver married stonecutter Daniel Pittenturff, whose wife, Cynthia Powers Pittenturff (daughter of Gettysburg granite cutter Solomon Powers), had died in April 1864. Henrietta and Daniel had two daughters. Henrietta left Gettysburg in the 1870s, died in 1916, and is buried in Glenwood Cemetery, Washington, DC.

The house, now a museum, has been a filming site for PBS, the History Channel, A&E, Discovery Channel, and others.

5. James Pierce House, 301 Baltimore Street, 39°49.603' N, 77°13.867' W

James Pierce, a fifty-five-year-old butcher, lived on the second floor of this home, above his butcher shop. Living with him were his wife, Margaret (age fifty-three),

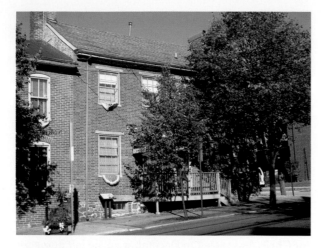

The Pierces' daughter Tillie wrote an acclaimed account of her experiences during the battle. The Pierce family lived in this house.

and his two daughters, Margaret A. (seventeen) and Matilda "Tillie" (fifteen). Also in the home at the time were Eliza Fetteroff (a fifty-one-year-old listed as a seamstress) and Franklin Culp (fifteen). The Pierces also had two sons in the Union army, both butchers in civilian life: James S. (age twenty-seven) and William H. (twenty-two).[9]

On the first day of fighting, James sent Tillie with neighbor Henrietta Shriver to the Jacob Weikert farm for her safety. The Weikerts were Mrs. Shriver's parents, and the farm was three miles outside town on the Taneytown Road, thought to be well out of the way of the fighting. The fighting would be far more widespread than the Pierces thought, however, and Tillie found herself in the midst of a large field hospital when she arrived at the Weikerts. For the next six days, she helped care for the wounded, returning

home on July 7. Tillie would go on to write a highly regarded account of her life during and after the war titled *At Gettysburg; or What a Girl Saw and Heard of the Battle.*

On July 2 and 3 Confederate sharpshooters positioned themselves outside the Pierce house, not knowing that Mrs. Pierce had five wounded Union soldiers receiving treatment in the home. Mr. Pierce had gone to warehouses in the northern part of town to assist with the wounded shortly after the fighting began and was unaware of the presence of the wounded men. On his way home, he was stopped by a Southern soldier who demanded that Pierce turn over his gun. When Pierce said he had no gun, the soldier shot at him but missed. It would not be Pierce's last encounter with a Confederate soldier.

Before arriving home, he was stopped again by five Confederates who ordered him to go home. When he said that was where he was going, they accompanied him. Once there, they demanded to search the house for Union soldiers. Pierce insisted that there were none, unaware of the presence of the Union wounded, but before he could enter the home, his accosters again insisted on searching it. Fearing that his family was probably frightened, he reminded the rebels that it was against the laws of war to break into private houses. After discussing the situation among themselves, the soldiers agreed to leave after reminding Pierce that Union sharpshooters were active and that he was in danger of being shot by his own side if he stayed outside. (This was not an idle comment. Tillie Pierce later counted seventeen bullet holes in the balcony of her home.) It was only when Pierce got inside that he learned of the five Union wounded in his home.[10]

Over the next several days, the family spent the daylight hours in the cellar to avoid stray bullets that found their way into the house and riddled the back porch. They came up only at night when the shooting subsided. Unfortunately, their horse remained outside and was taken by rebel soldiers. The Pierces occasionally saw the animal being ridden past their house over the next few days but never saw it again after the rebels retreated.

The family did not leave a record of the names of the men they treated, although one was known to be Corporal Michael O'Brien of the 143rd Ohio Infantry. He had been badly wounded in the arm. In 1888 he returned to Gettysburg for what would become known as the Grand Reunion. While there, he made it a point to visit the Pierces to thank them for their kindness, not realizing until his arrival at the home that Mrs. Pierce had died seven years earlier.

When the battle ended, a Methodist minister knocked on the door to tell the family that the rebels had gone. Mr. Pierce rushed outside, where he found a musket lying on the ground. As he picked it up, he saw a lone Confederate soldier running toward the alley. Ordering the man to stop, he learned the man was a deserter. As he marched his captive back to the house, he spied two more who also claimed to be deserters. Pierce took the three to the front street, where he handed them over to passing Union soldiers. He would go on to capture three more Confederates before realizing that the gun he had found was not loaded.[11]

A few days after the battle, Colonel William Colvill of the First Minnesota was brought to the house on a litter. Colvill had been at Nathaniel Lightner's farm since he had been wounded in the ankle and shoulder, with the latter wound affecting his spine. Surgeons had tried to amputate his foot above the wounded ankle but Colvill had adamantly refused to allow it. Colvill's sister came to the Pierce home to assist in his treatment, and two men from his regiment, Musician Milton L. Bevans and Private Walter S. Reed, also stayed behind to help.

Colvill remained at the Pierce home for several months before he was pronounced well enough to leave. He left on crutches, still in possession of his foot. Three years later, he returned to the house while he was in town to tour the battlefield.

6. Henry Comfort House, 241 Baltimore Street, 39°49.656' N, 77°13.872' W

Also known as the Sweney house, this home was occupied by Henry Comfort and his family during the battle. Little is known about the Comfort family or the extent to which their home was used as a temporary hospital.

The number of wounded who were treated here is unknown, but at least one Union officer, believed to have been Captain John Costin, Company F, Eighty-Second Ohio Infantry, is known to have died in the house. Costin was wounded on July 1 but lingered until July 11 before succumbing to his wounds. Costin's wife and son were said to have come to the Comfort house to help with his treatment, and other records indicate that there was probably at least one more wounded man here at the same time.

The Comforts were neighbors of Jennie Wade, whose birthplace and home were across the street. Charles Comfort was a coachmaker and a carpenter and is credited with being the person who finished the coffin that was used to hold Wade's remains when she was interred. Marie Comfort commented on her

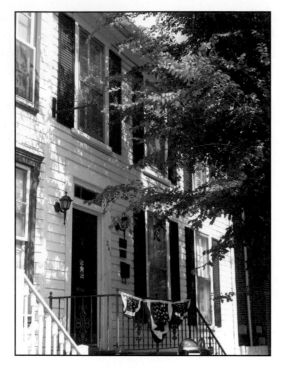

The Henry Comfort House.

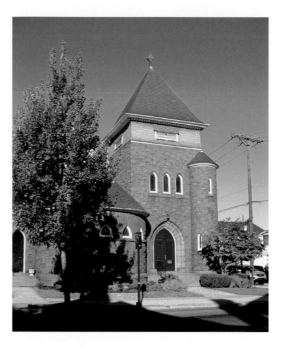

The David McCreary House sat on the site now occupied by the Prince of Peace Episcopal Church.

death: "When poor Jennie was killed my son Charles furnished the coffin that Jennie was buried in. What a sad day that was. She was only 20 years old." She went on to say, "In 1861 I had my likeness taken and had the Wade girls accompany me. It has turned out to be the only photo of Jennie Wade ever taken."[12]

7. David McCreary House Site, 20 West High Street, 39°49.623' N, 77°13.872' W

Now the Prince of Peace Episcopal Church, this is the site of the home of David McCreary and his family. The fifty-nine-year-old McCreary was a widower,

his wife, Ann, having died just three years earlier. McCreary worked as a harness and saddle maker, with his shop adjacent to his house. He lived with his children James (age thirty-one, also a harness maker), Louisa (twenty-nine), John F. (twenty-two), William S. (a printer's apprentice, age nineteen), Francis F. (seventeen), Albertus (fifteen), and Mervin J. (twelve). A domestic worker, fifty-nine-year-old Sarah Claud, also lived here.[13] Another daughter, twenty-five-year-old Georgie Ann, was not living at home at the time of the battle.

McCreary also had a free black domestic worker named Elizabeth Butler who was taken captive by

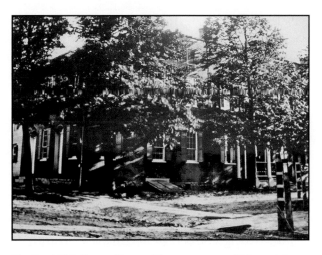

The David McCreary House. (Photo courtesy of Memorial Church of the Prince of Peace, the Rev. Dr. Herbert Sprouse, Rector)

the Confederates when they overran the town on July 1. She was marched with the rest of the captured blacks down the street, and there was such a crowd that when they were opposite the Christ Evangelical Lutheran Church, Butler slipped into the church without being seen. Once inside, she climbed up into the belfry, where she stayed for two days with nothing to eat or drink.[14]

McCreary's son Albertus spent a great deal of his time observing the events taking place around town and wrote several accounts of the battle. He was proud to be able to say that he learned from a friendly rebel soldier how to identify the various types of bullets and shells by the noises they made.

Albertus documented much of what happened in his home, including the fact that every bed in his house was filled with wounded. He also noted that several Confederates entered the house at one point

and captured several Union soldiers who had taken refuge there, including some of the lesser wounded, even though a red flag designating the house as a hospital was prominently displayed.

The adventuresome Albertus nearly lost his life the morning of July 1 while observing the activities from a door to the roof of the McCreary house. Nearly every surrounding rooftop held a sharpshooter and, as he watched, two bullets struck the McCreary roof just a short distance from him. The close call made him decide to quickly abandon his position.[15]

Not long after, Albertus, wearing a Union kepi, stood on his front porch watching Confederate troops march past. Some of the rebels spotted his hat and an officer, believing Albertus was a Union soldier, ordered the young McCreary arrested. It took a great deal of persuasion from the elder McCreary and his neighbors to convince the Confederate officer otherwise.[16]

The house and shop were torn down in 1888 and construction of the Prince of Peace Episcopal Church began. The cornerstone of the church was laid on July 2, 1888, for the twenty-fifth anniversary of the Battle of Gettysburg.

Episcopal services in Gettysburg had been conducted at the courthouse beginning in 1867, followed by a move to an abandoned Methodist church on East Middle Street (which later became the local hall of the Grand Army of the Republic). In December 1876, the congregation occupied a new small wooden church on Stevens Street.

For the twenty-fifth anniversary of the Battle of Gettysburg, in 1888, the official program of the Army of the Potomac and the Army of Northern Virginia publicized a project for a church "to be named the

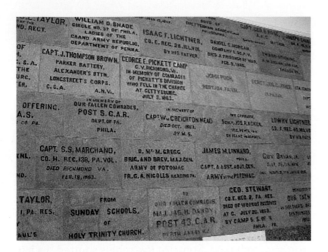

The Prince of Peach Church's Memorial Wall is made up of more than 150 stones and plaques in honor of fallen Union and Confederate soldiers.

National Memorial Church of the Prince of Peace. That Church upon whose loving unity the terrible events of the Civil War made no mark, is surely the one above all others to embrace the memorials of both sides in rearing a lasting Temple to the Prince of Peace." And with that statement the church became more than just a house of worship. It is also a battle-field memorial and a symbol of reconciliation, where survivors from both armies placed more than 150 plaques inside the large tower in memory of their fallen comrades, no matter where they fell.[17]

In addition to those plaques are six stones in the columbarium, including one dedicated to a marine killed at Manassas, one referencing the Baltimore riots, and one honoring a soldier mortally wounded at Fair Oaks while rescuing his regimental colors. Also included is the wooden grave marker of Lieutenant Manning Livingston of the Third US Artillery, killed

on July 2 at Gettysburg. In the choir area are four large plaques donated by the Military Order of the Loyal Legion of the United States between 1901 and 1902, dedicated to General George Meade, General John Reynolds, General Winfield Scott Hancock, and Colonel Harry Goodman.

In 1970 a disastrous fire gutted the church, but the tower room and memorial stones were largely untouched. The few memorials that were damaged have been replaced.

8. St. Francis Xavier Roman Catholic Church, 25 W. High Street, 39°49.718′ N, 77°13.918′ W

The first church for the St. Francis Xavier congregation was on South Washington Street. When the congregation outgrew that building, they purchased this lot on West High Street in 1849, laying the cornerstone in 1852. The six pillars on the front are not original, having been added in 1925.

The church became a hospital during the battle, treating more than 250 from both sides. Most of those were from the fighting during the second and third days of the battle. The sick and wounded filled the church, leaving scarcely enough room to walk through. Every inch of available space was taken. They lay in the pews, in the aisles and sanctuary, beside the pulpit and the altar, and in the gallery, many lying in their own blood. With no available space in the church, cooking was done at the nearby Peter Myers house.

When it became apparent that more wounded were coming than could easily be accommodated, every other pew was removed to expand the available space. Later, bunks were made by placing doors

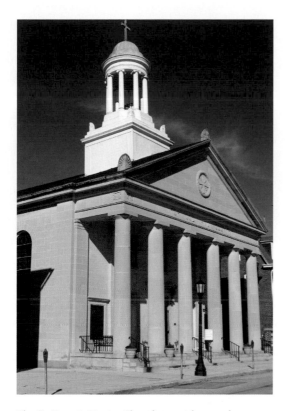

The St. Francis Xavier Church treated more than 250 wounded.

across the pews to raise the wounded from the floor, and the musty, bloody straw was removed and fresh bedding put down. The churchyard became strewn with amputated arms and legs that had been thrown out windows. Blood splattered the walls, where it remained for nearly a year until the church could dedicate funds for cleaning and renovation.

The entrance doors were opened to provide additional light, and windows were left open to provide fresh air. The open windows, however, also had the unwelcome side effect of allowing the moaning and cries from the wounded to drift outside for passersby to hear. An operating table was set up just inside the main entrance; another was placed in the basement, which also served as a temporary morgue where the dead were taken for preparation for burial or transport.

The doctors stayed in the two rooms adjoining the altar, with Dr. Philip Quinan of the 150th Pennsylvania Volunteer Infantry in charge. Other doctors who served here included Assistant Surgeon James Fulton (143rd Pennsylvania Volunteer Infantry), Surgeon F. C. Reamer (also of the 143rd Pennsylvania), Dr. W. G. Hunter (149th Pennsylvania), and a Dr. Gates, who may have been a civilian doctor. The doctors were captured when the Confederate Army of Northern Virginia took the town, but were kept at the church to continue to treat the wounded. Most of the doctors shuttled between St. Francis Xavier and the United Presbyterian and Reformed Church across the street.

As the battle drew to a close, twelve Sisters of Charity arrived from Emmitsburg, Maryland, bringing bandages, sponges, clothing, and food. On their arrival, Sister Serena Klimkiewicz found her brother among the wounded. They dressed wounds and sat with the dying. In 1953 eight new stained-glass windows were dedicated, including one commemorating the work of the Sisters of Charity. A bronze plaque on the front of the church also recognizes their efforts.

On July 2 Confederate general Richard Ewell and his men came to the church to use the cupola as an observation post. The soldiers climbed into the cupola and called the progress of the fighting down to Ewell, who could not climb the ladder because of the loss of

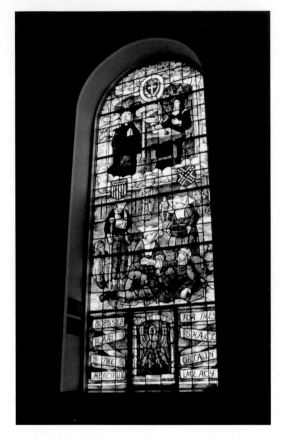

A stained-glass window commemorating the work of the Sisters of Charity.

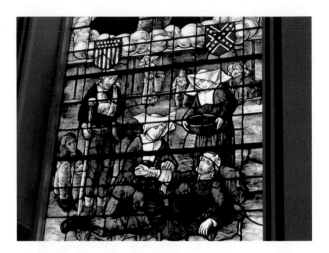

A closer view of the stained-glass window commemorating the work of the Sisters of Charity.

his leg a year earlier at Brawner's farm near Manassas, Virginia.

One of those treated at the church was Lieutenant Colonel Henry S. Huidekoper of the 150th Pennsylvania, wounded twice in the first day's fighting near the McPherson barn. Huidekoper's right arm had been shattered at the elbow and, with the arm wrapped with cord above the elbow to stem the loss of blood, he walked from McPherson Ridge to the church, a distance of more than a mile. There, surgeons removed his arm.

On July 2 local civilian nurse Sallie Myers brought Huidekoper a cracker and some wine when she learned that he had not eaten since early the previous morning. The next day, Huidekoper walked to the Myers house, staying until July 9, when he lay on the wet floor of a freight car that had just brought ice to Gettysburg. That freight car took him to a hospital in Baltimore, a trip that took twelve hours.

Huidekoper, who served as president of the Gettysburg Battlefield Memorial Commission until his death in 1918, sent a letter of appreciation to the Sisters of Charity for what they had done for him.[18] On May 27, 1905, Huidekoper was awarded the Medal of Honor for his actions at Gettysburg. His citation reads, "While engaged in repelling an attack of the enemy, received a severe wound of the right arm, but instead of retiring remained at the front in command of the regiment."[19]

The church remained an active hospital until late in July, when the patients were moved to the newly opened general hospital on York Road.

9. United Presbyterian and Associated Reformed Church, 30 W. High Street, 39°49.710' N, 77°13.920' W

The congregation of this church first worshipped in a small log church along Rock Creek, beginning in the 1750s. They moved to this location and built a small church in the early 1800s.

Like the St. Francis Xavier Roman Catholic Church across the street, the church became a hospital during the battle. It served the Third Division, First Corps, in conjunction with its Catholic neighbor.

The same doctors and nurses served both church hospitals, shuttling back and forth across the street to treat the wounded as well as they could. Surgery was performed in the yard outside the church, and the dead were buried in two nearby trenches. Civilian John Burns, who walked to McPherson Ridge to fight on July 1, became a member of this congregation in January 1866.

Little is known about the hospital or the men who were treated here. However, its location adjacent to the David McCreary house provided young Albertus McCreary with an excellent vantage point to view what was happening. "I spent hours on the fence watching them operating on the wounded," he said. "I got pretty well hardened to such sights."[20]

The church was razed circa 1890 and now is the site of the Gettysburg United Methodist Church.

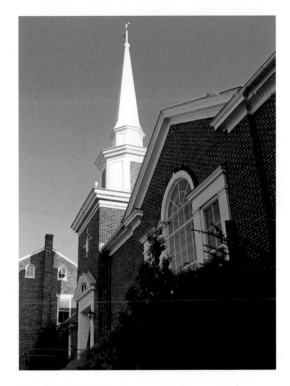

Site of the United Presbyterian and Associated Reformed Church. Surgery was performed in the yard outside the church.

10. Peter Myers House, 55 W. High Street, 39°49.716' N, 77°13.970' W

This home housed the family of Peter Myers, a cabinetmaker who also served as justice of the peace and judge of elections for the town of Gettysburg. Peter and his wife, Hannah, lived here with five of their seven children. A young son, Peter Jr., had died in 1847 at age three, and their oldest son, Jefferson, had recently married and moved into a separate home. The oldest daughter, Elizabeth Salome, better known

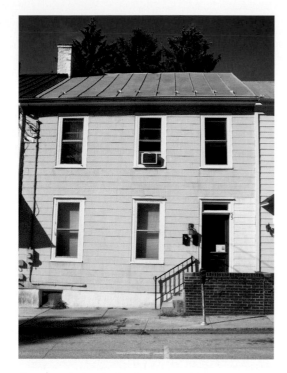

During and after the battle, this small house held the Myers family, eleven wounded soldiers, and a number of family members of the wounded for several weeks.

from our house," she said. "I was a teacher, not a nurse! I got sick at the sight of blood. I told them they didn't want me. I ended up going to the church anyway, and oh, how awful. There were men everywhere—on the pews, under the pews, between the pews."[21]

Kneeling beside the first man she came to, she asked what she could do for him. "Nothing," he said. "I am going to die." Sallie said she immediately went outside and cried. Regaining her composure, she returned later and had the man (Sergeant Alexander Stewart, 149th Pennsylvania Infantry) moved to her home. At one point while she was tending to Stewart, Sallie stood up to stretch. Seconds after she arose, a minié ball passed through two walls and struck the floor where she had just been sitting. Despite her care, Stewart, who had been wounded in the lungs and spine, died on July 6.[22]

In addition to Stewart, Lieutenant Colonel Henry S. Huidekoper (150th Pennsylvania), Major Thomas Chamberlain (150th Pennsylvania), Captain Bruce Blair (149th Pennsylvania), Captain James Ashworth (121st Pennsylvania), Captain Henry Eaton (Sixteenth Vermont), his brother Sergeant Eugene Eaton (Sixteenth Vermont), Private William Sheriff (142nd Pennsylvania), Private Andrew Crooks (149th Pennsylvania), Private A. R. Wintamute (143rd Pennsylvania), and Private Charles Decker (142nd Pennsylvania) were treated here. Some of the men had their mothers or servants present to help in their treatment. The wounded all insisted on paying the Myers family for their care.

Huidekoper and Blair both lost arms, and Crooks had his leg amputated. Wintamute survived but was killed in his first battle after returning to his regiment. Decker also met an unfortunate end, drowning a few years later.[23]

as Sallie, was twenty-one years old and was an assistant to the principal at the High Street School. She and her sister Susan were destined to serve as nurses for the next several weeks.

On the first day of the fighting, a doctor from the 143rd Pennsylvania Infantry, probably either Assistant Surgeon James Fulton or Surgeon F. C. Reamer, came to the house and asked that Sallie and her sisters come to the nearby St. Francis Xavier Church to help with the wounded. "I was asked to help with the wounded at St. Francis Xavier Catholic Church a few doors

Alexander Stewart's father came to Gettysburg on July 16 to claim his son's body. The next summer, Alexander's mother and his brother, Henry, came to visit the Myers family. While there, Henry and Sallie fell in love. They married in 1867. Sadly, Henry died the next year, in September 1868, just a month before his son was born. Sallie never remarried, but her son, named Henry after his father, became a well-known doctor and historian in the area. Sallie died on January 17, 1922, and is buried in Evergreen Cemetery.

11. Gettysburg Academy, 68 W. High Street, 39°49.706' N, 77°13.979' W

In 1810 the Pennsylvania state legislature allocated $2,000 to establish the Gettysburg Academy. The state's grant stipulated that $1,000 was for construction of the building and the purchase of books. The other $1,000 was to pay for the free instruction of up to four indigent children. The building opened in 1813 as the home for the Gettysburg Academy, with two large rooms on each floor.

The building later served as the first home for both the Lutheran Theological Seminary (1825–1832) and the Pennsylvania (now Gettysburg) College (1832–1837). In 1856 Rev. David Eyster moved into the building and, with the help of his wife, established the Gettysburg Young Ladies Seminary. When Eyster died in 1861 at the age of fifty-nine, his widow, Rebecca Reynolds Eyster, took over the duties as principal. During the battle it became a hospital.

When the Army of Northern Virginia appeared on June 26, 1863, Mrs. Eyster called the girls to the front porch to see what she perceived to be an event they would never forget, then apparently thought better of

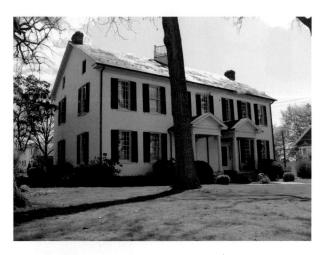

Gettysburg Academy had four large rooms filled with wounded.

it, saying, "Children, run home as quickly as you can!" The girls returned to class the next day but classes were disrupted again around noon. When Union troops marched past on June 30, the girls ran to the corner of High and Washington Streets and sang "The Union Forever" repeatedly as they passed.[24]

Tillie Pierce, a fifteen-year-old student, talked of her experiences, saying, "Within the same walls had been placed some of the wounded and dying heroes of the struggle; and as we passed from room to room we would speak in subdued tones of the solemn scenes which imagination and report placed before our minds as having transpired when the conflict was over."[25]

Just below the roof line and immediately adjacent to the third window from the right while looking at the building from West High Street, a shell can still be seen in the wall. The projectile is a Reed shell and

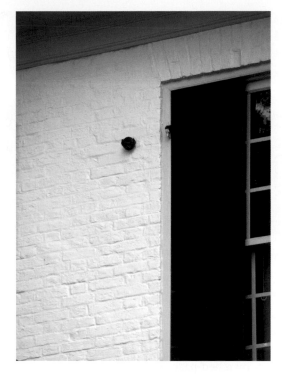

A shell from the first day of the battle remains embedded in the wall near the top corner of this window of the Gettysburg Academy.

would have come from a ten-pounder Parrott rifle somewhere within the Confederate lines, most likely from the Oak Ridge area on the first day of fighting.

12. Solomon Powers House, 65 W. High Street, 39°49.716' N, 77°13.992' W

Solomon Powers (age sixty), Catherine (fifty-nine), Ann J. (twenty-seven), Mary D. (twenty-six), Elizabeth V. (twenty-four), Alice (twenty-two), and Elizabeth L.

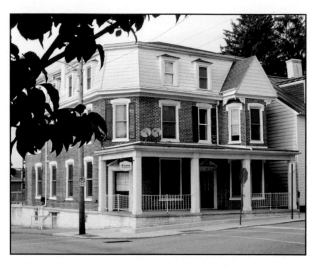

As many as sixteen wounded were treated here in the Solomon Powers home.

(eighteen) lived in this West High Street house that also served as the home of Solomon's granite-cutting business. Ann J., Mary D., and Elizabeth V. were all teachers. Joshua Haphold, a twenty-two-year-old stonecutter's apprentice who was learning the trade from Solomon, also lived in the home, and during the battle Catherine (age forty-five) and Lizzie (twenty) Sweeney came to the Powers home when their own house at the foot of the Baltimore Street hill had come under heavy fire. Catherine was separated from her husband, Harvey, who lived in what is now the Farnsworth house.[26]

Solomon was reputed to be the best stonecutter west of the Susquehanna River. The stones for the base of the Evergreen Cemetery gatehouse came from his quarry, and when the national cemetery opened, the State of Massachusetts contracted with Powers to help transfer remains of 158 Massachusetts soldiers to the cemetery.

J. Howard Wert, a chronicler of much of the battle, wrote that Powers was a "great, uncouth, elephantine man" and that "his clothes hung on him as if most unskillfully thrown into their places with a pitchfork." He also noted that he "had a heart ten times larger than his massive frame. Blunt of speech, unmerciful in his excoriation of all shams, hypocrisies, and false pretences, it was the glory of his life to pour balm upon sorrow and alleviate suffering, and all of his large family of daughters had inherited the gift of the Good Samaritan soul."[27]

His profitable business on High Street provided the capital to give his daughters a fine education, and Solomon often spoke glowingly about his five well-educated daughters. Alice taught in one of the country schools in 1863 and was home for summer vacation during the battle. She and her sister Sallie nursed the wounded and dying inside the Catholic church.

Jane Powers McDonnell, Alice's older sister, was married to one of the civilians seized by the Confederates on July 1, but Henry McDonnell's fate was more fortunate than most prisoners'. A Confederate officer ordered him released on July 4, and he was able to rejoin his wife and two small children. Some of the captured men from Gettysburg spent significant time in Southern prisons.

There were fifteen or sixteen wounded in the house, tended to by Dr. James Fulton (143rd Pennsylvania). Catherine Sweeney, Lizzie Sweeney, Alice Powers, Catherine Powers, and Jane Powers all helped with the wounded at the Powers house. The granite yard, which was fenced in, was a temporary holding pen for Union prisoners of war.

The Powers home was the scene of a tragedy in November 1863. After the death of his parents, four-teen-year-old Allen Frazer had moved in with the Powers family. The youth was watching an adult named Russell M. Briggs attempt to open an unexploded artillery shell on Powers's porch when it exploded. The blast badly injured Briggs and tore young Frazer nearly in two, killing him instantly.

Briggs had come to town from his Philadelphia home to retrieve the body of his son, George, of the Seventy-Second Pennsylvania Volunteer Infantry, who had been mortally wounded on July 3 near the Angle during Pickett's Charge. Briggs had planned his visit in conjunction with his attendance at the dedication of the national cemetery, and he had the coffin containing his son's body on the front porch with him when the accident occurred. He was taken to Camp Letterman, where both hands and a leg were amputated. He also lost both eyes. Frazer was buried in Evergreen Cemetery.[28]

13. James and Catherine Foster House, 155 S. Washington Street, 39°49.718' N, 77°14.008' W

Elderly couple James and Catherine Foster, who had been married in 1817, lived here with their only daughter, Catherine Mary White Foster (thirty-seven years old at the time of the battle). The Fosters' niece, Belle M. Stewart, a student at the Eysters' Young Ladies Seminary, was visiting with them during the battle.

On July 1, when the skirmishing began, Catherine Mary and Belle went to their western balcony to watch. Later in the morning, General John Reynolds dashed down the street, calling for everyone to go to their cellars. James, a seventy-nine-year-old veteran of the War of 1812, would have none of that. Confusing his wars, he protested, "If those 'Hessians' were only here now we would make a pot-pie of them."[29]

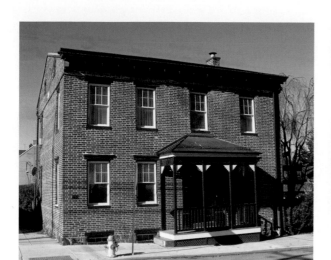

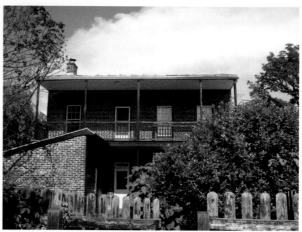

The home of James and Catherine Foster. Union general John Reynolds warned the Fosters to take cover in their cellar just minutes before he was killed near Herbst Woods.

The Foster family narrowly escaped death or serious injury when a shell struck the balcony located here shortly after they left to get water for passing soldiers. This balcony is a replacement for the damaged balcony.

Catherine also described her close call that same morning: "On July 1 we went to our rear balcony to watch as skirmishing began west of town. When we heard pleas for water, we carried water to the front door and poured it into the soldiers' cups. Moments after we left the balcony, a 12-pound shell demolished the roof and ceiling."[30]

One of the wounded who only spent a short time at the Foster home was Corporal Leander Wilcox of the 151st Pennsylvania Volunteer Infantry. The Fosters hid his gun in the stovepipe; his knapsack was hidden in the ashes of the fireplace. Wilcox hid in a potato bin and covered himself with kindling just as a rebel captain and two privates burst into the cellar. Catherine stood between the soldiers and Wilcox, since the Fosters had not had enough time to sufficiently cover him. When

the Confederates left the cellar to search the rest of the house, the kindling was rearranged, allowing better concealment. During the night, two Louisiana Tigers came and demanded entry to search again. When they also demanded fifty dollars, James Foster told them he only had three dollars, which they took before leaving. Wilcox eventually escaped undetected.[31]

Two surgeons stayed with the Fosters, Theodore J. Heard of Boston (assistant surgeon of the Thirteenth Massachusetts and medical director for the First Corps) and Richard M. Bache of Philadelphia (surgeon on General Reynolds's staff). They had been captured but were allowed to perform hospital duty. Both likely treated the few wounded who came to the house, as well as the wounded in some of the surrounding homes. They also may have treated some Confederate wounded on the last night of the battle after ambulance officers from North Carolina used the front porch to supervise removal of their wounded from the southwestern part of the field. The two doctors used the home for two days.

Both came very close to becoming casualties themselves. The guns began before dawn on July 3, forcing the family to the cellar once again. As daylight broke, Mrs. Foster gave the two doctors a light breakfast, after which they left to assist wounded in other locations. Shortly after their departure, a shell entered the room in which they had slept, blasting away the mantel and tearing all the bedclothes from the bed. Young Catherine and Belle rushed to the cellar as a second shell passed through the breakfast area, demolishing everything in its way and carrying the clock weights into an opposite partition.[32] Throughout the course of the battle, three artillery shells hit the house, the most of any home in town.

Daughter Catherine moved to Johnstown, Pennsylvania, after the battle, living with her cousin, Belle. Both were there in 1889 when the infamous flood struck that city, killing at least 2,209 people. During the flood, Catherine and Belle were forced to leap from the roof of the Stewarts' frame house, which was being swept away, to a flat roof nearby to avoid being drowned. Despite near-death encounters in both the Battle of Gettysburg and the Johnstown Flood, Catherine lived to the age of ninety-one.

14. Samuel Weaver House, 108 W. Middle Street, 39°49.780' N, 77°14.018' W

Drayman and photographer Samuel Weaver shared a home on this site with his wife, Elizabeth A. (age forty-six); his eldest son, Peter, an artist from Maryland (twenty-seven); his younger son, Rufus B.

(twenty-one); and Edward Boehme, a photographer (twenty-five). Henry Redding, a black male who would have been eighteen at the time of the battle, is shown on the census as living in the house in 1860 but was not known to be there in 1863.[33] It is likely that he fled before the Confederates arrived.

The fifty-one-year-old Samuel was the first full-time photographer in Gettysburg and operated a studio on the second floor of his home. Known as the Sky Light Ambrotype Gallery, the studio operated at this location from approximately 1857 to 1860. Weaver was active in

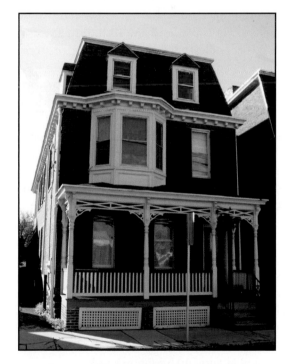

Samuel Weaver supervised the exhumation of more than 3,500 Union soldiers for reburial in the new national cemetery.

community affairs and was a member of the Order of the Red Men, which assisted widows and children. He also became a battlefield guide after the battle.

Elizabeth and some of her neighbors rolled bandages in the early stages of the battle but had to abandon their effort when the house became filled with wounded, forcing them to redirect their efforts to using the bandages they had just rolled.

After the Battle of Gettysburg, Samuel was appointed by Pennsylvania governor Andrew Curtin to oversee the exhumation of Union soldiers from graves scattered across the battlefield and prepare them for proper burial in the Gettysburg National Cemetery. He supervised the disinterment of more than 3,500 bodies, including those buried from the Battle of Hanover.

Weaver examined bodies meticulously so he could identify them. He was even known to study the material of the dead man's underwear in a final effort to determine whether the deceased was Union or Confederate (Union men normally wore wool underwear; Confederates wore cotton). Weaver would proudly say, "I firmly believe that there has not been a single mistake made in the removal of the soldiers to the Cemetery by taking the body of a rebel for a Union soldier."[34] History, of course, would prove otherwise.

The information he gathered on Southern dead was shared with Dr. John W. C. O'Neal in their common efforts to reunite Southern families with their loved ones. When Weaver died in a railroad accident in 1871, his son, Rufus Weaver, by then the demonstrator of anatomy at Hahnemann Medical College in Philadelphia, took up his father's task.

While Rufus continued the exhumation of Confederate soldiers after the death of his father, Samuel's son Peter and nephew Hanson continued the photography business for several more years.

15. Michael Jacobs House, 101 W. Middle Street, 39°49.787' N, 77°14.007' W

Michael Jacobs taught mathematics and natural sciences at Pennsylvania College while living in this home on West Middle Street. A man of many interests, he developed a process for canning fruit, recorded weather conditions three times a day throughout the battle that have been used extensively by historians, and published the first full book-length account of the battle's effect on Gettysburg's citizens. Jacobs also became a battlefield guide.

Built in the 1830s, the house looks much as it did in 1863 except for the rear addition, which is postwar. Michael, fifty-five years of age at the time of the battle,

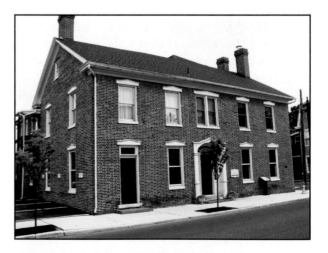

The Michael Jacobs House. Jacobs recorded weather conditions throughout the battle that are widely referred to by historians today.

lived here with his wife, Julia M. (age fifty-one); son Henry E. (eighteen); daughter Mary J. (sixteen); son Michael W. (thirteen); and son George E. (nine).[35]

Henry was a student at the Lutheran Seminary and shared his father's passion for writing. He kept an account of the battle in a journal. He wrote, "As I stared from the window, I saw a Union soldier running, his breath coming in gasps, a group of Confederates almost upon him. He was in full flight, not turning or even thinking of resistance. But he was not surrendering, either. 'Shoot him, shoot him,' yelled a pursuer. A rifle cracked and the Fugitive fell dead at our door. One after another fell that way in the grim chase from the Carlisle Road."[36]

The family spent most of their time during the battle in their cellar, except for one poorly timed excursion that Michael and Henry took to the backyard to hear the cannonade on July 2. Henry noted that the bullets came so frequently that they deemed it prudent to get back into the cellar as soon as they could.

On July 3 Michael ventured to the garret to observe the activity on Seminary Ridge. It was not long before he yelled down to Henry, "Come! Come! You can see now what in all your life you will never see again."[37] Michael was right, and Henry made it up to the garret in time for both to witness Pickett's Charge.

16. Adams County Courthouse, 111 Baltimore Street, 39°49.768′ N, 77°13.871′ W

Gettysburg was chosen as the county seat for Adams County in 1800, and the first court met in the home of Isabella Gettys, mother of town founder, James Gettys. By 1804 the need for a formal courthouse became obvious, and the original courthouse, a two-story building with a bell tower, was constructed in the town square, adjacent to Thaddeus Stevens's law offices.[38]

In 1859 this structure on Baltimore Street was built to replace the old courthouse. On June 26, 1863, Confederate troops occupied the new building, and when the battle began, the courthouse became a hospital. Wounded were scattered throughout the building, with the furniture thrown out the windows to make room for more. The courtroom was converted into an operating theater, and the building's cupola was used as a signal station on at least two days.[39]

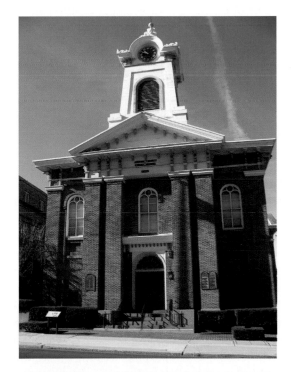

The Adams County Courthouse. About 250 wounded were treated here.

Some 250 wounded from both sides were treated here, with most of them from the Union army's First Division, First Corps. Of the 250 hospitalized here, 77 had amputations, the severed limbs tossed out of the windows. Several loads of amputated limbs would be carted outside town to be burned or buried. Somehow, many amputated limbs were missed, and several were dug up in 1906 during a renovation of the building.

The cries of the wounded wafted through the open windows. The sound was so disturbing to those outside the building that a band came every afternoon to play patriotic songs and drown out the pitiful pleas for relief from the pain. Fannie Buehler, who lived across the street from the courthouse, noted that the smells and sounds emanating from it, as well as the sights, were "too horrible to describe."[40]

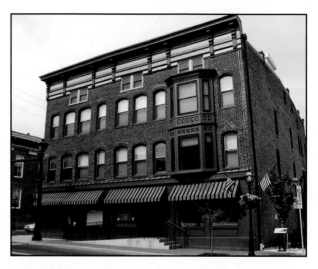

The Fahnestock Store served both as a supply depot and as a hospital.

17. Fahnestock Store, 47 Baltimore Street, 39°49.788' N, 77°13.871' W

This structure was built as a private home and tavern by Bernhart Gilbert in 1810. Samuel Fahnestock purchased the building in 1833 and converted it to a general store that became the largest retailer in town. In 1863 it was operated by brothers James, Henry, and Edward Fahnestock. Today's building does not resemble the 1863 structure, although the original structure is still there, surrounded by alterations.

When it became obvious that a battle was likely, the Fahnestocks shipped much of their stock out of town for protection. Because of its size, the building quickly became a field hospital, treating the wounded of both sides. At battle's end, it was taken over by the Union. At that time, wounded Confederate soldiers were sent to Pennsylvania College and Fahnestock's became a Union hospital only.

On July 7, when the White Run School storehouse closed, the US Sanitary Commission moved into the store, using the Fahnestock facility as a distribution center for supplies. So many supplies were brought in that some had to be stored on the street, according to attending physician H. H. Douglas. Every morning, representatives from all the hospitals came to Fahnestock's to pick up supplies from the Sanitary Commission. Many local citizens, as well as thousands of wounded soldiers, received supplies from here.[41]

The store had steps leading from the third floor to the roof via a trap door. There, an eight-foot-square observatory provided officers, including Union general O. O. Howard, an unobstructed view of the terrain west and south of town. Howard was on the observation deck when he received word of the death of General John Reynolds.

18. Stoever-Schick Building, 1 Baltimore Street, 39°49.838' N, 77°13.879' W

Built in 1819 by local attorney John McConaughy, this building was owned by Martin Stoever at the time of the battle and is believed to be the oldest building on the square. Stoever, a professor at Pennsylvania College, had married McConaughy's daughter Elizabeth in 1849, and they lived here with their two children, Susan Elizabeth and William. A domestic worker named Catherine Kolbflein lived with them.[42] The Stoevers lived in the upper floors and leased the first floor to John L. Schick, who operated a dry-goods business in the space.

The Stoever family stayed in their home during the battle, and three Union soldiers hid in their basement during the July 1 retreat. On the night of July 3, they were discovered by the Confederates, who immediately woke the Stoevers by pounding on their door. They told Stoever he was being taken prisoner for harboring Union soldiers, but he steadfastly refused to leave his family unprotected. After some negotiation, he promised to go with them in morning. The Confederates agreed.

However, the Union controlled the town by the next morning, saving Stoever from capture. With the building being one of the tallest in own, the Federals told the Stoevers they all had to leave because Union sharpshooters were going to move into the top floors and would likely attract enemy fire. The family left for a week and when they returned, William (age thirteen) found a sword belonging to Cap-

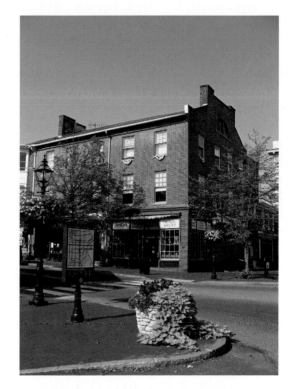

The Stoever-Schick Building served as a hospital and as a base for the US Christian Commission.

tain M. R. Baldwin in the cellar. William kept it for several years until he eventually returned it to the owner.

Early in the battle, the house became a hospital for about twenty wounded, who were placed in the Stoevers' dining room. Stoever's recitation room became the amputation room.[43] The Stoevers, with Schick's agreement, allowed the US Christian Commission to work from the house, and the commission fed large numbers of Union soldiers in the backyard.

Just as the Fahnestocks had done, Schick had sent his merchandise to Philadelphia. The open space that created in his store was perfect for the needs of the Christian Commission, and Schick was immediately agreeable to relinquishing the space for their use. It would become the commission's main supply depot. For his part, Schick would spend the battle in the cellar, telling a reporter from the Philadelphia *North American* on July 7, 1909, that it was so tense that he smoked twenty-one cigars in a single day.

Doctors here included Assistant Surgeon Abraham Stout (153rd Pennsylvania Infantry), Surgeon M. Watson (Alabama), and Surgeon Andrew J. Ward (Second Wisconsin).

19. Smith S. McCreary House, 20 Chambersburg Street, 39°49.848' N, 77°13.921' W

During the battle, hatmaker Smith S. McCreary (age fifty-six) lived in this building with his four daughters, Agnes (twenty-five), Louisa (twenty-three), Kate (nineteen), and Minnie, who was also known as Jennie (seventeen).[44] McCreary's wife, Harriet, had died a few years earlier. The 1863 building still stands, but it has been extensively modified for commercial use, including the addition of a third floor.

Several wounded were treated here, including Colonel Samuel H. Leonard (Thirteenth Massachusetts), who had suffered an arm wound; Assistant Surgeon Edgar Parker (Thirteenth Massachusetts), who had received a head wound while walking down the Christ Evangelical Lutheran Church steps; and General Gabriel Paul, commander of the First Brigade, Second Division, First Corps, who had been horribly

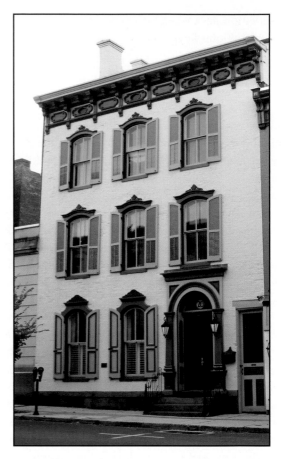

The home of Smith S. McCreary, a local hatmaker.

wounded on July 1 when a bullet passed through both of his eyes, an injury so severe that he was not expected to live. Understanding the wound to be mortal, the general's son had come to Gettysburg with a coffin to take his father home. In an effort to make the general more comfortable in his last hours, McCreary had given up his own bed.

Paul defied the odds and recovered, and was able to travel to Washington, DC, where he eventually made his home. He would suffer from seizures for the rest of his life as a reminder of his time in Gettysburg.

McCreary's youngest daughter, Jennie, related an incident that made her laugh, although she admitted it could have been very serious. She said, "The chaplain, a couple of surgeons, and the colonel were standing on the porch when a shell came and struck just above their heads."[45] She noted that even the men involved laughed at what they must have looked like when the shell hit.

The doctor here was Surgeon William F. Osborne (Eleventh Pennsylvania Volunteers), assisted by the wounded Parker, who helped as his condition permitted. The McCreary daughters served as nurses.

20. Robert McCurdy House, 24 Chambersburg Street, 39°49.847' N, 77°13.932' W

Robert McCurdy, forty-nine years old, and his thirty-eight-year-old wife, Mary, lived here with their son and five daughters, ranging in age from three to sixteen. Domestic worker Lucy Irvin and her three-year-old son also lived here.[46] McCurdy was the president of the Gettysburg Railroad, and he would go on to assist with the disinterment of Confederate dead in 1871.

His son Charles, who was ten years old at the time of the battle, recalled that he stole out of his house without permission when he saw Confederate soldiers enter Philip Winters's confectionary store across the street. Curious to see what an enemy soldier looked like, and even more curious to see what they were doing, he was shocked when they came out and gave

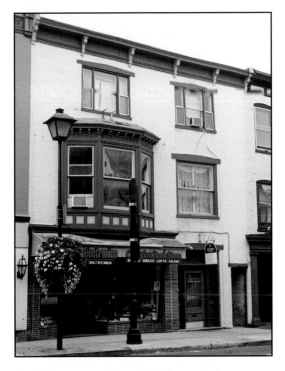

Confederate general Isaac Trimble received treatment at the McCurdy house, raising protests from local citizens.

him some of the candy they had just taken. He had another experience that was not so pleasant, however, when two of his friends were killed several months after the battle while trying to open an unexploded artillery shell.[47]

The family went to Robert's mother's home on July 1, returning in the evening. On their return, they found two dead Union soldiers beside their porch. The stable had been looted but, fortunately, the house had not been disturbed. The next day they took in wounded soldiers from both sides.

Their most famous patient was Confederate general Isaac Trimble, who had been badly wounded in Pickett's Charge. His leg had been amputated at Samuel Cobean's farm before he was moved to the McCurdy home, and he was placed on a cot on the first floor the first night he was there, before being moved to a second-floor bedroom the next day. The room next to Trimble was occupied by a Union officer with a shattered arm. He adamantly refused to let the surgeons amputate the limb, and he died as a result.[48]

Trimble's presence brought an outpouring of protests from local citizens who thought he was being treated too well for an enemy combatant. After two weeks, he was moved to the hospital at the Lutheran Seminary to ease the tensions. Apparently, the cantankerous Trimble did not include the McCurdy family in his contempt for the citizens of Gettysburg. After his recovery, he sent Mrs. McCurdy a silver soup ladle to show his appreciation for his treatment. The ladle contained the inscription "To Mary McCurdy, from a grateful heart."[49]

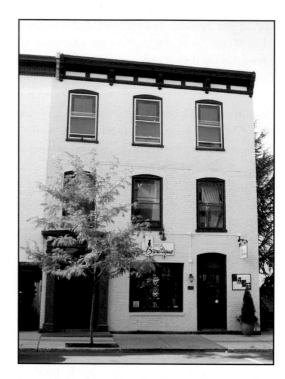

Margaret Ziegler and her daughter took in some of the overflow of wounded from the neighboring Christ Evangelical Lutheran Church.

21. Margaret Ziegler House, 28 Chambersburg Street, 39°49.848' N, 77°13.938' W

Sixty-one-year-old widow Margaret Ziegler lived in this home next to the Lutheran church with her brother John Chritzman and her two sons, David and Charles, all three of whom were carpenters. Her daughter-in-law Ann and granddaughter Ida rounded out the family.[50] The home had originally been owned by Margaret's deceased parents, Christian and Anna Chritzman.

Margaret had been married to Charles Ziegler, who had died at the age of thirty-two in 1832. She had a second brother, George, who was a well-known builder in town, having built the Evergreen Cemetery gatehouse.

When the neighboring Christ Evangelical Lutheran Church became overcrowded, Margaret took in some of the wounded from the church to lighten the burden, and she and Ann served as nurses. No surgeon has been specifically found to have been at the home, but it is likely that neighbor Dr. Robert Horner visited the wounded at least once.

22. Christ Evangelical Lutheran Church,
     30 Chambersburg Street, 39°49.848' N,
     77°13.950' W

Built in 1836, Christ Evangelical Lutheran Church is
the oldest structure in Gettysburg continuously used
as a church, and it appears as it did in 1863. It was the
primary assembly hall for the Lutheran Theological
Seminary and for Pennsylvania College, giving rise to
its sobriquet "the College Church." As such, it hosted
numerous graduation ceremonies and other meetings
for both the college and the seminary. It was one of the
first hospitals established during the battle, and at its
peak it accommodated approximately 150 wounded
soldiers. The church had only been open as a hospital
for a short time when an artillery shell struck the roof.
Those inside were hardly fazed.

More than one hundred men crowded into the
central portion of the church. The pews quickly filled,
some men lying, others leaning against the person
next to them. Other wounded lay on the floor or on
boards crudely placed across open pews. Amputees
were forced to lie on the wooden floors with only a
blanket beneath them. Seeing this, the Patriot Daughters of Lancaster went to their quarters across from
the church and retrieved pillows and blankets. They
also reached out to the US Sanitary Commission
for bedsacks filled with straw, and in a final gesture
of kindness, they provided handkerchiefs wet with
cologne.[51]

Sergeant Austin Stearns of the Thirteenth Massachusetts was among the wounded, sitting in a pew
waiting his turn for medical attention. When he was
touched on the shoulder by someone behind him, he
turned and "saw a reb who was wounded in the arm."

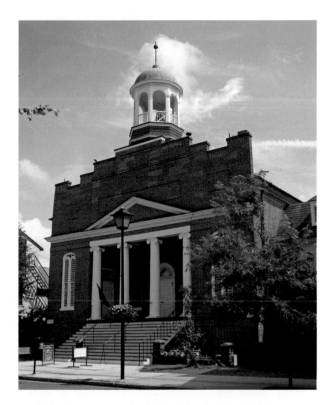

Horatio Stockton Howell, chaplain for the Ninetieth
Pennsylvania Infantry, was killed by a Confederate soldier at
the top of the steps when he refused to relinquish his sword.

The man was from a North Carolina regiment, and
Stearns found him "a very intelligent man." Stearns
recollected, "We entered into conversation immediately, he doing most of the talking."[52]

John Hill, a dentist, lived adjacent to the church,
and his home became a de facto supply warehouse.
There is a plaque on the east wall of the church commemorating his role.

Rev. Henry L. Baugher, president of Pennsylvania College, was pastor at the time of the battle, and he tried to maintain some semblance of normalcy by conducting a service for the wounded and any parishioners who could get there on the Sunday following the battle. Five men were said to have died during the service. It would be the last service in the church for more than six weeks.

Amputations were performed in a small anteroom off the main hall or in the basement, with limbs tossed into the churchyard through the nearest window. When the pile of amputated limbs became too large, it was hauled away by wagons to make room for more. Surgeons worked nonstop, some falling asleep at their operating table. Many of the wounded could not be saved despite the best efforts of the doctors, and each morning the dead were laid on a platform in a sheet or blanket and carried off.

On July 1 Horatio Stockton Howell, a Presbyterian minister from Philadelphia, was among those offering spiritual guidance to the wounded. Howell, chaplain for the Ninetieth Pennsylvania Volunteer Infantry, typically wore a soldier's uniform rather than regulation chaplain's attire. As he stepped outside, a Confederate soldier demanded that Howell give up his sword and surrender. When he tried to explain that he was a chaplain and a noncombatant, the Confederate shot him, killing him instantly. The Confederate claimed that Howell was about to shoot, but Sergeant Archibald Snow of the Ninety-Seventh New York, who had just been treated in the church and was in the doorway directly behind Howell, said that Howell had made no such threatening move, a position corroborated by other witnesses. An argument ensued, defused only when the rebels got on their horses and rode off. It is said that Dr. Francis Burger of the Thirteenth Massachusetts was also shot on the steps. He lived to become a well-known presidential portrait artist.

Physicians here included Gettysburg civilian doctors Charles Horner and Robert Horner, Surgeon J. D. Osborne (Fourth New Jersey), Assistant Surgeon William F. Osborne (Eleventh Pennsylvania Volunteer Infantry), and Dr. Franklin Grube (US Volunteers). In addition to the Patriot Daughters of Lancaster and the US Sanitary Commission, nurses here included Nancy Weikert and Mary McAllister, among others.

The columns on the front of the church are original, made of solid brick with a plaster covering. The main door, framework, and hardware are also original. The steps are not original, nor are the pews, which were damaged so badly that they could not be salvaged. The six-hundred-pound church bell, cast in 1788, has been in the cupola since 1836. The church served as a hospital until August 15, 1863, when the wounded were all moved to the Camp Letterman General Hospital on York Pike.

The building was so contaminated by human waste and other diseased conditions resulting from six weeks of intense use as a hospital that the church trustees filed damage claims of $1,200. When they did not receive any compensation, three members of the church went to Philadelphia to raise funds for repairs. They got $1,500.

23. Lazarus Shorb House Site, 100 Chambersburg Street (Southwest Corner, Chambersburg and Washington Streets), 39°49.849' N, 77°14.010' W

Little is known about this site, but a letter written by Chaplain William C. Way of the Twenty-Fourth

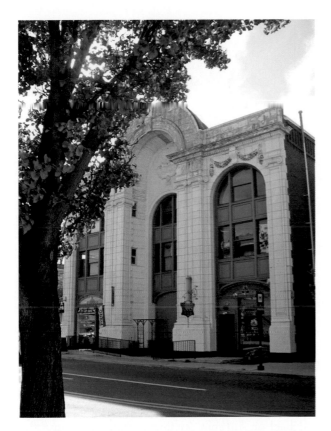

At least two men from the Twenty-Fourth Michigan Infantry received treatment here.

Michigan confirmed its use as a hospital, with at least two of the regiment's men treated here.[53]

Lazarus Shorb, fifty-five years old at the time of the battle, lived here with his wife, Sarah, also fifty-five years old, and six of their eight children.[54] The two who were not living with the family at the time were both serving in the Union army. Their eldest son, Thomas, was serving with the 101st Pennsylvania

Volunteer Infantry and would be captured at Plymouth, North Carolina, nine months after the Battle of Gettysburg. He would survive a year's incarceration at the infamous Andersonville Prison in Georgia.[55] His younger brother, twenty-one-year-old Joseph, had enlisted as a musician with Company E, 165th Pennsylvania Volunteer Infantry, in October 1862. He was serving as a substitute for Adam Deardorff and was mustered out twenty-five days after the battle in his hometown.[56]

A coachmaker, Shorb and his family probably did not own the property, and were probably renting from Alexander Cobean. The Shorbs stayed in their cellar during the fighting.

24. John Burns House Site, 252–254 Chambersburg Street, 39°49.848′ N, 77°14.196′ W

One of the great characters associated with the battle was local citizen John Burns. Born in 1793, he had served in the War of 1812, but there is no record that shows he saw combat. He returned home and married Barbara Hagarman. The two had no children of their own, but they did adopt a young girl, Martha. Martha was an adult at the time of the battle.

Burns had served as the town's constable, and he and his wife had purchased the house that originally sat on this site from Jesse D. Newman just a few months before the battle. He worked as a cobbler at town council president David Kendlehart's boot and shoe shop.

Hearing the noise of battle on July 1, Burns told Barbara that he was going to go see what was going on. He took his musket and walked to McPherson

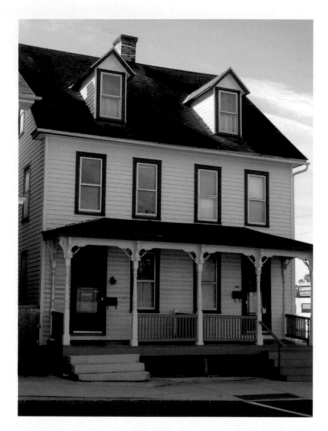

John Burns, the only local civilian known to have fought in the battle, lived in a house on this site.

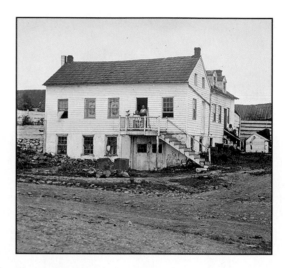

The wartime home of John Burns. (Courtesy of Library of Congress, Reproduction Number LC-DIG-cwpb-01662)

Ridge, where he fell in with the First Corps. The men of the corps supposedly gave him a more modern gun and twenty-five rounds of ammunition. At this point, the story becomes a bit murky, as Burns was given to embellishment and his story often changed when he perceived the need for more dramatization.

What is known is that he actually did fight. He said he knew he killed at least three Confederates, and he was wounded anywhere from three to seven times, depending on when he told the story. He was left on the field when the Union had to fall back.

He made his way to the home of Alexander Riggs and was eventually taken to his own home by either Michael or Anthony Zellinger. There, he found the house filled with Confederate wounded. He was taken upstairs, where his wounds may have been dressed by a Confederate surgeon from North Carolina. (Other accounts say that Burns had already been treated while he was at the Riggs house. Still other accounts indicate that he was treated by Union doctors. The identification of the location of his treatment also varies.) Burns would later say the rebels tried to assassinate him by shooting at him as he lay wounded in his own home, but the validity of this story is not certain.[57]

After the battle, Burns became known as the Hero of Gettysburg. Even Lincoln asked to meet him when the president came to town to deliver his speech at the dedication of the national cemetery in November 1863, and the two attended a patriotic rally together at the Presbyterian church in town later that day. Burns became a much-sought-after battlefield guide after the war.

His home was razed and replaced with the current building in 1890, and a statue to Burns was erected on McPherson Ridge near the area where he fought. The only citizen of Gettysburg to take up arms and fight in the battle, Burns had nothing but unkind things to say about his fellow townsmen, whom he considered cowards for not joining in the fray.

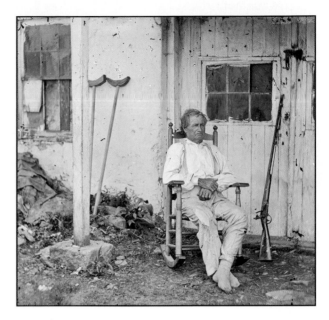

John Burns recovering after being wounded in the first day's fighting. (Courtesy of Library of Congress, Reproduction Number LC-DIG-cwpb-01659)

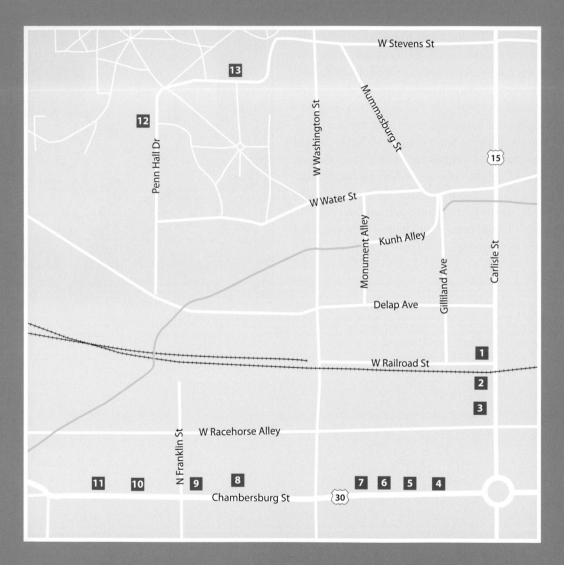

Chapter 4 sites: in town, northwest of square. (Map by Bill Nelson)

1. Spangler's Warehouse Site, 104 Carlisle Street, 39°49.935' N, 77°13.872' W

Unfortunately, not much is known about the Spangler warehouse, which stood on this site. One thing that is known is that it treated wounded from both sides, Union men from the First Division, First Corps, and Confederates from Early's Division.

The *Detroit Advertiser and Tribune* reported that at least five men from Michigan were treated at the hospital, probably from the Twenty-Fourth Michigan Infantry, a regiment that had many of its wounded treated in the area around the railroad station.[1] The only doctor listed for this hospital was Surgeon Abram William Preston of the Sixth Wisconsin.

The building was owned by Alexander Spangler. Spangler was one of sixteen children. Forty-one years old at the time of the battle, he had married Maria Hayward in 1857 and the couple had four children. In a stroke of bad timing, Spangler had just purchased Hoke's warehouse after moving to Gettysburg from Dover in York County. Spangler also served as a vice

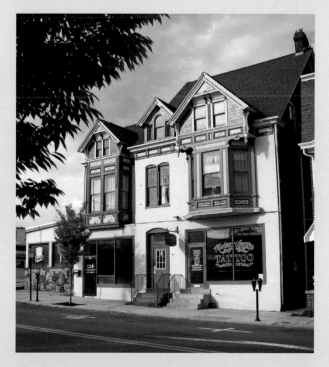

The site of Alexander Spangler's warehouse.

president of First National Bank. He died in 1910 at age eighty-seven, after asking his daughter Laura to raise him up on his pillow.[2]

2. Washington House Hotel Site, 32 Carlisle Street, 39°49.921' N, 77°13.872' W

Built in 1860, the three-story building that occupied this site served as the Washington House Hotel during the battle. About sixty New Yorkers from the First and Second Divisions of the First Corps were treated here.

On July 1 the building was already filled with wounded when the Confederates captured the town and, with it, the hotel. That same day, the building was struck by artillery fire, adding to the woes of the wounded. Located directly across the street from the railroad station, it had served as the railroad ticket office while the passenger station and ticket office were being completed. Its location also made it a good place for an embalming station, which was placed adjacent to the hotel building.

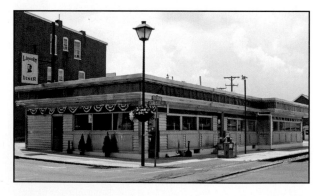

The site of the Washington House Hotel, where an embalming station was set up.

As with most of the hotels in Gettysburg that served as hospitals, few records were kept about those who were treated here. However, it is known that Theodore Dimon, former surgeon for the Third New York Artillery, and Surgeon James Farley of the Fourteenth New York State Militia were attending physicians here.

In May 1890, the remains of a Union soldier were dug up by workers working on the hotel. The building was razed in 1930.

3. McConaughy's Hall, 18 Carlisle Street, 39°49.898' N, 77°13.872' W

The year before the battle, the building that sat here was owned by attorney David McConaughy and housed Company H of the Tenth New York Cavalry. A social and business hall, it had also served as the site of an organizational meeting for the establishment of Evergreen Cemetery. During the battle, it served as a hospital for the Union's First Division, First Corps. The building that replaced the original once housed the *Gettysburg Times*, but it is now a general office building. McConaughy did not live here, as some believe. His home was at what is now 13 Chambersburg Street.

After Evergreen Cemetery was established, McConaughy served as president of the board of directors and had tended to the burial of some one hundred soldiers. In that position, he proposed to Governor Andrew Curtin that all Pennsylvania soldiers from the battle be buried in Evergreen at the state's expense, with the cost offset by a public fundraiser. He also suggested that a national monument be erected in Evergreen.[3] At about the same time, local attorney David Wills was proposing a central national

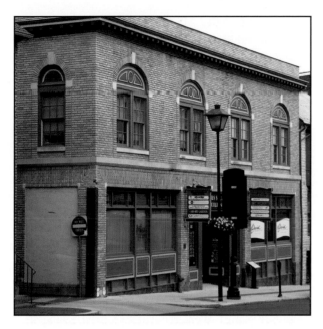

McConaughy's Hall became the site of the organizational meeting for the establishment of Evergreen Cemetery.

munity, he helped organize and served as captain in the Adams Rifles, a local militia. Upon the June 1863 invasion, McConaughy offered his services to the government and was assigned to the secret service.

The medical director for the First Corps was Theodore J. Heard (US Volunteers), and the surgeon in chief was George W. New (Seventh Indiana Infantry). Both probably spent at least some time here. Dr. George W. Ramsey of the Ninety-Fifth New York Infantry was also at this location. The number of men treated is unknown.

4. Union Hotel, 27 Chambersburg Street, 39°49.859' N, 77°13.936' W

This is one of the facilities in town that may or may not have been a hospital. Two sources confirm that it was: the history of the hotel itself, and the Gettysburg Chamber of Commerce, so it is included here.

In 1787, John Troxell Sr. bought this plot of land from James Gettys, the founder of Gettysburg. In 1804, Troxell opened a tavern and roadhouse, the Sign of the Buck, to accommodate travelers. In 1827 former Pennsylvania state senator Zephaniah Herbert purchased the facility, by then known as the Indian Spring Tavern. Herbert renamed the tavern the Union Hotel in 1854, and in 1863 the hotel was said to be a field hospital, with an operating room in the basement.

By the time the twenty-fifth anniversary of the battle took place, tourists were already flocking to see the battlefield. Many, including veterans, chose to stay at what was now known as the City Hotel. The name remained the same until the 1960s, when the hotel closed. It later reopened as an apartment building.

cemetery, as did Theodore Dimon, former surgeon for the Third New York Artillery, who was then serving as relief agent for New York. Curtin eventually accepted the proposal submitted by Wills. McConaughy, a political rival of Wills, would soothe his feelings by becoming a major player in the founding of the Gettysburg Battlefield Memorial Association in April 1864, serving as the association's secretary.

A staunch Republican, it was McConaughy who reported *Gettysburg Compiler* editor Henry Stahle, just as staunch a Democrat, for turning in the locations of Union wounded. McConaughy was also a member of the 1860 National Convention that nominated Lincoln for president. Always active in the com-

fifty-one; his wife, Martha (forty-three); their five children; and Martha's sister, forty-one-year-old Mary McAllister. McAllister supported herself by purchasing bacon and other cured meats from area farmers and reselling them to the people of the town. Domestic worker Mary Walker (twenty-six) also lived with the family.[4] The original house still exists, changed only by the addition of a third story.

Scott's son Hugh, age seventeen, was the town's telegraph operator, making him vulnerable to capture. He remained at his post around the clock on June 25 until the rebels began entering the town. As they came in from the west, Hugh and his father dismantled their equipment and fled to the east. The Confederates were said to be furious that Hugh and his telegraph equipment had evaded them.

As the battle progressed on July 1, McAllister and neighbor Nancy Weikert went to Christ Evangelical Lutheran Church to nurse the wounded. When a badly wounded officer was brought into the church, a doctor instructed McAllister to go get some wine or some other stimulant. She rushed to neighbor George Guyer, who fearfully told her that the rebels would come to his home if they saw her. She convinced Guyer to give her some wine, however, which she hid in her apron, and returned to the church. The wine was poured into the officer's mouth but it failed to help the man, and he soon died.

When a shell struck the church roof, McAllister decided to return to her home. Outside the church, she saw that the steps were filled with wounded. Other wounded were streaming up the street, with those who were least hurt carrying others on their backs. Picking her way through the crowd, she crossed the street to her home, where she saw the door standing

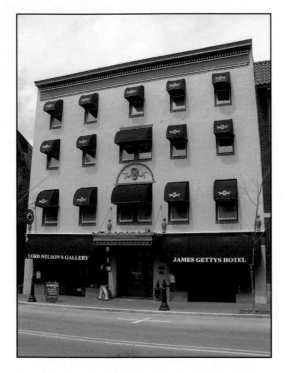

The Union Hotel, today's James Gettys Hotel, is believed to have had an operating room in the basement.

In the 1980s the building became a youth hostel until, in 1995, the building was renovated and took on the current name: the James Gettys Hotel. No records have been located naming physicians, nurses, or regiments served during the time it may have been a hospital.

5. John Scott House, 43–45 Chambersburg Street, 39°49.860' N, 77°13.950' W

In 1863 this building contained a residence, a tenant residence, and a grocery store. A brewery was located behind the house. Living here were John Scott, age

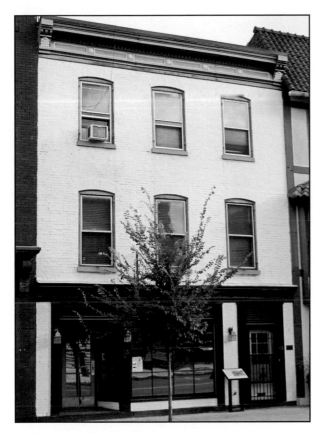

The John Scott House. A large number of Union wounded were captured here when the Confederate army overran the town on July 1, 1863.

open and the front step covered with blood. Fearing for her family's safety, she rushed inside. There, she found her family uninjured, but the house was now filled with wounded soldiers. Martha had hung a red shawl out an upstairs window to designate the house as a hospital, which acted as a beacon for those desperate for help.

McAllister described the ordeal: "Such sights I had never seen before and hope to never see again!" She went on: "I worked almost all day but was overwhelmed and wanted to go home. That was not as easy as it sounds! By the time I got home, it too was full of wounded. Those days were so hard and we were all so frightened. I slept on the windowsill keeping watch over our home."[5]

A wounded Lieutenant Dennis B. Dailey of the Second Wisconsin had Confederate general James J. Archer's sword, which Archer had surrendered to him. Outside, Confederate soldiers were tearing down a fence to get into the home. Dailey asked McAllister to hide the sword before the rebels got in. She placed it under some wood near the kitchen fireplace.

Colonel Henry Morrow of the Twenty-Fourth Michigan had received a slight head wound but was still coherent despite his pain. At his direction, McAllister also hid Morrow's diary in her dress and Dailey's pocketbook behind a small red cupboard. When she offered Morrow a coat belonging to her brother-in-law John Scott, to put on over his uniform, Morrow refused, saying he would not hide the fact that he was a Union officer. Morrow also ordered all soldiers in the house to give their real names when they were taken prisoner. They also gave their names and addresses to McAllister so she could contact their families.

When the rebels broke in, they captured all those who could still walk. The seriously wounded were given paroles and left behind. The house would serve as a hospital until after the Confederate retreat.

On July 3 several Confederate soldiers entered the home and asked for food. Martha brought a freshly baked pie into the entrance hall and offered it to the men, but the rebels, fearing she had poisoned it, insisted she eat some first. Despite Martha's assurances, the hungry men left without eating.

On July 4 Morrow returned, having escaped from being held prisoner at Gettysburg College. He had made his escape by wearing a green surgeon's sash and walking out with several doctors. McAllister gave Morrow his diary and Dailey's pocketbook. She also gave him Archer's sword to return to Dailey.

Five surgeons stayed with the Scotts but were unavailable when a seriously wounded man required immediate surgery. Dr. Robert Horner, who lived just a few houses from the Scott house, was summoned to perform the operation. He spent most of his time during the battle moving from home to home, rendering assistance wherever it was needed. The surgery at the Scott house, not an unusual gesture by Horner, was successful.

6. Dr. Robert Horner House, 51 Chambersburg Street, 39°49.859' N, 77°13.964' W

In 1863 the original building on this site served as Dr. Robert Horner's residence and drugstore. The thirty-eight-year-old doctor occupied it with Mary (thirty-three), John (eleven), Annie (seven), and two domestic workers, Catherine Storick (twenty-eight) and Annie Odle (twenty-nine).[6]

The original house, which once had belonged to former senator Thaddeus Stevens, was razed in 1923. Stevens, a noted champion of civil rights and public education, was instrumental in getting the Thirteenth and Fourteenth Amendments added to the United States Constitution. He lived in the original home from 1816 until 1842. The Horners moved into the home in 1858.

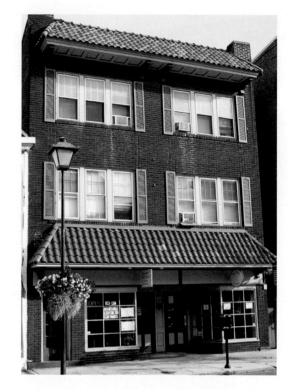

The site of Dr. Robert Horner's home. The original house had belonged to Senator Thaddeus Stevens.

At the beginning of the battle, all occupants of the homes on the west side of town were ordered to evacuate. Dr. Horner chose to remain behind to assist with the anticipated wounded while Mrs. Horner and her children set out for Dr. Henry L. Baugher's home at Pennsylvania College. The shelling became so bad, however, that they were called into banker T. Duncan Carson's house by Mrs. Carson. There, they joined sixteen others, plus two dogs and a cat, inside the bank vault, where they remained for the rest of the day.

Shortly after their arrival, a shell came through a window but failed to detonate. The danger they had been in became even more apparent after the fighting stopped, when it was noticed that there were bullets in the wall where a baby had been sleeping.

Mrs. Horner returned to her home on July 2. Her first glimpse of the house revealed a dead horse in front of her door, dead soldiers in the street, the debris of battle everywhere, and the wounded being taken anywhere there was an open doorway, including her own home.

The wounded were placed in the halls and rooms of the first floor, and it was not long before the carpets were saturated with blood, the walls bloodstained, and books that were used as pillows ruined.[7] Cornelia Hancock and several other nurses came to render assistance, and Hancock stayed at Horner's home until September.

On July 4 as the Confederates were retreating, Mary Horner spent much of the day scraping mud and blood from her pavement. The wounded remained in her home for about two weeks, until their removal to Camp Letterman.

7. Nancy Weikert House Site, 53 Chambersburg Street, 39°49.859' N, 77°13.961' W

Nancy Weikert became one of the first civilians to help with the wounded when she and Mary McAllister went to Christ Evangelical Lutheran Church on July 1 to volunteer their services. In fact, she had to obtain

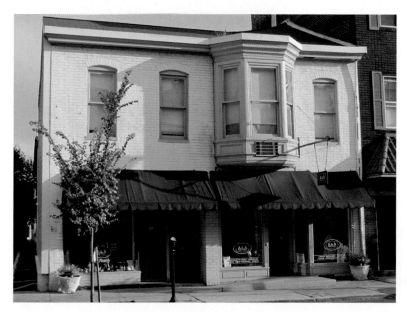

The site of Nancy Weikert's home. Weikert was one of the first civilians to help treat the wounded.

the keys from the sexton of the church to open the doors so the wounded could be treated.

The forty-four-year-old widow of Peter Weikert operated a boarding house in her home for students from Pennsylvania College and the seminary. She shared her home with her twenty-two-year-old niece, Amanda Reinecker, who supported herself by making mantuas, ladies' elaborate outer dresses popular in the era.[8] Both treated the wounded.

On July 4, several Confederate sharpshooters remained active despite the fact that the Army of Northern Virginia was already in retreat. As McAllister approached the Weikert home to assist the wounded there, one of the Weikerts' boarders, Amos Moser Whetstone, spied a sharpshooter and shouted a warning to her. The young seminary student's alert may have saved McAllister's life, but it came at a cost, as he was shot in the thigh. His wound was treated and bound by Sarah "Sallie" Broadhead, who lived nearby and helped treat the wounded both in her own home and at the Lutheran Seminary. Whetstone survived his wound and served thirty years as a Lutheran minister.[9]

The original home was razed and replaced with the existing structure circa 1900.

8. Dr. Charles F. Schaeffer House, 133 Chambersburg Street, 39°49.858' N, 77°14.058' W

Fifty-six-year-old Dr. Charles F. Schaeffer was a professor of German at both the Pennsylvania College and the Lutheran Seminary, and he operated the German Evangelical Ministry from his home. He lived with his wife, Susan S. (age fifty-two), and their children

Georgianna C. (twenty-six), Amelia M. (twenty-four), Charles H. (twenty-two), and Virginia S. (seventeen). Mary Snyder (twenty-nine), a domestic worker, also lived with the family.[10]

Colonel Lucius Fairchild of the Second Wisconsin Infantry Regiment was badly wounded in the same encounter that resulted in the death of General John Reynolds on July 1, when a minié ball shattered Fairchild's left arm just above the elbow. He was taken to the Schaeffer home, where his

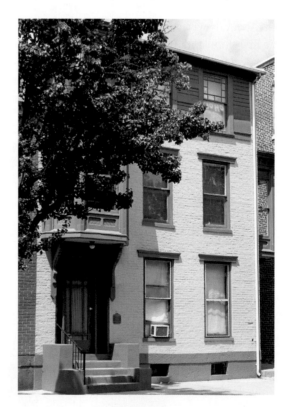

The home of Dr. Charles F. Schaeffer, a professor at both the Lutheran Seminary and the Pennsylvania College.

arm was amputated just below the left shoulder by his friend, Second Wisconsin regimental surgeon Andrew J. Ward. Fairchild was captured by the advancing Confederates, but when they realized he was too badly injured to be moved, they accepted his parole, allowing him to remain with the Schaeffers.

Amos Moser Whetstone, the Lutheran Seminary student boarder at Nancy Weikert's home who was wounded by a sniper, also received treatment here.

All the Schaeffer women assisted with the wounded in the home, and Mrs. Schaeffer and her seventeen-year-old daughter, Virginia, also went to David McMillan's house and helped treat wounded.

9. David McMillan House, 153 Chambersburg Street, 39°49.859' N, 77°14.091' W

David McMillan, a seventy-eight-year-old veteran of the War of 1812, lived in this small home with his sixty-five-year-old housekeeper, Sarah Hafely.[11]

Despite the house's small size, at least fifteen men were treated here. Hafely tore up all the sheets and pillowcases to use as bandages and began treating the wounded as quickly as they came in. She was helped by at least five neighbors: Catherine Neinstead and her daughter Catherine, who lived to McMillan's immediate right; Sarah Eichelberger, who lived on McMillan's immediate left; and Susan Schaeffer and her daughter Virginia, who lived at Dr. Schaeffer's, on the opposite side of Eichelberger's.

No records have been found listing most of the names of those treated, although Private Richard Laracy of the Ninety-Fifth New York noted that he received treatment for a foot wound there.

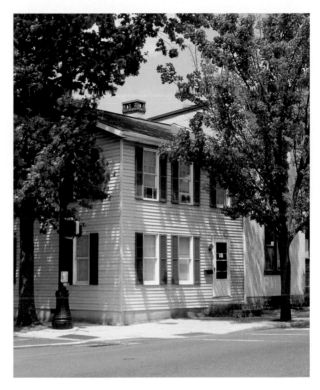

This small home belonging to David McMillan took in as many as fifteen wounded.

10. Jacob Gilbert House, 213 Chambersburg Street, 39°49.857' N, 77°14.123' W

Jacob Gilbert's home is part of a group of four connected houses known as Warren's Row, named for the builder, Thomas Warren. The row remains today and looks much as it did during the battle. The house was occupied at the time of the battle by Jacob (age twenty-eight); his wife, Elizabeth (twenty-eight); Jacob's mother, Ann (fifty-one); and two of Jacob's sisters, Elizabeth (fifteen) and Sarah (eleven). The 1860

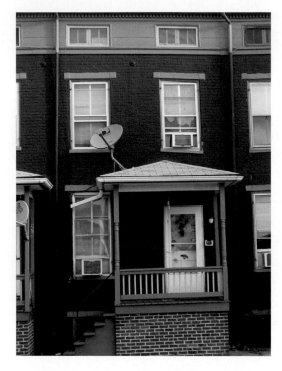

The Gilbert family spent the daylight hours in a neighbor's cellar, going home only after dark.

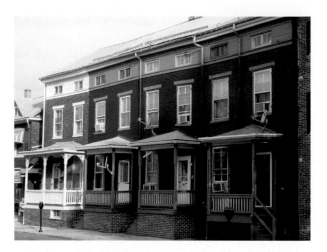

The Gilbert family lived in the second home from the right in what was known as Warren's Row.

census also shows that Jacob had a younger brother living in the home, but he is unaccounted for in 1863, as is an infant son, Frank, who may have died. Jacob's father, Samuel, had enlisted in the Union army and also was not in the home in 1863.[12]

Years after the battle, Elizabeth said in an interview with a local newspaper that Jacob had also enlisted as a horn player in the Eighty-Seventh Pennsylvania Regimental Band when the war broke out but had been discharged when the band was incorporated into the brigade band.[13] There is also evidence that Jacob served in the Adams Rifles in 1861.[14]

The morning of July 1, Union soldiers told the Gilberts they should leave because they expected the Confederates to begin shelling the town at any minute. Jacob and Elizabeth went to Henry Stahle's home on Baltimore Street, while Jacob's mother and sisters took refuge in another home. At Stahle's, Elizabeth helped roll bandages until that evening, when she and Jacob returned home.

There they encountered a Confederate officer who asked them where they were going. Told that they were going to their home, he said they would be safe there if they stayed inside. He said their belongings would not be disturbed, but if they left, the house may be ransacked. He suggested they go to their cellar during any fighting. Just as the man had told them, their home was not bothered, although the Gilberts had to share what little they had with the rebel soldiers, who occasionally searched the house for Union soldiers.

On July 2 and 3 the Gilberts went to neighbor David Troxell's, where they huddled in his cellar with twenty others each day. They spent the nights in their own home after the sounds of the fighting had subsided.

On July 4, believing the fighting was over, Jacob went up to Middle Street and was caught between Union sharpshooters in town and rebel sharpshooters on Seminary Ridge. He was shot in the arm, receiving a minor flesh wound. He worked his way through alleys and yards to Dr. Charles Horner's, two blocks from the Gilbert house, where Horner attended to the wound. Jacob then returned home.

That same day, a wounded Confederate soldier came to the house and asked to be treated, offering his horse to Jacob as payment. The man was brought in, the saddle was removed from horse, and the horse was taken to a barn at the corner just two doors away, where it was taken by another soldier and never seen again. The wounded man was later taken prisoner when Union soldiers searched the Gilberts' house.[15]

After the battle, the Iron Brigade band remained in town and invited Jacob to join them, playing from July 6 to July 29. When the band left town, Jacob went with them and was sworn in when the band reached Washington. He remained with them until the end of the war, perhaps making him the only Pennsylvanian to serve in the Iron Brigade.[16]

After the war, Jacob became a battlefield guide.

11. Joseph Broadhead House, 217 Chambersburg Street, 39°49.857' N, 77°14.129' W

Also part of the four interconnected row houses known as Warren's Row, the Broadhead home was

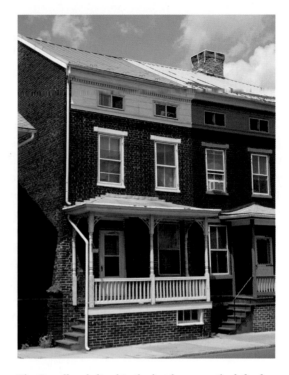

The Broadheads lived in the last home on the left of Warren's Row. Sarah Broadhead kept a diary during the battle that historians often rely on for information about the civilians.

just two doors away from the Gilberts'. Joseph Broadhead (thirty-two years old) and his wife, Sarah (thirty), lived here with their three-year-old daughter, Mary. English-born Joseph worked as an express messenger for the Gettysburg Railroad.[17]

Sarah followed the war in the South more closely than most, since her brother Paul was serving in the Union army. She maintained a daily journal for several weeks, detailing her activities and thoughts. That journal has been cited by historians as one of the best accounts of the reactions of the civilians to the sights and sounds of the battle. She may have been thinking of her brother when she wrote, "The sounds of the shells and bullets made me so sad because I knew that it meant that some soldier was leaving this earth in agony."[18]

The first day of the battle, Sarah bathed the wounds of passing Union soldiers at her doorstep. As the situation intensified around her home on July 2, she went to the cellar for safety. Joseph, however, chose instead to pick beans from the family garden as bullets whizzed past, insisting that the rebels were not going to get any of his beans. Later that day, the family went to the adjoining home, owned by David Troxell, where they were among the twenty-two who huddled there in safety. That became their routine for the next few days during the daylight hours, until around ten o'clock at night, when they returned to their home and stayed there until the cacophony resumed the next morning.

On July 5 Sarah walked to the Lutheran Seminary to help with the wounded, carrying food, blankets, and quilts with her. At the seminary she cleaned and dressed wounds, fed the most severely wounded, and wrote a letter for a dying soldier when she returned home in the evening. On July 8 she helped move nearly one hundred men who had been too badly wounded to move themselves, carrying them out of the rainwater that was beginning to flood the seminary basement and up to the fourth floor.

On July 9 she wrote that the flooding in the streets from the incessant rain prevented her from reaching the seminary, so she visited some of the closer hospitals in town. She was so impressed with the work she saw the US Sanitary and Christian Commissions doing that she entered her admiration in her journal: "The merciful work of the Sanitary and Christian Commissions, aided by private contributions, was to be seen at every hospital. Without the relief they furnished, thousands must have perished miserably, and thousands more have suffered from want of the delicacies, food and clothing their agents distributed, before the government even could bring assistance."[19] Later in the day, in response to a request, the Broadheads took three wounded men into their own home.

Sometime between July 9 and July 11, one of the wounded in Sarah's care died. The next day, his widow arrived to see him, not knowing that he had passed away. It fell on Sarah to give her the sad news that her husband was dead. She also wrote that another of her patients was worsening, and that local citizens were getting many requests to house visitors. She noted that there would be no church that day; all the churches were being used as hospitals.

On July 14 her patients were removed from her home to Camp Letterman. Among the final entries in her journal was this poignant comment: "Had any one suggested any such sights as within the bounds of possibility, I would have thought it madness."[20]

Sarah had seventy-five copies of her diary printed and offered for sale at a sanitary fair in Philadelphia as a fund-raiser for the Sanitary Commission.

12. President's House, Pennsylvania College, 39°50.043' N, 77°14.104' W

Rev. Dr. Henry L. Baugher, age fifty-nine, was living in this home and serving as president of Pennsylvania College in 1863. The house was relatively new, having been completed just three years before the battle. The

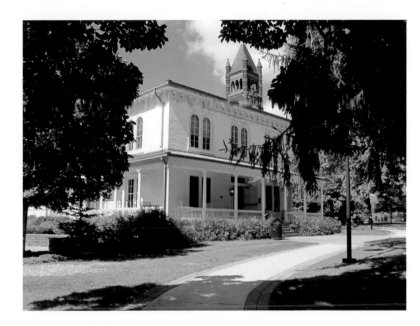

The home of the president of Pennsylvania College served as a Confederate hospital but treated men from both sides.

house was the third building constructed on campus, after the College Edifice (today's Pennsylvania Hall) and Linnaean Hall, a science building constructed in part with student labor. In addition to serving as the college president, Baugher was also a Lutheran minister, and his wife, Clarissa, and their daughter, Alice, lived in the home with him. All three stayed in the house during the battle.

The Baughers had already felt the intense personal pain of war a year earlier, when their son, Nesbit, was killed at Shiloh. Serving with the Forty-Fifth Illinois Infantry, Nesbit had been wounded seven times and had the dubious distinction of being the first Gettysburg resident to die in the war. Dr. Baugher had been with him when he died and had accompanied his son's body home for burial.[21]

The President's House served primarily as a Confederate hospital, but there were also at least eighteen Union men from the Second Division, First Corps, treated there. Clarissa and Alice served as nurses, treating the men from both sides equally. Henry Fraser, from Heth's Division of the Army of Northern Virginia's Third Army Corps, was the surgeon in charge. Dr. James K. Shivers and Dr. Thomas L. Smiley, also from Heth's Division, assisted.

During the fighting, shell fragments hit the house and tore limbs from the trees in the yard. Despite the damage, the Baughers refused to file damage claims. Rev. Baugher would gain a measure of fame on November 19, 1863, when he pronounced the benediction for the dedication of Soldiers' National Cemetery.

Given the nickname "the White House" in 1863, today the building is known as Gettysburg College's Norris-Wachob Alumni House.

13. Pennsylvania Hall (College Edifice), Pennsylvania College, 39°50.085' N, 77°14.058' W

Depending on the source, an estimated five hundred to nine hundred wounded were treated in this building. Whatever the real number, it was a major hospital that treated Union soldiers from the Eleventh Corps and from the Confederate divisions of Early and Heth. Dozens of men were buried on the north-side lawn, and each morning eight to ten more bodies lay at the entrance for burial.

Classes were in session when the battle began, and Dr. Henry L. Baugher was giving a lecture when Union soldiers entered to use the cupola as an observation

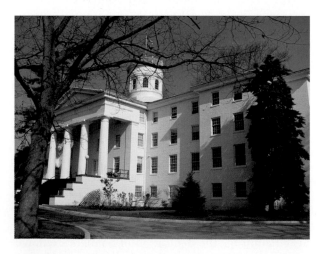

Pennsylvania Hall treated as many as nine hundred wounded.

station. The students became so distracted that Baugher eventually gave up, saying to his class, "We will close and see what is going on, for you know nothing about the lesson anyhow."[22] General Robert E. Lee would also use the cupola for the same purpose later in the battle.

At least eight Confederate soldiers had graduated from the college, and student Michael Colver, who would soon graduate with the class of 1863, remained at the school to help with the wounded, earning him the title of "Doctor" to many of the men he treated.

With the battle's opening salvo taking place less than a mile from the college, it was only a short time before the wounded began pouring into the building. Soon every room and hallway were filled. Books were used as pillows in the building students affectionately referred to as Old Dorm. Students moved their trunks and personal belongings to the president's office to make room for the wounded. The portico soon became an amputation theater.

Surgeon Hugh Lennox Hodge (Pennsylvania Reserve Corps of Surgeons), Acting Assistant Surgeon James K. Shivers (unknown regiment), Surgeon Henry Fraser (Heth's Division), and Dr. Thomas L. Smiley (Heth's Division) were among the surgeons who worked here.

Nurses came from the US Sanitary Commission and the Sisters of Charity. Initially the Sisters had only two members of their group present, but when the number of wounded became almost, overwhelming they were joined by more. Soon the Sisters found themselves being called on to settle disputes when the men involved refused to listen to anybody else.

Individuals who served as nurses here included Euphemia Goldsborough, Hettie McCrea, and

Maggie Branson. There were, of course, many more whose names were not recorded. Many of those were said to have been Confederate sympathizers from Maryland who brought civilian clothing with them to help the more mobile wounded to escape their Union captors.

Goldsborough made a name for herself with her passion for doing the extra things to help the wounded. Known to them as Miss Effie, she hailed from Baltimore and was said to be particularly partial to the Confederates. Nevertheless, she performed yeoman duty.

One of her patients was Colonel Waller Tazewell Patton of the Seventh Virginia Infantry, the great-uncle of famed World War II general George S. Patton III. Colonel Patton was a graduate of the Virginia Military Institute, where he had later served on the faculty. He had been shot in the face by artillery fire on July 3 during Pickett's Charge. His jaw gone, he was brought to the college, where he lay for two weeks.

Patton's condition was such that he was unable to eat, and he had to sit upright to avoid suffocation. On the night of July 20, the starving Patton lapsed into unconsciousness, too weak from hunger to sit up any longer. Although she weighed only ninety-eight pounds, Miss Effie took it upon herself to use her own body to support the colonel. She sat back to back with him, tethered together with her legs extended. She sat in that position all night without moving, fearing any movement could be fatal to her patient, despite the cramping and numbness that set in. Despite her efforts, Patton died the next morning. Apparently, this was not an unusual act for Miss Effie. When the wounded were relocated to Camp Letterman, she was given a book of letters and signatures of one hundred of her patients as a show of appreciation for her work.[23]

While the exterior of the building did not suffer much damage, the interior did. The college made a public appeal for donations to aid in repairing the damage, receiving $1,864.51.

For years after the battle, construction workers turned up remains while digging, and the building was honored with a congressional decree that allows a reproduction of the 1863 flag to fly over the cupola twenty-four hours a day.

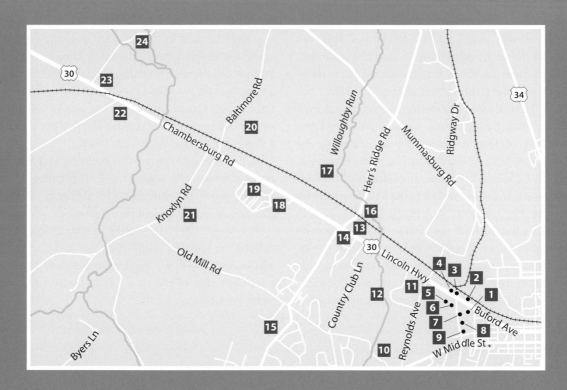

Chapter 5 sites: Seminary Ridge/Chambersburg Road. (Map by Bill Nelson)

Chapter 5

Seminary Ridge/Chambersburg Road

1. Samuel K. Foulk House Site, Buford Avenue, 39°50.019' N, 77°14.608' W

This long-gone home sat on what is now part of the Lutheran Seminary campus. On July 1, 1863, it was filled with wounded, and would be for the next several days. During the battle, the home was occupied by fifty-five-year-old blacksmith Samuel Foulk; his wife, Hanna; and their four children, ranging in age from five to twelve, along with a twenty-one-year-old apprentice blacksmith named Cornelius Beecher, who was learning the trade from Samuel.[1] Samuel was proud to be a charter member of the Good Samaritan Lodge No. 200 of the Free and Accepted Masons.[2]

As the fighting moved from McPherson Ridge to Seminary Ridge on July 1, wounded men from both sides began showing up on the doorsteps of homes around the seminary, including the Foulks'. As the fighting drew nearer and the Foulks began bringing in the wounded, the children were sent to the cellar for their safety. In addition to treating the wounded, Hanna baked bread that she took to her mother's home not far away. Her mother was Mary Thompson,

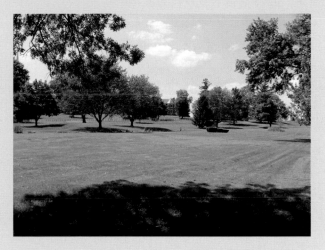

The Samuel K. Foulk home sat in this area of the Lutheran Seminary campus.

whose home would become Robert E. Lee's headquarters during the battle. Hanna would continue to do this throughout the battle, despite the danger of leaving her home. The Foulk house would become known as the White Hospital.[3]

In his damage claim, Samuel Foulk noted that his home was used as a hospital from July 1 through July 4. He claimed that it was inside rebel lines the entire four days and that his fencing was destroyed, several acres of grass and corn trampled, his potato crop destroyed, and his barn and hog pen also damaged. His claim was in the amount of $237.25; he was awarded $170.25 for his losses.[4]

2. Elias Sheads House, 331 Buford Avenue, 39°50.037' N, 77°14.578' W

In July 1859, Edward McPherson sold three acres of land to Carolyn "Carrie" Sheads for $135 an acre. On that parcel of land, either Carrie Sheads or her father, Elias, built a residence that also housed Carrie's Oak Ridge Seminary for Girls.[5] Carrie, who taught music and French, opened her school for girls shortly after construction on the house was completed, attracting students from as far away as Baltimore. The home contained twelve rooms and was completed in March 1862.

The family consisted of Elias; his wife, Mary; and their three daughters and four sons. All four sons served in the Union army, and all four would die as a result of their service. Elias Jr. was killed at the Battle of Monocacy. The youngest son, Jacob, who ran away to enlist after his father had forbidden him to do so, contracted mumps and died at a hospital in City Point, Virginia. Robert was seriously wounded in the neck at the Battle of White Oak Swamp and died of complications from his wound four years later, never having been able to speak again after being wounded. The oldest son, David, died of tuberculosis ten years after contracting the disease while in the army.

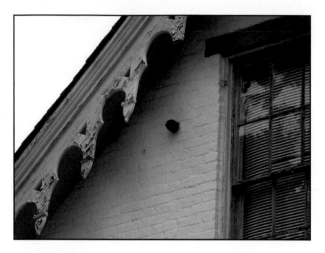

A shell, one of more than sixty to strike the house during the battle, remains embedded in the front wall of the Sheads House.

During the first day of the battle, the two armies went toe to toe for hours just a few hundred feet from the house. With the fighting practically on their doorstep, it was inevitable that the house would soon become a hospital, and before the last wounded man left several days later, seventy-two wounded soldiers would be treated here. The building was hit by shells in more than sixty places, and one of those shells, a ten-pounder Parrott shell, remains embedded near the top window on the house's front.

Hundreds of Union soldiers were captured within feet of the Sheads home, including Lieutenant Colonel Charles Wheelock of the Ninety-Seventh New York. On the afternoon of July 1, Wheelock and several of his men took refuge in the Sheads basement. When Confederate soldiers entered the cellar and demanded his surrender, Wheelock refused, and a Confederate officer pointed his pistol at him and insisted that

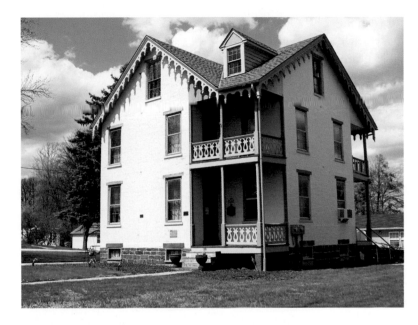

Some of the window frames in the Sheads home still contain the initials of wounded men treated here.

Wheelock give up his sword. Elias and Carrie begged the man not to shoot, saying that there was already too much bloodshed. When the rebel's attention was diverted by the arrival of more prisoners, Carrie hid Wheelock's sword under her skirt. When the officer returned, she said another officer had come and taken the weapon. Five days after the battle, Wheelock returned, having escaped his captors, and retrieved his sword.

Carrie, her mother, and her sisters spent several days caring for the wounded, assisted by some of the girls enrolled in the school. Five Union prisoners also helped.

As tragic as the battle was, one happy story came from the Sheads house, albeit only temporary. One of the five Union prisoners who remained behind to assist the wounded was Private Sleath Hardman of the Third Indiana Cavalry. He eventually returned to the Sheads home and married one of his nurses, Louisa Sheads, in 1866. Unfortunately, Louisa would die just one month later. To compound the sadness in the Sheads home, Elias's wife, Mary, died just four years after Louisa. The losses of his wife, daughter, and all four sons within a few years of one another were said to have left him a broken man.[6]

To add to his woes, Elias was a coachmaker, and a significant amount of his business was with Southern states. The war caused major losses of business and severely hurt the family financially. Possibly because of his family's service and losses, Elias was awarded a pension in 1886, and his daughters Carrie and Elizabeth were given clerkships in Washington, DC. He was also awarded $180 for damages to his fences, wheat, trees, and shrubbery.[7]

The house fell into disrepair but was restored in the 1950s and converted into apartments. It was returned to a single-family home in 1979 and now looks nearly identical to its 1863 appearance except that dormers have been added to its roof. Some window frames still contain the carved initials of soldiers from both sides.[8]

On December 8, 1976, the Sheads house was placed on the National Register of Historic Places.

3. Casper Henry Dustman Farm, Chambersburg Road, 39°50.103' N, 77°14.681' W

Widower Casper Henry Dustman, who listed his occupation as a bootmaker, lived on this site in 1863. All that remains is the foundation of his barn. His property extended northward to the railroad cut. The house sat just south of the barn, toward Chambersburg Pike, and served as a hospital on at least the first day of fighting. At least two Union soldiers were buried on the property. The barn suffered heavy damage from shot and shell, with several holes in the roof.

Dustman's wife, Evelyn, had died before the war, and Dustman had at least one child living at home at the time of the battle. His five other children had reached adulthood and their whereabouts are uncertain. One of them, twenty-eight-year-old John Henry, is known to have been with the Eighty-Seventh Pennsylvania Infantry and would not have been home at the time. An apprentice shoemaker, eighteen-year-old Daniel Kitzmiller, was also in the home.[9] Kitzmiller and Dustman's daughter had left the farm before the outbreak of fighting, but Dustman remained behind.

On the afternoon of the battle's first day, a soldier told Dustman of an old man lying on a cellar door across the road. The old man was John Burns, who was

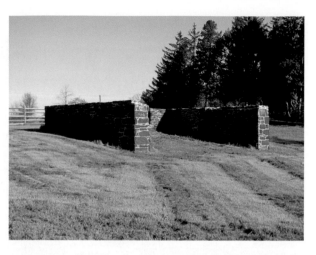

The barn foundation is all that remains of the Dustman farm.

lying on the exterior cellar door of a property owned by Dustman but rented by Alexander Riggs and his family. Burns asked Dustman to get Burns's wife to bring a carriage to take him home, but Barbara Burns told Dustman that she had no wagon and could not come for him. Dustman then unsuccessfully tried to get ambulance drivers to take Burns home. That evening a passing resident, believed to be either Anthony or Michael Zellinger, stopped and took him home.

Dustman would file a claim in the amount of $370.90 for damages to his fences, crops, and a carriage. He would be awarded $350.90.[10]

4. Mary Thompson House, Chambersburg Road, 39°50.096' N, 77°14.705' W

Fighting in this area was deadly. On the first day, this ground was occupied by the 143rd Pennsylvania Volunteers and three guns of James Stewart's

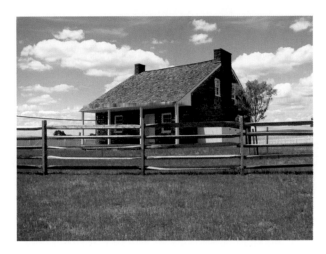

The Mary Thompson House served as Robert E. Lee's headquarters, as well as a Confederate hospital.

Battery B, Fourth US Artillery. When the Union right on Oak Hill collapsed, the 143rd Pennsylvania had many men taken captive. Meanwhile, the Thirteenth North Carolina advanced toward the house, losing 150 of their 180 men in the process, with every field officer except one either killed or wounded. That evening, Lee established his headquarters here.

The home was occupied by seventy-year-old Mary Thompson. Mary had married Daniel Sell in 1818, a marriage that lasted only four years, as Daniel died in 1822 at age thirty. Six years later Mary married Joshua Thompson, who would leave the family in the late 1830s. In 1841 Mary and her daughters went to court and had Joshua declared unfit to manage his affairs, and shortly after, Mary and her family moved into the stone house. In 1846 the house and three acres of land were obtained at auction by Thaddeus Stevens,

trustee for Mary Thompson, at a cost of $16.00.[11] Some sources have also noted that the farm was an integral part of the Underground Railroad, with Mary receiving slaves from J. Howard Wert and moving them to York Springs.

On July 1, 1863, with the dead and wounded of both sides scattered throughout the property, Mary's home quickly became a Confederate hospital, although it treated men from both sides, as did most of the hospitals. Mary stayed in the house the entire time of the battle, treating the wounded. She also cooked for the soldiers, baking pies that they took out of the oven before they were done. With her son, James Henry, serving with the 165th Pennsylvania Volunteers in Suffolk, Virginia, her daughter-in-law, Mary Jane, and Mary Jane's two children spent their time at the Thompson house when their own home filled with wounded. Mary Jane's youngest child was only one day old.

Mary Thompson filed a claim for damage to the house and property, as well as bedding and clothing used as bandages, and eighteen yards of carpet used to wrap the dead for burial.[12] Mary died of consumption in May 1873.

The house burned in 1896, suffering extensive damage to the inside. Fortunately, it was able to be restored. The stone exterior was not damaged.

Mary's home gained a degree of notoriety in 1907 when fifty-three-year-old Emaline Feister, who was living in the house at the time, was charged with keeping a bawdy house. She received a suspended sentence after pleading guilty.

At about the same time, Henry S. Moyer published a controversial article claiming that Lee had never been at the Thompson house and that his headquarters had actually been in the orchard owned by Samuel Hartzell, which sat across the road from the Thompson house. Nothing has been found to support Moyer's claims. Opinions vary, and we will probably never know for sure. However, despite the controversy, there is little doubt that Lee did use the house in some manner during the battle.

5. Alexander Riggs House Site, Chambersburg Road, 39°50.072' N, 77°14.716' W

The outline of this home is easily seen in the accompanying photo, which was taken not long after an archaeological dig. Dirt has been replaced and straw placed over the grass seeding. Those who have not visited Gettysburg in several years may remember the location of this house as being a parking lot across Chambersburg Pike from the Lee Headquarters and the former Quality Inn. The foundation of the house was under the parking lot.

Riggs, sixty-six years old, was a shoemaker. He and his wife, Mary (age forty-eight), had five children, two of whom lived here with their parents as tenants in the property owned by Casper Henry Dustman. Riggs's son Joseph was in Virginia as a member of the 165th Pennsylvania Volunteer Infantry at the time of the fighting in Gettysburg.

The family left their home the morning of July 1 when fighting erupted all around them. When they returned, they found that the house was being used as a field aid station, with the loft full of wounded. Their carpets were soaked with blood and everything of any value in the structure was destroyed.

Riggs was a good friend of John Burns, the civilian who had taken his musket and joined the First Corps

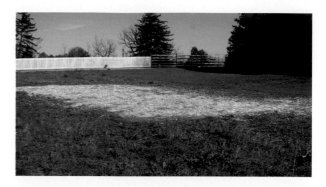

Civilian John Burns crawled or walked to the Riggs house after being wounded on July 1. He was eventually moved to his own home.

in the early fighting. It was only natural for Burns, after being wounded, to try to reach the Riggs house, not far from where he had been wounded. He walked or crawled approximately a half mile, only to find that his friend had left the house, which was now filled with wounded. He lay on an outside cellar door, hoping for someone to summon his wife to take him home.

Casper Dustman noted that he had been approached by a soldier who told him that a man was lying on a cellar door across the road from Dustman's farm and wanted to see him. Burns asked Dustman to go tell Burns's wife that he was wounded and that she should come for him with a wagon to take him home. Mrs. Burns, however, had no means of getting to the Riggs home, and Dustman eventually hailed a wagon coming down the pike and had him taken home. Burns would later confirm that Dustman's house was filled with wounded Confederates.

The length of time that the Riggs property was used as a hospital or aid station is not known, but it is unlikely that it was for more than a few days.

6. James Henry Thompson House, Seminary Ridge, 39°50.069' N, 77°14.698' W

James Henry Thompson was the son of Mary Thompson, who lived on the opposite side of Chambersburg Pike. James was serving with the 165th Pennsylvania Volunteer Infantry in Suffolk, Virginia, at the time of the fighting around his home. He would be discharged less than a month after the battle.

James, who was a laborer before he was drafted into the army, was married to Mary Jane (Arendt) Thompson. At the time of the battle, the couple had a small son, Elias, and a daughter, Jeannie Meade, who was born the day before the battle started. Jeannie Meade would not survive infancy. James and Mary Jane would eventually have three more children.

The house filled with Union First Corps wounded, with so many of them crowded into the house that Mary Jane decided to cross the road with her two children and spend the next several days at the home of Mary Thompson, her mother-in-law.

The small stone wall on the opposite side of the Seminary Ridge road is the site of Mathew Brady's famous photograph of three Confederate prisoners.

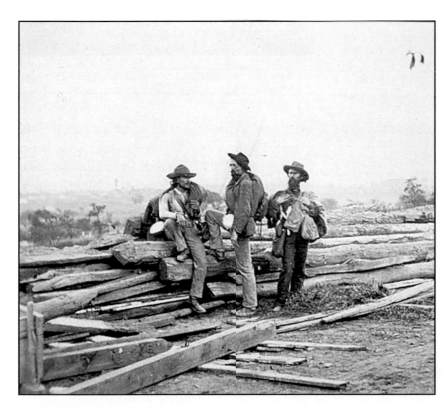

This famous photo of three Confederate prisoners was taken across the road from the James Thompson House. (Courtesy of Library of Congress, Reproduction Number LC-DIG-cwpb-01451 and LC-DIG-cwpb-01450)

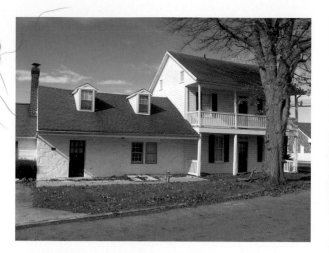

James Thompson's family, including a one-day-old infant, left their home during the battle.

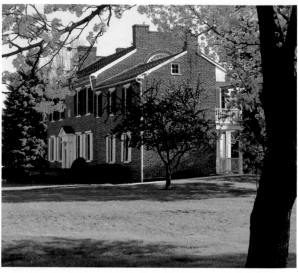

When the Krauth house filled with wounded, tents were set up in this grassy area to accommodate additional injured.

The photographer would have had his back toward James Henry Thompson's house. The prisoners' names are not known.

Only the center portion of the house, with the two dormers, was here during the battle.

7. Rev. Dr. Charles Krauth House, Seminary Ridge, 39°50.010' N, 77°14.681' W

This house was owned by the Lutheran Seminary but was occupied by sixty-five-year-old Rev. Dr. Charles Krauth; his wife, Harriet (fifty-three years old); their two children, John (seventeen) and Sarah (fourteen); and sixty-three-year-old domestic worker, Elizabeth Sharps.[13] Krauth was a professor and former president of the seminary.

The house was built in 1834, and the property's rear butted against the property of Samuel Foulk, Krauth's brother-in-law. In the July 1 fighting, the house was taken over by the Union army as a hospital, with wounded enlisted men on the first floor and officers on the second. When the Confederates overran Seminary Ridge, it began treating men from both sides. Tents were set up between the house and the seminary's main building, now named Schmucker Hall.

Forced to leave their home, the Krauths walked to the Jacob Hankey farm on Mummasburg Road. When they returned, they found their floors and carpet saturated with blood and the house in ruin. All their mattresses and bedding were torn and bloody, the matting had to be burned, and bloodstains covered the walls. Many items were also missing, although a silver coffee urn was eventually returned to them from Virginia.[14]

Only two surgeons, Richard M. Bache, a surgeon on General John Reynolds's staff, and Medical Director

M. J. Asch of the US Volunteers, were documented for the Krauth home, although there likely would have been at least one other from the Army of Northern Virginia.[15]

Krauth died on May 30, 1867, and a damage claim was filed by his wife, Harriet in the amount of $1,10.00. She was awarded the full claim.[16]

Seven unidentified sets of Confederate remains were disinterred from behind the house a few years after the battle.

8. Lutheran Seminary, Schmucker Hall, Seminary Ridge, 39°49.924' N, 77°14.675' W

Also referred to as the Old Dorm, this building served as the main academic building for the seminary and was pressed into service as a field hospital shortly after the battle began. Built in 1826, its cupola was used as

an observation post by both General John Buford and General John Reynolds. Nearly seven hundred men were treated here, from both sides, and it was the last temporary hospital to close after Camp Letterman was established. The most seriously wounded were housed in the basement until flooding required nearly one hundred men to be moved to the fourth floor. The east side of the building (the side facing town) was used as a supply staging area.

Several high-ranking Confederate prisoners were housed here, including General Isaac Trimble (brought from Robert McCurdy's home), Colonel Charles Grogan (Trimble's aide), General James Kemper (brought from Bream's Mill), and Major Henry Kyd Douglas. Also treated here was Colonel Robert M. Powell, who was wounded on July 2 while leading the Fifth Texas in the assault on Little Round Top, and

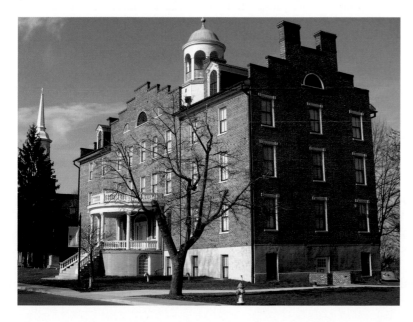

Nearly seven hundred men were treated here, including several high-ranking Confederate officers.

Lieutenant James E. Crocker of the Ninth Virginia, valedictorian of Pennsylvania College's class of 1850, who was wounded at Pickett's Charge. The officers were confined to three rooms and kept under heavy guard. It was said that several female Confederate sympathizers visited Kemper and Trimble.

While most of the prisoners caused little trouble, Trimble was not a model prisoner. He habitually complained about his food, often sending his meal back to the kitchen. For reasons that can only be speculated on, he only stayed at the seminary about three weeks. He was then sent to Baltimore and ultimately to prison at Johnson's Island.

Union doctors began treating the wounded early in the battle until the Confederates pushed the First Corps back. At that time, Surgeon Robert Loughran (Twentieth New York State Militia), Surgeon Amos Blakeslee (151st Pennsylvania), and several others remained behind to continue treatment of the wounded. Taken captive when the Confederates arrived, they were held as prisoners of war for three days. Loughran reported that a Confederate took his clothing and two horses, as well as his instruments as he was in the midst of an operation. With no instruments, surgeons were unable to operate until a local citizen named Lizzie Critzman smuggled some in on the evening of July 3.

The Union regained control on July 5, and the wounded who had been left on the battlefield continued to be carried into the seminary. Two Confederate surgeons were captured, and they treated the wounded while in captivity. Tents were set up on the grounds to accommodate the overflow of wounded from the building itself. Supplies resumed and surgery continued for several days.

Initially, twelve medical officers treated the wounded, but by mid-August most of the surgeons had returned to their own units. Civilian doctors took their place, including local physicians Robert and Charles Horner. From the time the hospital opened on July 1 until it was closed in mid-August, the following doctors are also known to have served the wounded here: Surgeon James R. Reiley (179th Pennsylvania Volunteers), Surgeon Amos Blakeslee (151st Pennsylvania Volunteers), Dr. Cram, Dr. Day (New York), Dr. Ellis, Surgeon Charles Fuller (civilian contractor), Surgeon James L. Farley (Fourteenth New York State Militia), Assistant Surgeon James Fulton (143rd Pennsylvania Volunteers), Assistant Surgeon Abraham Haines (Nineteenth Indiana), Assistant Surgeon John M. Hayes (Twenty-Sixth Alabama, captured July 5), Surgeon Robert (Henry) S. Huber (civilian contractor), Surgeon John N. Jacobs (civilian contractor), Dr. Henry Janes (chief surgeon, Gettysburg area field hospitals), Assistant Surgeon Jonas Kauffman (151st Pennsylvania Volunteers), Surgeon Henry Leaman (civilian contractor), Chief Surgeon Robert Loughran (Twentieth New York State Militia), Surgeon John B. McAffery (civilian contractor), Surgeon Murdock M. McGregor (Thirty-Third Massachusetts), Surgeon Henry K. Neff (Eighth Pennsylvania Reserves), Chief Surgeon George W. New (Seventh Indiana), Surgeon Charles J. Nordquist (Ninth New York State Militia), Assistant Surgeon William F. Osborne (Eleventh Pennsylvania Volunteer Infantry), Surgeon Abram William Preston (Sixth Wisconsin), Assistant Surgeon William R. Ramsey (Ninety-Fifth New York), Surgeon William Rulison (Ninth New York), Surgeon John R. Shreve (Ninetieth Pennsylvania Volunteers), Surgeon Robert G. Southall (Sixth Alabama, captured

July 5), Assistant Surgeon Warren Underwood (151st Pennsylvania Volunteers), Chief Surgeon Andrew J. Ward (Second Wisconsin), and Surgeon W. W. Welch (civilian contractor).[17]

Among the nurses at the seminary were Ellen Orbison Harris (Ladies' Aid Society of Philadelphia); the Ziegler family on their return to the seminary, Sarah Broadhead, Fannie Buehler, and Sallie Myers (all local citizens); the Patriot Daughters of Lancaster; and four from the Sisters of Charity from Emmitsburg, Maryland (Sisters Gabriella, Mary Ellen, Annie, and Melia).[18]

Even families who arrived to care for their own loved ones helped. Among those was the "Colonel's Lady," Addie McFarland, who arrived July 10 with her one-year-old son to treat her husband, Colonel George F. McFarland (151st Pennsylvania Volunteers). Addie treated her husband and several others until the end of August. At one point, the colonel narrowly escaped death when the room he had just been lying in was struck by an artillery shell, shattering furniture just after he had been moved.

As soldiers healed, they returned to their units. Those who could no longer fight but had healed enough to travel were sent to a general hospital in Baltimore. Others were taken to Camp Letterman.

Emanuel Ziegler (age twenty-nine) was serving at the seminary as its steward, and he occupied several rooms on the first floor with his wife, Mary (age twenty-eight); their six children; and a domestic worker.[19] The family was forced to leave, not returning until July 5. Their daughter Lydia (age thirteen) later wrote that they first went into town for safety, then to Culp's Hill, then to Spangler Spring, then to Wolf's Hill, then finally to Two Taverns. At each stop they were forced to move because of the battle. They had

to carry their dog, Sport, the last few miles because he was too exhausted to go any farther.[20]

On the Zieglers' return, family members spent the next two months helping with the wounded. Even ten-year-old Henry pitched in, carrying amputated limbs away to provide space for more.

The family filed a claim for $2,300 for damages to bedding, clothing, food, and so on. They lost everything except two cows, which somehow had been spared. They were never reimbursed for their losses.[21]

The building itself was pierced by several artillery shells, and the northeast gable corner had several pieces knocked out. A large crack in the wall extended two stories, and all the fencing around the fields and along Seminary Avenue had been destroyed.[22]

There were at least twenty-three Confederate burials behind Schmucker Hall and the Krauth House, and another two from North Carolina behind and west of Schmucker Hall.[23] The last man to die at the seminary was Sergeant Joseph Lifflith of the 104th New York Infantry.[24]

9. Lutheran Seminary, President's House, Seminary Ridge, 39°47.847' N, 77°14.642' W

Called the First Professor's House, the president's house was built in 1833 shortly after completion of the Old Dorm. Upon its completion, it was occupied by Rev. Dr. Samuel Schmucker and his family. Schmucker and his first wife had seven children from 1833 to 1848, and in the 1840s an addition was built to accommodate the growing family. Schmucker would eventually have three wives and thirteen children. He was an outspoken abolitionist, and some sources indicate that this home was used as a station on the Underground Railroad.

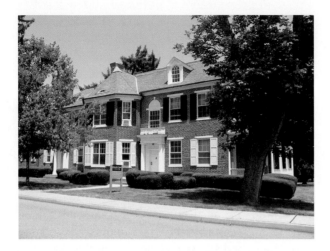

A ten-pounder Parrott shell remains lodged in the wall on the porch side of the seminary president's house.

By the time of the battle, all of his children had married or moved away. The only residents of the home were Schmucker, then age sixty-four, and his third wife, Esther M. (Wagner) Schmucker, age forty-eight.[25] The empty house was destined to become a hospital, as did the other two buildings on the campus. Ten wounded are believed to have been cared for in the home.

During the afternoon of July 1, 1863, Seminary Ridge became a defensive position for the Union army. Fighting raged around the seminary buildings, and the Confederates ultimately took the ridge from the Northerners. They would hold it for the next two days, placing artillery around the seminary buildings on July 2 and 3. These artillery pieces naturally attracted artillery fire from the Union artillery, and the house had thirteen cannonballs or shells pierce the walls, making holes two to three feet in length and

nearly as broad. A ten-pounder Parrott shell remains lodged in the wall on the porch side of house. Window frames were shattered and sashes were broken, and most of the glass was destroyed throughout the house. The fences were nearly all broken.

Schmucker would later accuse the Confederates, who occupied his home following the afternoon of July 1, of destroying much of the furniture, slitting an oil painting of Schmucker's father with a bayonet, and scattering his papers and books inside and outside the house. Some had been trampled into the mud, including the family bible. A repentant Confederate soldier retrieved the bible and placed it back on its shelf, complete with a handwritten note on the back page saying that the bible should not have been treated in such a manner.

It is said that, for years after the war, bloodstains could still be seen on the hardwood floors. To repair the extensive damage, donations were solicited from the public, and within a year most of the damage to all three buildings had been repaired.[26]

10. John Herbst Farm, 45 Old Mill Road, 39°49.724' N, 77°15.326' W

Considered by many historians to be the bloodiest piece of land on the battlefield, the 160-acre John Herbst farm saw more than two thousand men killed, wounded, or captured on the first day of fighting. Among them was Union general John Reynolds, who was killed in the area now known as Herbst Woods. In the general's honor, it is often referred to as Reynolds's Woods. Not quite as serious, but still an important loss to the Confederates, was the capture of General James Archer. Sent to the Fort Delaware

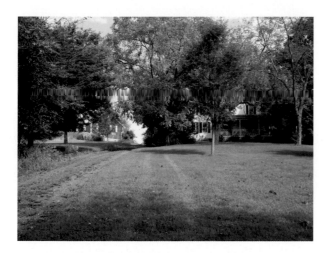

Wounded soldiers convinced a Confederate officer not to burn the Herbst home. The barn, however, was not spared.

the day, the two Union men and the Confederate soldier had been shooting at each other. Now, however, they were united in their appeal to the officer that he not burn the house. Their pleas did not fall on deaf ears. The house was spared.[27]

Herbst filed a claim for $2,689.36, claiming losses for a wagon, ladders, a reaper, a mower, a winnowing a mill, a cultivator, a plow, and all the wheat, corn, hay, straw, rye straw, and corn fodder in and around the barn. He received $2,606.75.[28]

The year 1863 was not a good one for Herbst. The battle took an economic and emotional toll, and later that year his wife, Susan, died. He eventually remarried and lived until 1904. He is now buried in Evergreen Cemetery in Gettysburg.[29]

prisoners-of-war camp, Archer was later moved to Johnson's Island before being exchanged in August 1864. By then, his health had deteriorated to the point where he collapsed after the Battle of Peebles's Farm and died in October 1864.

During the fighting, Herbst and his family stayed in their cellar. As the fighting began to quiet down, Herbst cautiously left his place of safety to survey what had happened. He immediately spied a Confederate officer, who told Herbst that he had orders to burn every building on the farm to prevent Union soldiers from using them for cover. The barn was already burning, and the officer now planned to order his men to burn the house.

Despite Herbst's protests, the Confederates entered the house, where they saw two wounded Union soldiers and one wounded Confederate. One man was so badly wounded that he could not be moved. Earlier in

11. Edward McPherson Farm, Chambersburg Road, 39°50.215' N, 77°15.082' W

Farm owner Edward McPherson (age twenty-eight) resided in Washington, where he served as deputy commissioner of internal revenue. He was a former congressman who had lost his reelection bid in 1862 and had just inherited the farm from his father a few months earlier. The farm consisted of 119 acres, 95 of which were planted in crops, the remainder in woodland, pasture, and an orchard. The barn, built from 1811 to 1820, is the only original structure remaining on the farm.[30]

During the July 1 fighting here, the barn was a prominent landmark and was used to shelter various Union regiments from artillery and small arms fire. Sharpshooters occupied the barn and fired from embrasures located in the gable walls. Confederate general Henry Heth later believed he was wounded

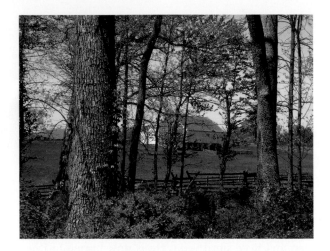

The wounded were packed so closely together in the McPherson barn that visitors had to step on them to move through.

by a shot from this barn. The position was overrun by overwhelming numbers of Confederate infantry on the afternoon of July 1, stranding scores of wounded Union soldiers. These men lay unattended until the barn and other McPherson buildings were hastily transformed into an emergency field hospital. Officially, the hospital was for the Union First Corps, but other Union soldiers were also treated here, as were several Confederates.[31] Union general John Reynolds was killed just south of the McPherson homestead.

Among those treated here was Colonel Roy Stone (149th Pennsylvania), who had been wounded in the hip and arm. He would recover and eventually attain the rank of brigadier general. A Private Foot, also from the 149th Pennsylvania, had been shot through the neck and was brought to the barn. He recovered well enough to be sent to Baltimore via freight train, where he could receive better treatment in one of the general

hospitals there. The move, however, proved fatal when the jostling of the train reopened his wound, causing him to bleed to death.[32]

A medical attendant, visiting the barn on July 2, found that the wounded were packed so closely together that he had to step on them to move through. A similar comment was made by Attorney William McClean when he brought food to the barn on July 4 after learning that the men had not eaten since the beginning of the battle.

John Slentz, age thirty-five at the time of battle, became McPherson's tenant in 1858, along with his wife, Eliza, and two school-age daughters and an infant daughter. At least two sons were born before the battle, bringing the family's total number of children to five.

Slentz owned three cows, six calves, four horses, four hogs, three turkeys, and at least forty chickens. He planned to remain during the battle so he could

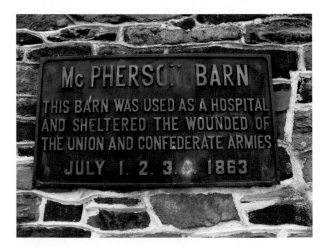

A tablet on the exterior wall of the McPherson barn.

keep the soldiers from stealing his stock but had to leave when the fighting got too intense. He planned to take the livestock to Culp's Hill or the Round Top area but was forced to abandon them when they panicked from the gunfire. The family tried to get to town but fighting forced them back, leading to their taking refuge in the seminary cellar, where they stayed for the entire three days of the battle. Eliza Slentz said that all that the family could save was the clothing they were wearing when they fled.[33]

When the family returned, they found the house ransacked and being used as a hospital. Amputations were taking place in the nearby wagon shed. They returned to the seminary, where they lived for three months while the farm was repaired.

Slentz filed a damage claim for $1,080.69, saying that seven of his nine head of cattle were killed, the other two crippled. All his horses had been taken by the rebels, as well as the family bible, beds and bedding, hogs, chickens, farming utensils, household goods and furniture, provisions, and clothing. No record has been located that indicates that he received any compensation.[34]

McPherson returned from Washington a week after the battle. After taking inventory, he filed a damage claim of $581.60 for fences, rails, boards, and posts. He also was never compensated.[35]

On April 6, 1895, a fire destroyed the house. Abandoned, the outbuildings fell into a state of disrepair and were removed by the War Department in 1904–1905. The barn was refurbished to its current appearance at the same time. It is the only structure remaining on the farm from 1863.[36]

Basil Biggs (age forty-four) and his wife, Mary, had lived on the McPherson farm when they first arrived

in Gettysburg in 1858. They were active in the Underground Railroad, concealing runaway slaves on the farm during the day and taking them to Quaker Valley at night as part of the slaves' flight to the North.[37]

12. Hospital Woods, Stone-Meredith Avenue, 39°50.103' N, 77°15.358' W

Little is known about this field aid station that arose out of necessity on the first day of fighting along the banks of Willoughby Run. More than forty Confederates and an unknown number of Union men received treatment here. It was located near the spot where Confederate general James Archer was captured, and the description of Surgeon LeGrand Wilson of the Forty-Second Mississippi places it in the area of Katalysine Spring.[38]

Water from the spring fed into Willoughby Run and was said to have medicinal properties and curative

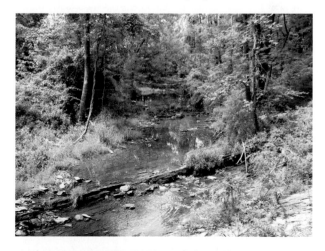

An outdoor hospital was hastily set up in these woods in the midst of the first day's fighting.

powers, although the soldiers were not likely to have known of that claim. Rather, the site for the hospital was likely chosen because it was close to the July 1 fighting on McPherson Ridge, the geography offered some physical protection, it was on the Confederate side of the battle line, and it provided a good water source in a shady location.

Rev. Charles G. McLean, on whose ground the springs were found, attempted to interest local residents in them as early as the 1830s. In 1868, the Gettysburg Lithia Springs Association began bottling and selling the "medicinal waters."

Tourists visiting the battlefield after the war wanted to visit the spring and enjoy its healing powers. Soon, Katalysine Springs Hotel (a.k.a. the Gettysburg Springs Hotel) was opened in 1869 to accommodate both battlefield visitors and those seeking relief from the many aches and pains the water was said to heal.

Veterans returning to reunions or on group visits to the battlefield often used the hotel as their headquarters. A trolley brought visitors from the town's railroad station to the hotel. The hotel closed in 1901 and burned down in 1917, with the property eventually becoming the Gettysburg Country Club.

Amanda Reinecker, a local citizen, volunteered as a nurse at this site on July 2 and 3.

13. Abraham Spangler Farm Site, Chambersburg Road, 39°50.528' N, 77°15.629' W

Not much is known about this site either, although there are records that indicate that Surgeon William Altman (Twenty-Eighth Pennsylvania) and Dr.

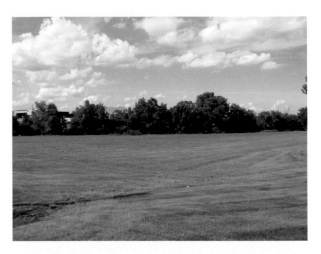

Period maps place the Abraham Spangler farm in this vicinity.

Cornelius M. Campbell (150th New York) both served the wounded at the Spangler farm. Unfortunately, however, Spangler also owned a farm on Baltimore Pike that was occupied during the battle by his son Henry, leaving some doubt as to which Spangler farm the two doctors attended.

It is known that the Baltimore Pike farm was a hospital, but there are indications that the farm on Chambersburg Pike may have also served as a field aid station. Confederate brigadier general Joseph R. Davis's Mississippi Brigade passed over this farm in their advance on July 1, so any wounded who may have been treated here would likely have been from the Second, Eleventh, or Forty-Second Mississippi Infantry or the Fifty-Fifth North Carolina Infantry.

Abraham Spangler (age seventy-six) also owned the land on which Spangler Spring sits on Culp's Hill. Spangler was married to Mary Knopp Spangler until her death in 1819. A year later he married Elizabeth Lady Spangler. He had two children with Mary and seven with Elizabeth. The youngest child, Levi, was twenty-one when the battle broke out at Gettysburg, so it is possible that none were at home at that time, although Levi enlisted in the 101st Pennsylvania Infantry in 1865, so he may have still been residing with Alexander and Elizabeth in 1863 with his wife and infant son. The second to the youngest son, William, was definitely not at home, as he was serving with the 165th Pennsylvania Infantry and was not discharged until three weeks after the battle. The remaining children were known to have been living elsewhere by 1863. Abraham and Elizabeth stayed in their cellar during the battle and found themselves behind Confederate lines when they came out.

Family records indicate that Abraham died in May 1876 from injuries suffered in a fall.

14. Frederick Herr Tavern and Farm, 900 Chambersburg Road, 39°50.541' N, 77°15.714' W

The tavern was constructed in 1815 by Thomas Sweeney. Frederick Herr purchased the ninety-five-acre property in 1828. Although the tavern honorably served as a stop on the Underground Railroad, there are also unsubstantiated reports that it had a more nefarious history, with a counterfeiting operation in the basement and a brothel operating on the second floor.

Its location on the Chambersburg Pike lent itself to becoming one of the earliest field aid stations on July 1, when it became an aid station for Pettigrew's

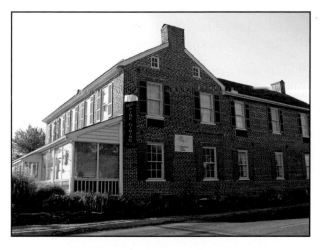

Frederick Herr's property became one of the first Confederate hospitals.

Brigade. Herr's farm is one of four possible locations that General William Dorsey Pender may have been brought to for treatment for a thigh wound suffered on the evening of July 2 when he was struck by shrapnel. Other possibilities include the David Whisler farm (Pender's Headquarters), Lohr's farm, or Heintzelman's farm.

Pender was evacuated to Staunton, Virginia, where he showed signs of recovering. However, an artery in his leg ruptured on July 18. Surgeons amputated his leg in an attempt to save him, but he died a few hours later.

Bloodstains are still visible on the second floor of the tavern, and at least six Confederate burials were found on the farm.

The Herrs claimed damages of $1,045.56 and received an award of $805.56 for two cords of wood that were burned and lost oats, boards, nails, and fencing.[39]

15. Dr. Samuel Hall Farm, 1619 Herr's Ridge Road, 39°49.863' N, 77°16.266' W

This 138-acre farm was occupied by Samuel Hall and his wife, Ellen. The sixty-seven-year-old physician had moved to the area in 1837 and set up his practice. He never claimed that his home was a hospital or aid station, although he did say that wagon trains from the Army of Northern Virginia camped on his property.

Two of Pettigrew's men were interred east of the house, in woods near the county road. John H. Hancock and James D. Leaman, both of the Fifty-Second North Carolina Infantry, died on July 1. Hancock was said to have been killed, while Leaman was wounded and died later in the day.[40] Because the men were on Hall's property, it is not a stretch to believe that he may have treated Leaman before the North Carolinian passed away.

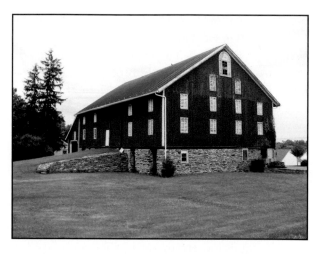

Dr. Hall's barn. The wounded may have been housed here.

In a history of Cumberland and Adams Counties, Hall was described as a good physician, but "impulsive and sometimes warm in discussions."[41]

After the war, Hall and his wife sold the farm and moved west.

16. Michael Crist Farm, 1130 Herr's Ridge Road, 39°50.642' N, 77°15.543' W

Michael Crist purchased this 141-acre farm just months before the battle. Michael is believed to be related to John Crist, who owned an adjoining farm. The house and barn were used by Major General William Dorsey Pender's Division of Lieutenant General A. P. Hill's Corps. Both the house and the barn are still standing.

Dr. John Henry McAden (Thirteenth North Carolina) is shown in various sources as serving at Heintzelman's, Lohr's, Herr's, John Crist's, Michael Crist's,

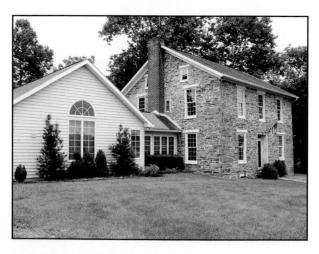

Dr. Hall is believed to have treated at least two men from North Carolina in his home or barn.

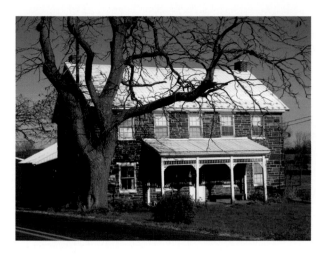

Michael Crist's house and barn were both used to treat Confederate wounded from Pender's Division.

or George Stoever's farm. It is possible that he moved among all of them, considering their proximity to one another.

There were three burials on the property. Festy Joyce (Richmond Letcher Artillery) was buried under a large oak tree. The other two burial locations were not recorded as specifically. They were of Jesse Franklin Slade, who was buried as JS, Thirteenth North Carolina, and a Corporal Wells from Georgia.[42]

In his damage claim, Michael Crist listed losses of hay and wheat, fence rails, bacon, lard, apple butter, saws, hatchets, shovels, a saddle, a Rockaway buggy, and many blankets, sheets, towels, and pillowcases. He said the damages totaled $1,269.51. He was awarded nearly the entire amount, $1,257.51.[43]

John Q. Allewelt was living on the Crist farm at the time of the battle but fled with the horses to keep them out of Confederate hands. Crist's family also left before

the fighting began, and Michael Crist was the only person on the farm during the battle. Allewelt claimed damages of $560.37 for sheets, coverlets, and other items of bedding. He received full compensation.[44]

17. John Crist Farm Site, Herr's Ridge Road, 39°50.942' N, 77°15.778' W

At about the same time that Michael Crist was buying his farm, his relative John Crist purchased the adjoining property. The latter property covered 125 acres and served as a field aid station or temporary hospital for the Louisiana Tigers.

As noted in the discussion of the Michael Crist farm, Dr. John Henry McAden of the Thirteenth North Carolina may have treated the wounded here.

John Crist filed a damage claim for $1,887.60 and received an award of $1,829.60, indicating a significant amount of damage. He filed for damages and losses of wagons and gear, rails, livestock, grain, beds and bedding, clothing, farm equipment, stove, and

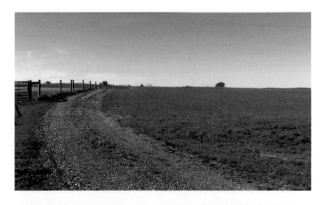

John Crist's farm became a hospital for the Louisiana Tigers. Five of their number were buried on the property.

tools. Among the livestock he said he lost was a horse taken on July 1.[45]

There were five confirmed burials on the property, all members of the Louisiana Tigers. Major Henry L. N. Williams (Ninth Louisiana) had been wounded by a bayonet on July 1. He died on July 5, the highest-ranking officer to die at the Crist farm, and was buried under a gum tree. The other burials were of Sergeant John Gibson (Seventh Louisiana), Aristides L. Lague (Eighth Louisiana, who died July 3), W. H. Williams (Fifth Louisiana, who was wounded on July 2 and died on July 4), and Lieutenant WTP (Seventh Louisiana), who was actually Wallace P. Talbott.[46]

18. George B. Stoever Farm Site, Chambersburg Road, 39°50.701′ N, 77°16.186′ W

Period maps place this now vanished farm on or near the ground occupied today by the Gettysburg airport. Stoever's name is also spelled Stover in some sources, and the farm is believed to have served as a hospital or field aid station for Henry Heth's Division. As noted in the discussion of the Michael Crist farm, Dr. John Henry McAden of the Thirteenth North Carolina may have treated the wounded here.

Little is known about the farm or the family, although a George B. Stoever is listed as a plaintiff, among others, against the National Homestead regarding treatment of the children. That George B. Stoever is shown as working as a butcher, which would be a natural occupation for a farmer. No other references have been found.[47]

Stoever filed a damage claim in the amount of $922.95 and was awarded $891.02 for an extensive list of items that were either damaged or lost. Stoever's neighbor C.

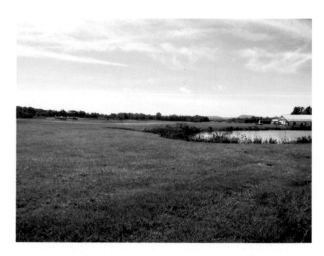

Period maps place the Stoever farm in the area of the Gettysburg airport.

Dougherty signed a statement witnessing Stoever's claim in which he said that Stoever's house and barn were completely plundered and that the rebels had stayed on Stoever's farm for eight days.[48] If the Confederates actually did occupy the farm for that long, it would indicate a larger operation than a temporary aid station.

19. Mary Jane Buser House Site, Unknown Location, Chambersburg Pike Area

What little is known about Mary Buser comes entirely from her damage claim, which was witnessed and verified by George W. Erb. She is not listed in any tax records of the period and is believed to have been a tenant on an area farm, possibly in the area around the George B. Stoever farm.

In her claim, sworn before Zachariah Myers, Esq., she stated that the house was used for the wounded during the battle and that she had fled on July 1 with her two young children. She filed a claim for damages amounting to $960.05 and was ultimately awarded $716.95.[49]

20. David Whisler Farm Site, Chambersburg Road, 39°51.155' N, 77°16.505' W

This small farm served as both the headquarters and one of three wagon parks for Pender's Division, the other two parks being at the Andrew Heintzelman farm and the Samuel Lohr farm. It was also a small aid station, probably only used for a few days. The Whisler farm is one of four possible locations that General William Dorsey Pender may have been brought to when he was struck by shrapnel on the evening of July 2. Other possibilities include Lohr's farm, Heintzelman's farm, and Herr's farm and tavern (see section 14 of this chapter, where there is more on Pender).

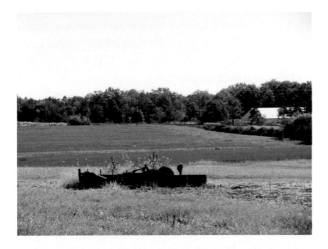

Whisler's farm served as a wagon park, Pender's headquarters, and a small aid station during the battle.

One general who definitely was brought here was Isaac Trimble. He subsequently was moved to the Samuel Cobean farm, where his leg was amputated, then to the Robert McCurdy home in town, and finally to the Lutheran Seminary hospital.

At the time of the battle, the farm contained a two-story house and a large log barn, plus some out-buildings and a small orchard. None of the wartime buildings remain, although a modern home now occupies the property. The current owner states that occasionally he finds Civil War–era bullets around the home.

Dr. Joseph Holt of the Eleventh Mississippi helped treat the wounded here.

21. E. D. Kellar (or Keller) Farm, 206 Knoxlyn Road, 39°50.613' N, 77°16.925' W

Dr. John W. C. O'Neal, who kept a comprehensive tally of Confederate burials, stated that this was formerly the Charles Polly farm. Burial records for four of those Confederates indicate some confusion as to whose farm it was, stating that the individual was "buried on E.D. Kellar's farm (also shown as Charles B. Polly's Farm)."[50] It is possible that the farm had recently changed hands or that Kellar was a tenant on Polly's farm. Period maps also are of little help, with Polly's name appearing on some maps, Kellar's on others. Several attempts to contact the current owners in person have been unsuccessful, and it is possible that the farm is currently unoccupied.

The farm was described as containing 228 acres, with 40 acres in woodland with prime meadow. It had a two-story weatherboard house with wash house, springhouse, large bank barn, wagon shed, corncrib,

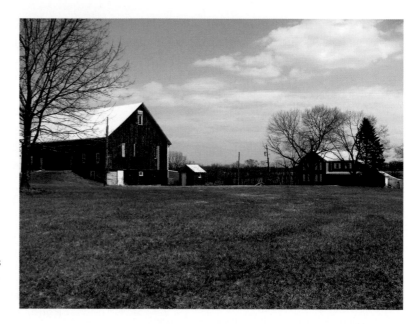

At the time of the battle, the Kellar farm was also referred to as the Charles B. Polly farm, creating some confusion for those in charge of burial records.

carriage house, hog pen, orchard, and a well near the house.

There were seven confirmed burials on the property, one of them being an unknown soldier who was buried under two apple trees. The four who were shown as "buried on E.D. Kellar's farm (also shown as Charles B. Polly's Farm)" were Captain Campbell Tredwell Iredell (Forty-Seventh North Carolina), who was wounded July 1 and died the next day, Captain William Westwood McCreery of Pendleton's staff, Second Lieutenant William W. Richardson of the Twenty-Sixth North Carolina, and Captain William Wilson, also of the Twenty-Sixth North Carolina. McCreery was shot through the heart and killed instantly on July 1. Richardson and Wilson were killed the same day, with Wilson being killed in "McPherson's Woods,

near the spot where Colonel Burgwyn fell." The remaining burials were of Lieutenant Colonel William Terrell Harris (Second Georgia), who died on July 2; and Captain Cecil Ballard (Macon Guards), who was wounded on July 1 and died on July 2.[51]

No statements have been found by either Kellar or Polly that indicate that the farm was a hospital or aid station, and with several of the dead having been killed in other locations, those would have received no treatment here. However, at least two of those (Ballard and Iredell) survived until the day after their injuries. They may have been left on the field until their bodies were found, or they may have been brought to Kellar's and received some level of treatment, even if only palliative. It is unlikely that they would have been moved from another location simply to be buried, because most Confederate burials took place either where the bodies were found or nearby in mass graves. The fact that they were buried in individual graves a day after being wounded makes it likely that the Kellar/Polly farm served as some type of temporary aid station early in the battle, even if only informally.

22. Samuel Lohr Farm Site, 1899 Lincoln Highway, 39°50.352' N, 77°17.547' W

Samuel Lohr's 125-acre farm served as the main hospital for Henry Heth's Division, as well as some of Pender's Division and possibly some of Anderson's Division. It was one of the largest Confederate hospitals along the Chambersburg Pike. From the first day of the fighting, the wounded filled the road, the yard, and Lohr's field, where they lay on the bare ground or a thin layer of straw.

Among those treated here were Colonel William J. Hoke (Thirty-Eighth North Carolina), Colonel John Kerr Connally (Fifty-Fifth North Carolina), and Colonel John M. Stone (Second Miss). Pender himself may have been treated here before being transferred to Staunton, Virginia, where he died after an amputation of his leg. Other possible sites for Pender's early treatment include the David Whisler farm (Pender's headquarters), Herr's farm, and Heintzelman's farm.

The house was made of solid chestnut logs. There were several outbuildings, including a springhouse, and every building was filled with wounded. The house was lost in a fire in the early 1980s, and only the foundation and some of the rubble remain, as well as the springhouse. All the current buildings on the farm, with the exception of the springhouse, are replacements. The Lohr family, except for son Aaron,

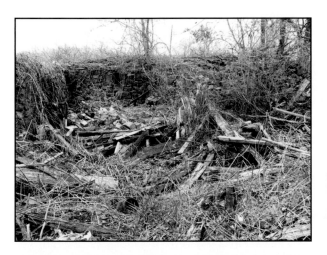

A fire destroyed the Lohr farmhouse in the 1980s. Some of the charred beams are visible in the center of the picture.

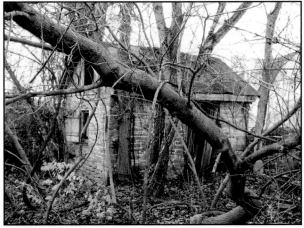

The spring house is the last building remaining on the Lohr farm.

who was serving in the Twenty-First Pennsylvania Cavalry, left the farm and did not regain possession until September 1.

More than seven hundred were treated here, and there were sixty-six burials around the farm, including forty-five sets of remains buried around a pear tree opposite the house. One unidentified Mississippi soldier was buried in an unspecified woodlot. There were also twelve burials in the woods on the north side of the farm, as well as eight burials in unspecified areas of the farm. Most of the remains were removed to Hollywood Cemetery in Richmond in 1873.[52]

Doctors on the Lohr farm included Benjamin Green (Fifty-Fifth North Carolina); L. P. Warren (Twenty-Sixth North Carolina), who asked to remain behind because his brother Lieutenant John Christian Warren of the Fifty-Second North Carolina had fallen on July 3 and was still unaccounted for; Spencer Welch (Thirteenth South Carolina); LeGrand Wilson (Forty-Second Mississippi); B. F. Ward (Eleventh Mississippi); and H. H. Hubbard (Second Mississippi). The on-scene chaplain was Rev. Dr. Thomas Dwight Witherspoon (Second Mississippi).

Others who assisted in treating the wounded were members from both the Eleventh and Twenty-Sixth North Carolina bands. When they were not assisting with the injured, they were asked to play tunes to keep up the morale of the men being treated.

Lohr's damage claim for $3,382.20 said the rebels occupied his land for several weeks and that the house, barn, and outbuildings were badly damaged. He asked for reimbursement for losses of rails, pilings, posts, and other fencing, as well as nearly forty-eight acres of grains and crops, damages to buildings and

the farm, five cords of wood, 242 bushels of wheat and oats, ten tons of hay, linens and bedding, carpet, livestock, buggy and harness, food, tools, and farm implements. He received $2,155.12.[53]

23. Andrew Heintzelman Farm and Tavern, 1980 Lincoln Highway, 39°51.493' N, 77°17.849' W

Andrew and Elizabeth Heintzelman owned this eighty-two-acre farm and tavern, which had been built in 1817 by George Arnold. Their son William lived with them. The tavern's name was Sign of the Seven Stars, and Seven Stars remains a local name for the area today. The primary clientele were railroad employees working on the bed of the nearby railroad. Andrew had been a county commissioner and postmaster for the village of Seven Stars before the war.

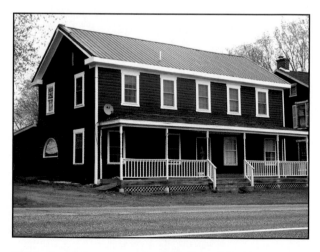

Heintzelman's tavern was named the Sign of the Seven Stars at the time of the battle. It became a Confederate hospital.

The house and barn were used for about ten days as a hospital for Pender's Division, and the farm is one of four where Pender may have been treated for his leg wound before being moved to Virginia. There, shortly after the amputation of the leg, Pender died. Other local farms where he may have been treated before being moved include the David Whisler farm, Herr's farm, and Lohr's farm. There were more than one hundred burials on the farm.

Doctors who served here, as well as at other farms in the vicinity, included John Henry McAden (Thirteenth North Carolina), John Tyler McLean (Thirty-Third North Carolina), W. M. Scarborough (Fourteenth South Carolina), and W. P. Hill (Thirty-Fifth Georgia).

Heintzelman filed a claim of $1,193.75 for the loss of six thousand shingles, sixteen cords of wood, grain crops, two wagons, harness, household goods, shop tools, and farm implements. He was eventually awarded $985.85.[54]

24. Christian Shank Farm, 240 Crooked Creek Road, 39°51.819' N, 77°17.494' W

Christian Shank owned this three-hundred-acre farm, which was used as a Confederate hospital for about two weeks. The Army of Northern Virginia actually occupied the farm longer than that, camping in the fields from June 16 until July 6. Shank, seventy-two years old, lived here with his sixty-eight-year-old wife, Anna, and their young son, Christian. The Shanks had six other adult children, with thirty-four-year-old Aaron helping on the farm.

The house, built in 1847, was used primarily by Pender's Division, although the barn and other outbuildings were also used to house the wounded.

Christian and his son Aaron both filed damage claims. Christian noted that the rebels ravaged the area, stealing a bay mare and bridle, jack screw, and log chain. He said they also trampled his hay, corn, and oats, as well as eighteen acres of crop grass; damaged two trees and a spreader; and burned or destroyed six hundred fence rails. Christian also claimed that his outbuildings had been torn down and used for firewood.[55]

Aaron's damages were similar, saying the Confederates took his dark bay horse, sorrel mare, three sets of gears and collars, five bridles, a wagon, two halters and harnesses, a leather fly net, a buggy, a dung and hay fork, and his carpenter tools. He must have had a portion of the farm to operate as his own, claiming damages to his hay, corn, and oats.[56]

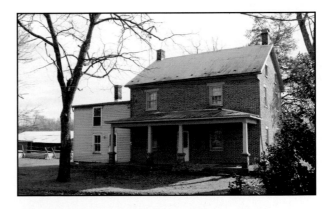

Shank's farm served as a campsite and hospital for the Confederate army before and during the battle.

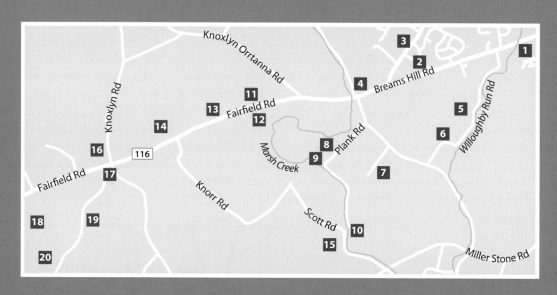

Chapter 6 sites: Fairfield Road area. (Map by Bill Nelson)

MOST OF THE DOCTORS AT THE HOSPITALS along Fairfield Road and the surrounding area moved between the hospitals and are not associated with any one facility. Where a doctor remained at one site, his name is listed with that hospital. "Floating" doctors included Benjamin Cromwell (First North Carolina), Lucious C. Coke (First North Carolina), DeWilton Snowden (First Maryland Battalion), Caspar C. Henkel (Tenth Virginia), Charles W. MacGill (Second Virginia), Robert A. D. Munson (Second Virginia), John A. Hunter (Twenty-Seventh Virginia), Edwin Latimer (Andrews's Battalion), and Bushrod Taylor (Jones's Brigade).

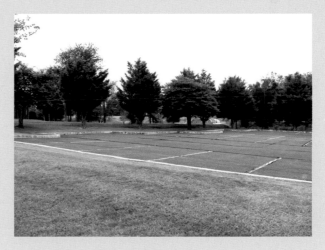

A small business park now sits on the site of the Arnold farm, which was occupied by tenant John Horting.

1. George Arnold Farm Site, Fairfield Road, 39°49.484' N, 77°15.432' W

This 124-acre farm was owned by George and Mary Arnold but occupied by a tenant farmer named John Horting. The farm consisted of 124 acres, 10–12 acres of which were in timber, plus 30 acres of meadow bottom. There were also two orchards: one of apples, one of peaches. The weatherboarded house was two stories and a cellar, with a back building, bake oven, smoke house, large bank barn, corncrib, outbuildings, a pump at the door, and what was described at the time as a "never failing spring of water" close by. Willoughby's Run formed the western boundary of the farm.[1] Nothing remains of the farm today, and the property is now the home of a small business park.

Rather than farming himself, Arnold was a businessman, preferring to let Horting handle the farm. Arnold had started the Gettysburg Iron Foundry in 1837 with Thaddeus Stevens. He also owned a clothing store on Chambersburg Street and was considered to be one of the town's most influential residents. At the time of the battle, Arnold was an officer of the Farmers and Mechanics Savings Institution he helped found in 1857. He was described as an ardent Unionist and active in politics. In a touch of irony, he had traveled to Harrison's Landing, Virginia, the summer before the fighting took place in Gettysburg to help care for the wounded from the Peninsula Campaign.

Dr. John W. C. O'Neal showed sixty-six burials on the farm, indicating that it was a fairly large facility. Most of those interred here were from Georgia, with some from Tennessee, Alabama, Texas, Arkansas, Mississippi, North Carolina, and South Carolina. Several were officers.[2]

Horting left the farm with his family on July 1 and returned on July 6. The farm served as a hospital from July 1 to July 7. As would be expected, he suffered significant losses and filed a claim of $517.00 for the loss of a horse, livestock, carriage and harness, tools, flour, bacon, salt, poultry, and a blanket. He included the cost of boarding the soldiers in his claim.

2. Adam Butt Schoolhouse, Fairfield Road, 39°49.300' N, 77°16.333' W

This small schoolhouse, owned by Adam Butt, served as a Confederate hospital for Cadmus Wilcox's and Ambrose Wright's Brigades of General R. H. Anderson's Division. The school consisted of only one room

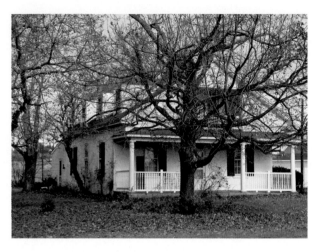

The one-room Butt schoolhouse is a part of the larger home that sits on the property today.

and is incorporated into the house that sits on the property today. It was often referred to as the Brick Schoolhouse and served as a hospital for six weeks.

The small schoolhouse was quickly overwhelmed with wounded, with some of the overflow taken to Allah and John Butt's property across Fairfield Road. Allah and John were relatives of Adam Butt.

There were nine known Confederate burials on the property, eight of them from the Third Georgia Infantry and one from the Forty-Eighth Georgia Infantry. The lone burial from the Forty-Eighth Georgia was William Davis. Those from the Third Georgia included T. W. Chapman, Charles N. Dean, Corporal William R. Gregory, Edward S. Aaron, Donald H. Montcrief, Council Wheeler, S. W. Stewart, and James Hodges. Most of these also appear on burial records for the Pitzer farm.[3]

3. Adam Butt Farm, Herr's Ridge Road, 39°49.435' N, 77°16.566' W

Adam Butt had purchased this farm, also known as the Samuel Herbst farm, just days before the battle. The fifty-three-year-old Butt, who worked as a carpenter, had just moved in with his wife, Nancy, and their four children. The 124-acre farm became a rather large hospital for Anderson's Division, with one thousand men treated in the house, bank barn, and yard. The farm also served as a wagon park for Anderson's Division and became an assembly point for ambulances and wagons on the retreat to Virginia. It would be in use as a hospital for about six weeks, although Butt would not be there to see it. He had taken ill and was recovering at a neighbor's home.

Doctors who treated the wounded here, in addition to any of those listed at the beginning of this chapter, included Henry DeSaussure Fraser (chief surgeon, Anderson's Division), Surgeon Henry A. Minor (Eighth Alabama and surgeon in charge), J. R. Woods (Second Georgia Battalion), W. F. Nance (Second Florida), James W. Claiborne (Twelfth Virginia), Samuel Dickinson (Twelfth Virginia), W. F. Richardson (Ninth Alabama), Assistant Surgeon John Madden (Perry's Brigade), and as many as ten others unnamed. The chaplain was Rev. Dr. J. O. A. Cook (Third Georgia).

Captain Charles W. Waddell of the Twelfth Virginia was assisting with the wounded here when he came down with typhoid fever. Considering the crowded conditions, quarantining was not a practical option. Despite the circumstances, Waddell recovered and lived until 1897. There is no record of any others who may have been infected before he was diagnosed.

There were six Union and thirty-one Confederate graves recorded on the farm. However, there were obviously some burials that were not recorded, as at least forty bodies were exhumed some ten years after the battle.[4]

John W. C. O'Neal's unofficial records indicate that there were three burials from the Eighth Alabama on the west side of the house at a road in the corner of the woods, three more from the Ninth Alabama buried north of the house under a cherry tree, and another six from an unknown regiment or regiments buried on the south side of the house near the road. O'Neal claimed that an additional thirty-one were interred between the farm and Bream's Black Horse Tavern.[5] His total of forty-three burials lines up better with the number of exhumations in the early 1870s.

Butt filed a claim for $5,163.50 for saddle bags, soap, land damage, furniture, bedding, leather goods, bees, livestock, fencing, a wagon, a rifle, and food.[6] It

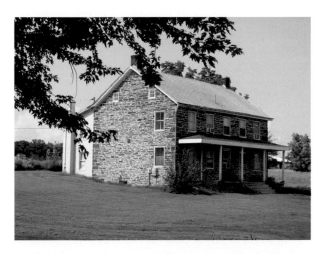

Butt's farm became a major Confederate hospital, treating as many as one thousand wounded.

is likely that his claim covered losses both at the farm and at the schoolhouse.

4. Black Horse Farm and Tavern, 82 Black Horse Tavern Road at Fairfield Road, 39°49.134' N, 77°17.017' W

The Black Horse Tavern and surrounding farm were the primary field hospital for Kershaw's Brigade. It was used for nearly three hundred wounded, including about seventy from other brigades in McLaws's Division. There were also a few from Brigadier General John B. Hood's Division buried here, indicating that some of his men were also treated at the farm.

The house had been built by the McClelland family circa 1803, and the property was owned by Francis Bream at the time of the battle. Bream was fifty-seven

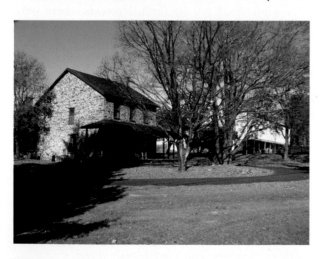

Before the war, visitors to the tavern often carved their initials or names on the tavern walls. When the farm became a hospital during the battle, a young wounded soldier found his parents' names on the wall.

years old and had served as the first sheriff of Adams County. He had purchased the property in 1845 from the heirs of William McClelland IV and operated a tavern in the house, which got its name from a large carved wooden black horse that stood in the front of the tavern. Using the horse as an advertising tool, Bream held horse races on the property that attracted visitors from several states, adding to his wealth and reputation as the wealthiest citizen in Cumberland Township. The former sheriff stayed throughout the battle, but his wife, Elizabeth, and their eight children all left.

The Fairfield Road had been a stagecoach route, and drovers used it to take cattle to Hagerstown. With such a built-in clientele, the farm was a natural location for a tavern. Over the years, it had become customary for travelers staying overnight at the tavern to carve their names and the date in the tavern wall, and during the battle a young wounded soldier convalescing at the tavern said he found his parents' names on the wall.[7]

Sitting on the north side of Fairfield Road, the four-hundred-acre farm contained a two-and-a-half-story stone house, a small log house, and a huge bank barn, along with the usual outbuildings associated with a farm of this size. The tavern made a perfect field hospital. There was plenty of room and, with two wells and the nearby Marsh Creek, there was an abundance of water. For several days the tavern, house, barn, and every outbuilding were filled with wounded. Passing generals stopped with their staff officers and met in the front yard.[8]

The night of July 1, General Cadmus Wilcox and his brigade of 1,200 men spent the night in the fields above the tavern. The next afternoon, ambulances began bringing in the wounded from the Peach Orchard and Wheatfield. Surgeons at the tavern began their round-the-clock effort, setting up makeshift operating tables by ripping doors from their hinges and placing them across dry-goods boxes and barrels. Pots in the fireplace were used to boil water, and bandages were torn from bedsheets. When it got too dark to see, surgeons worked by candlelight. Dawn on July 3 brought little respite, as the wounded continued to be brought in. It would be thirty-six hours before the surgeons got their first break.

Doctors here included twenty-three-year-old Simon Baruch from the Third South Carolina Battalion; Aristides Monteiro, H. Gray, and John Syng Dorsey Cullen of Longstreet's Corps; Landon C. Reeves of the First Virginia Cavalry; T. W. Salmond and Henry Junius Nott of the Second South Carolina; J. F. Pearce from the Eighth South Carolina; Acting Assistant Surgeon D. H. Ramseur from the Eighteenth Georgia; and a few unnamed civilian doctors from Baltimore.

Monteiro recalled that the wounded lay everywhere, on blankets, bare ground, or wherever there was space. Even the twenty-acre orchard and wooded lot sheltered them. The air was pierced with screams of delirium and calls for wives, sweethearts, and mothers. Chaplains moved among the wounded, offering spiritual comfort. Amputated limbs were tossed to the ground from the porch and then carried away. Only the seriously wounded would be given chloroform, which was almost gone. Food was in short supply, and olive oil was used in a desperate attempt to keep infection away. Large green horseflies were everywhere, and surgeons looked like butchers, with blood-spattered white shirts and navy trousers.

The orderlies were nearly all from Kershaw's Brigade, and they received assistance from two women from a wealthy Maryland family who came with an English nurse. The women took on a myriad of duties, caring for the wounded, preparing food and dressings, praying with the dying, writing letters home, and reading the burial services. They stayed in the attic of the tavern and remained until the men were moved to Camp Letterman in August.

Among those treated here were two colonels: William Davie DeSaussure of the Fifteenth South Carolina and John D. Kennedy of the Second South Carolina. DeSaussure died here, and although most of the burials from the farm were in the orchard or on a hill near the house, he was buried in the nearby McClelland Cemetery, which had served for decades as the family cemetery of the earlier owners of the farm.[9] DeSaussure was eventually disinterred and removed to Hollywood Cemetery in Richmond. He was disinterred once again in 1871 and finally reinterred in Columbia, South Carolina.

On July 3 conditions worsened, as acrid smoke from the Pickett's Charge cannonade covered the hospital, burning the eyes and lungs and reducing visibility. As chloroform supplies dwindled still further, the surgeons regretted the destruction of the barrels of the tavern's whiskey, smashed to prevent them from falling into the hands of the men.

Baruch had been operating for twenty-four hours when he finally dozed off. When he awakened he learned that the Confederates were going to retreat southward, and that he, Pearce, and Nott would stay behind with 222 wounded who were too badly injured to be moved. They would be assisted by ten orderlies.

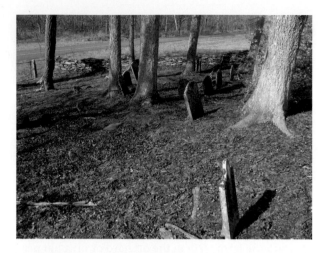

McClelland Cemetery, initial burial site for Colonel William DeSaussure, Fifteenth South Carolina Infantry.

When the Union cavalry approached the hospital on July 5, the doctors surrendered the farm and tavern, with them, the wounded, and the orderlies becoming prisoners of war. Baruch was instructed to go to the US Christian Commission depot in town for supplies, where he was also directed to try the US Sanitary Commission. All his requests for medical supplies were met.

The farm was the site of one of the most discussed events of July 2: Longstreet's controversial delay in attacking the Union left. As Hood and McLaws, commanding two divisions in Longstreet's First Corps, moved toward the battlefield via Fairfield Road, they passed the tavern behind the cover of Bream's Hill. At the top of the hill, they feared they could be seen by Union signal men on Little Round Top and had to reverse some ten thousand troops and march back past the tavern to find an alternate route. This action is often referred to as Longstreet's Countermarch.

Over the ten years following the battle, Bream filed three damage claims for a total of $7,102.00, noting that his property had been used as a hospital for six weeks and that he had lost all his crops, most of his fencing, household goods, and farm implements, in addition to the damage suffered to the tavern, house, barn, and outbuildings. His claims are believed to also include damage and losses at a nearby mill that he owned. He received nothing for his claim.[10]

5. George Culp Farm Site, Willoughby Run Road, 39°49.108' N, 77°15.939' W

This small farm no longer exists but was used for a short time as a hospital or aid station. Owned by George Culp, the farm may have been occupied at the time by a tenant named John Horner.

The farm was likely used by Hood's Division, and may have served to accommodate overflow from the adjoining John Edward Plank farm.

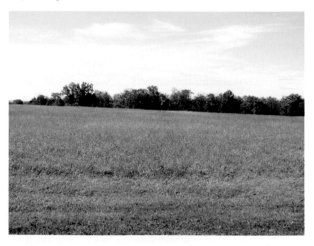

These fields once housed the George Culp farm.

There were eight burials listed on the farm, all of them along or near Willoughby Run. Their names are not known.

Both George Culp and his son George R. Culp filed damage claims for losses of crops, livestock, poultry, home furnishings, fences, and food. George filed for $1,107.07 and received $907.40. George R.'s claim was for $286.25 and he received the entire amount. George R. mentioned in his claim that the house and farm were used by the rebels as a field hospital from July 1 to July 5.[11]

6. John Edward Plank Farm, Willoughby Run Road, 39°48.898' N, 77°16.208' W

John Edward and Sarah Plank resided on this 220-acre farm that became a large hospital for Hood's Division. Their two children and John Edward's sister, Elizabeth "Lizzie" Plank, also lived here. Some earlier maps show the farm as belonging to Mrs. M. E. Plank, who is thought to have been John Edward's mother. The farm is also sometimes referred to as the Althoff farm, for Francis Althoff, who lived there in the late 1860s.

The hospital was established here on July 2 by Major Moses B. George, quartermaster for Hood's Division, and John Thompson Darby, the division's chief surgeon. Darby was initially in charge, assisted by ten to fifteen regimental surgeons and their assistants.

The 1,542 wounded who were treated here filled the two-and-a-half-story house, the brick bank barn, and the farm's outbuildings, one of which was used as a deadhouse. Here, the dead were held until they could be buried. Most were buried in shallow graves in the orchard, with additional burials every morning. There were more than one hundred burials over the

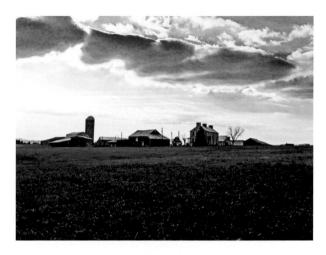

Used as a large hospital for six weeks, the Plank farm treated more than 1,500 wounded, including several Confederate generals and colonels.

six weeks the farm was in use as a hospital. To compound the misery, many of the horses that brought the ambulances to Plank's were so exhausted that they collapsed and died in the yard.

As the steady stream of wounded coming into the farm continued, the family was forced to leave. When they returned, they saw that the yard and garden fences were all gone, having been used for firewood. The flower and vegetable gardens were destroyed, the floors of the house were covered with bloody straw used for bedding, and most of their furniture had been thrown out into the fields. The room in the house described by the family as the Garner Organ room had been used as an operating room, with no attempt being made to contain the butchery. Their poultry, hogs, and cattle had all been consumed by the soldiers, and the house, porches, barn, and grounds were filled with wounded, and would continue to be until the second week of August.[12] Even the Confederate retreat left them with no relief, as 515 wounded were determined to be too badly injured to be moved.

Several officers were treated here, including General George T. "Tige" Anderson, General Jerome B. Robertson, Colonel F. H. Little (Eleventh Georgia), Colonel Robert M. Powell (Fifth Texas), Colonel John C. G. Key (Fourth Texas), Colonel Van H. Manning (Third Arkansas), Lieutenant Colonel William Luffman (Eleventh Georgia), Lieutenant Colonel Isaac B. Feagin (Fifteenth Alabama), Lieutenant Colonel W. M. Hardwick (Forty-Eighth Alabama), Lieutenant Colonel King Bryan (Fifth Texas), Major C. B. St. John (Forty-Eighth Alabama), Acting Major John R. Woodward (First Texas), and Lieutenant Colonel Benjamin F. Carter (Fourth Texas), who had been wounded in the face and legs in the attack on Little Round Top and Devil's Den the evening of July 2. Despite being considered mortally wounded, Carter survived and went on to become the mayor of Austin, Texas, after the war. The best-known patient, however, was Major General John B. Hood, who had been wounded on July 2 by shell fragments that ripped through his left hand, forearm, elbow, and biceps.

Surgeons here included Thomas A. Means (Eleventh Georgia), Thomas C. Pugh (Ninth Georgia), Henry W. Waters (First Texas), John Curtis Jones (Fourth Texas), William P. Powell (Fifth Texas), Karl H. A. Kleinschmidt (Third Arkansas), E. F. DeGraffenreidt (Fourth Alabama), W. H. Cole (Eighth Georgia), Thomas A. Rains (chief surgeon for Benning's Brigade), William O. Hudson (chief surgeon for Law's Brigade), John Thompson Darby (chief surgeon for Hood's Division), Surgeon J. R. Brown (Third

Arkansas), and John R. Bodly (unknown Georgia regiment). The chaplain was Rev. Dr. George E. Butler (Third Arkansas).[13] Elizabeth Plank said that she suspected that Bodly was actually a woman, and that the soldiers all referred to him as the woman doctor.

There were more than fifty nurses who assisted here, including Mary and Sally Witherow, who came each day from their home on Baltimore Street. At least three unidentified women arrived from the Baltimore area to care for the wounded here as well.

7. Samuel Johns Farm Site, Black Horse Tavern Road, 39°48.614' N, 77°16.870' W

Another farm that no longer exists is this one owned by John Crawford but tenant farmed by Samuel Johns, a forty-seven-year-old widower with two children. A housekeeper, Catherine Snyder, also lived on the farm. The farm consisted of a stone house, a small

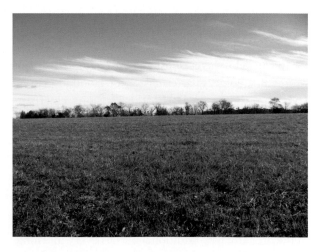

Only these rolling fields remain from the Samuel Johns farm.

barn, and one outbuilding, and it was part of a complex that included the John Crawford farm and the John Edward Plank farm.

The farm served as a hospital and wagon park for Semmes's Georgia Brigade and the artillery reserve. There were at least three physicians here to treat the wounded: S. P. Hobgood (Fifty-Third Georgia), James B. Clifton (Fifty-Third Georgia), and H. J. Paramore (Fifth Georgia). The chaplain was Rev. Crawford H. Toy (Fifty-Third Georgia).

There were ten burials on the farm, including Felix Ruleau of the Washington Louisiana Artillery, who had his foot amputated. He developed pneumonia and died on July 28, indicating that some form of aid station was in use here for at least a few weeks after the battle. He was buried behind the barn in a common grave with James B. Loughridge and Patrick McNeil, both of Parker's Richmond Battery. William P. Casey, a member of Brooks's South Carolina Artillery, died on July 4 and was buried east of the house, behind the barn. George Bryens of the Washington Louisiana Artillery was buried near the house with a misidentified companion from the same regiment who originally was believed to be William Creecy. However, Creecy survived the war, so the man buried with Bryens remains unknown. Another member of the Washington Louisiana Artillery, William Layman, who had been shot in the head, died on July 18 and was listed as being buried near the barn or at John Crawford's. Thomas J. Hayes, of Brooks's South Carolina Artillery, suffered a fractured femur, resulting in the amputation of his leg. He was buried in the woods east of the house, behind the barn. Andrew Martin, also of Brooks's South Carolina Artillery, was buried near the house east of the barn,[14] while Captain T. H.

Moore of the Eleventh Mississippi was buried at an unknown location on the farm.[15]

8. John Currens Farm, 143 Plank Road, 39°48.716' N, 77°17.219' W

This 105-acre farm with a two-story log house was the home of thirty-five-year-old John and thirty-three-year-old Elizabeth Currens and their two small children. The log house has been incorporated into the existing home and is said to still have bloodstains on the floor. Both the house and barn were used by Pickett's Division as a hospital. The Currens farm and the William E. Myers house were so close that they formed one large complex, treating as many as one thousand men.

There were thirty-four men from Pickett's Division buried here, including Lieutenant Colonel John

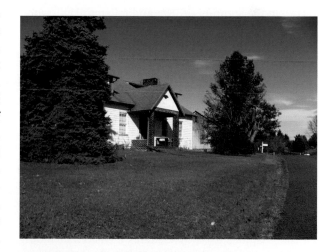

Bloodstains are still said to mar the floor inside the Currens house.

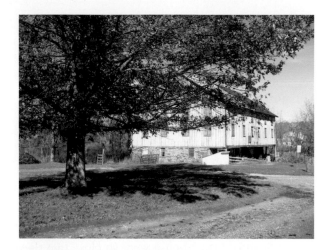

The barn held many who had been wounded in Pickett's Charge.

Thomas Ellis of the Nineteenth Virginia, who was interred southeast of the house under an apple tree in the orchard. Most of those buried here were disinterred in the summer of 1872 and taken to Hollywood Cemetery in Richmond for reburial.[16]

Men treated here did not lack medical attention. Among the doctors here were John Lewis (chief surgeon for Pickett's Division), Thomas A. Means (Eleventh Georgia), Thomas C. Pugh (Ninth Georgia), Henry Waters (First Texas), John Curtiss Jones (Fourth Texas), William. P. Powell (Fifth Texas), Karl H. A. Kleinschmidt (Third Arkansas), E. F. DeGraffenreidt (Fourth Alabama), W. H. Cole (Eighth Georgia), Thomas A. Rains (Benning's Brigade), and Wm. O. Hudson (Law's Brigade).

There were several other doctors who moved among all the hospitals used by Pickett's Division, including the Myers house, the Black Horse Tavern, Bream's Mill, and the Jacob Schwartz farm, in addition to the Currens farm. Those doctors were Surgeon F. W. Patterson (McLaws's Division), Thomas P. Mayo (Third Virginia), James W. Oliver (Seventh Virginia), Robert H. Worthington (Seventh Virginia), Charles E. Lippitt (Fifty-Seventh Virginia), John Mutius Gaines (Eighteenth Virginia), John R. Ward (Eleventh Virginia), William H. Taylor (Nineteenth Virginia), Alexander Grigsby (First Virginia), B. C. Harrison (Fifty-Sixth Virginia), William S. Nowlan (Thirty-Eighth Virginia), Charles B. Morton (chief surgeon, Kemper's Brigade), Landon C. Reeves (First Virginia Cavalry), Landon B. Edwards (Eighth Virginia), Dr. McAdams, and Dr. McCorky.

In addition to the doctors, there were nearly seventy-five nurses and stewards from Pickett's Division at the Currens-Myers complex. Several chaplains provided spiritual comfort as well, although only one, Rev. Dr. Peter Tinsley (Twenty-Eighth Virginia), was documented.

John Currens filed a claim for $1,558.71 for his losses, which included rails, boards, ladders, livestock, farm equipment, grain crops, seven cords of wood, fences, shingles, more than five hundred panels of snake fence, and unspecified damage to his orchard. He was awarded $1,440.50.[17]

9. Francis Bream Mill Site (William E. Myers House), 199 Plank Road, 39°48.658' N, 77°17.305' W

Francis Bream, who also owned the Black Horse Tavern, owned this property, which in 1863 consisted of a large three-story flour mill, sawmill, log house, blacksmith shop, cooper's shed, and other outbuildings. A small shed on the property was used for amputations.

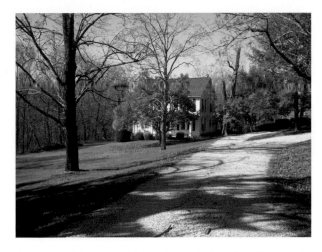

A portion of the original Myers house is thought to be part of this newer structure.

The mill was destroyed by fire in 1896 and nothing remains, although the original house may be a part of the existing structure. The mill, which sat on seventy acres, was operated by twenty-seven-year-old master miller William E. Myers, who also lived in the house.

Immediately beside the John Currens property, the mill formed one large hospital complex with the farm, sharing the doctors, nurses, and chaplains mentioned in the previous section.

Among the approximately one thousand treated here and at the Currens farm, the most prominent was General James L. Kemper, who was seriously wounded in the pelvis during Pickett's Charge. His wound was considered mortal, and he was placed in the house, where attendants tried to make him comfortable. Although he survived, he was considered too badly injured for further combat, and he took command of the Reserve Forces of Virginia.

The mill was also the receiving hospital for such other officers as Colonel William R. Aylett (Fifty-Third Virginia), Colonel William Dabney Stuart (Fifty-Sixth Virginia), Colonel Kirkwood Otey (Eleventh Virginia), Colonel Henry Gantt (Nineteenth Virginia), and Colonel Eppa Hunton (Eighth Virginia).

On July 4 Dr. Charles B. Morton from the Seventh Virginia stopped by with General Jubal Early to check on Kemper. With the retreat already starting, they warned the attending physicians that any of the wounded who were able to travel should get on the wagons as soon as possible. Shortly after Morton and Early left, the Union troops appeared and captured everyone who had stayed behind.

As would be expected, most of those who were interred on the property were from Virginia, with a few from North Carolina and Alabama. Most of the burials were at the dam that supplied water for the mill or at the edge of the woods near the property line. In 1870 more than forty sets of remains were removed from this area.

Bream filed three damage claims totaling $7,102.00. Those claims are believed to include losses here and at the Black Horse Tavern. His claims were all rejected.

10. John Crawford Farm, 500 Plank Road, 39°48.205′ N, 77°17.071′ W

The first settler on this land was Thomas McLean, who established a small farm in 1740 in an area inhabited by Lenape Indians. Subsequent owners were David Grier, then Abraham Usher, followed by William Crawford and his wife, Anne, who purchased the property in 1792. The farm included 225 acres with a log house and a well that still exists. Crawford, who

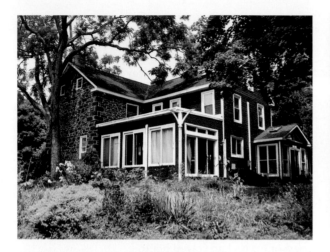

The dining room of the farmhouse on Crawford's farm, known as the Farm on the Ford, became an operating theater, and bloodstains remain visible on the floor.

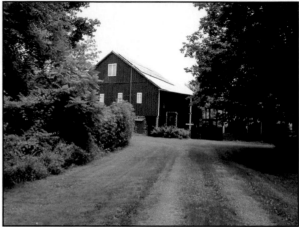

The barn was filled with Confederate wounded from McLaws's Division.

became a US congressman, built a two-story house with a well in the cellar. The farm ultimately became the property of Gettysburg attorney John Crawford.[18]

In 1863 the farm, now 289 acres and known as the Farm on the Ford, was occupied by tenant farmers, a free black veterinarian named Basil Biggs (age thirty-seven) and his wife, Mary Jackson Biggs (thirty-four). Basil was active in the Underground Railroad, and the house served as a stop for runaway slaves heading north.

Basil and Mary had come to Adams County in 1858 with their five children. With rumors telling of a buildup of Confederate forces, the understandably nervous Basil sent his family away but decided to remain at the farm himself. However, when the fighting began, he borrowed a horse and escaped to York.

During the battle, the farm became a major hospital for McLaws's Division, mostly those from Barksdale's

and Semmes's Brigades. The wounded were placed in the house, barn, shed, and outbuildings. When those became full, the adjacent grounds were utilized. The house's dining room became the amputation room, and bloodstains are still visible on the dining-room floor.

The surgeon in charge of the wounded was Francis William Patterson, of the Seventeenth Mississippi. Patterson was assisted by Henry Jones Parramore (Fiftieth Georgia), Assistant Surgeon Robert L. Knox (Seventeenth Mississippi), Taylor Gilmer (Barksdale's chief surgeon), R. L. Knox (acting assistant surgeon for the Seventeenth Mississippi), C. H. Brown (Eighteenth Mississippi), Aristides Monteiro (Alexander's Artillery Battalion), John Somers Buist (Henry's Artillery Battalion), and F. H. Sewell (Cabell's Artillery Battalion). Rev. Dr. William Burton Owen (Seventeenth Mississippi) and Rev. Crawford H. Toy (Fifty-Third Georgia) were chaplains.

The farm treated about three hundred wounded from July 2 through August 10. Among those treated here was Brigadier General Paul Semmes, whose leg had been mangled by shrapnel in the Wheatfield on July 2. He did not survive his wound, dying on July 10 in Martinsburg, West Virginia. Other officers treated here included Colonel William Dunbar Holder (Seventeenth Mississippi) and Colonel Thomas M. Griffin (Eighteenth Mississippi).

After the battle, Biggs buried nearly fifty men from Semmes's and Barksdale's Brigades. Officers known to have been interred included Colonel J. W. Carter (Thirteenth Mississippi), Captain J. W. Stamps (Company E, Twenty-First Mississippi), and Captain N. L. McDuffie (Company F, Thirteenth Mississippi).[19] Most of the burials took place around the house, barn, and orchard, with many near a large sycamore tree that remains on the property today.

When the national cemetery was established in Gettysburg, Biggs received a contract to exhume bodies from around the battlefield and bring them to the cemetery for reburial. Paid by the number of bodies, the business-savvy veterinarian got a two-horse wagon, enabling him to carry eight bodies, rather than the six that a one-horse team would allow.

Both Biggs and Crawford filed damage claims after the war. Biggs claimed $1,506.60 for forty-five acres of wheat, eight cows, seven other cattle, ten hogs, twenty-six yards of carpet, and $5.00 worth of jellies. He received the full amount.[20] Crawford was awarded $1,315.36 of his $1,440.36 claim for losses and damage to twenty-two acres of wheat, nearly ten acres of corn, oats, chestnut rails, oak rails, posts, picket fences, board fencing, and building damage (including blood on the dining-room floor from amputations).

Crawford claimed that his damage was compounded by the Union Sixth Corps, which he said tramped over his fields and crops in pursuit of the retreating Confederates.[21]

After the war, Biggs bought the Peter Frey farm on Taneytown Road.

11. Christian Byers Farm, Fairfield Road, 39°49.128' N, 77°18.131' W

Christian Byers (age sixty-six) lived on this 120-acre farm with his wife, Elizabeth (forty-six), in a house built by Christian's grandfather, Adam, nearly a century before the battle. The couple had nine children but most had died in childhood. One son, Christian Jr., was serving with the 138th Pennsylvania Volunteer Infantry near Harpers Ferry and was not in Gettysburg during the battle.

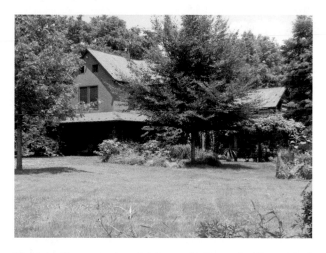

The Byers farm was a hospital for nearly five weeks. The original log house has been incorporated into the newer portion and is visible on the right.

Although the Confederates held the farm for only three days, the house and barn were used as a hospital for Isaac Avery's and William Smith's Brigades for about five weeks, serving approximately one hundred wounded for three of those weeks, of which fifty stayed for two additional weeks. The original house has been incorporated into the newer addition. The barn no longer exists.

John W. C. O'Neal found a total of twenty-six Confederate burials on the property, with only three of those identified. Those three were J. M. Gilbert, of the Fifty-Second Virginia, and L. C. Isley and George Moore, both of Company F, Sixth North Carolina. Moore is shown as having died on July 4.[22]

Byers said that he lost livestock, hay, a wagon, a carriage, and bridles; that one thousand rails were burned; and that there was damage to his house and barn. His claim totaled $1,007.00 and he received an award of $707.00.[23]

12. Jacob Plank Farm, Fairfield Road, 39°48.963' N, 77°18.020' W

This 184-acre farm was the home of Jacob (age fifty-nine) and Sarah Plank (age fifty-seven), along with several of their children. For about five weeks it served as a hospital for some five hundred wounded from Junius Daniels's Brigade of Rodes's Division. For about half that time the Planks were forced to share their house with the more severely wounded patients.

Only one doctor is documented as serving here, a Dr. Potts. His regiment is unknown. He was assisted by Chaplain Alexander D. Betts from the Thirtieth North Carolina.

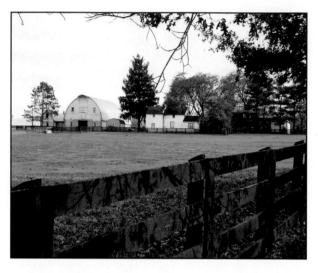

Jacob Plank's picturesque farm served as a hospital for five weeks. The most seriously wounded stayed in the house with the Plank family.

At least twenty-one officers and men of Rodes's Division were buried here, including five identified officers. Two men, Second Lieutenant William Henry Gibson (Thirty-Third North Carolina) and First Lieutenant Thomas W. Baker (Forty-Third North Carolina), were both buried under a walnut tree near the road. Two from the Second North Carolina Battalion were buried together behind the house: Second Lieutenant Joseph N. Duckett and Anthony Davers, who was misidentified as Anthony Dirge originally. It was fitting that Duckett and Davers were buried together. In one of those uncanny coincidences of war, both were wounded on July 1 in the thigh, both had their legs amputated, and both died on July 7. To finish off the strange sequence, both graves eventually were plowed over. A third man from the Second

North Carolina Battalion, Second Lieutenant Joseph W. Askew, was shot in the chest and lingered until July 15 before dying. He was buried behind the barn, and his grave was also plowed over.[24]

Jacob Plank filed a damage claim for $3,094.80, claiming losses of livestock, housewares, equipment, clothing, twenty cords of wood, seventy-one head of cattle, boards, grains, tools, farm implements, clothing, bedding, bee skeps, and foodstuffs. He was awarded $2,041.80.[25]

13. Andrew Weikert Farm, 2559 Fairfield Road, 39°48.949' N, 77°18.320' W

This ninety-seven-acre farm was purchased in 1834 by Andrew Weikert, who was sixty-three years old at the time of the battle. He lived with his fifty-nine-year-old wife, Susan, and their two children. Weikert and his family left during the fighting and returned on July 7 to be greeted by three hundred wounded men from Brigadier General John Brown Gordon's Brigade of Early's Division. The barn and orchard were used as a hospital for about six weeks.

There were twenty-two Confederate graves on the farm, with only two identified. A Lieutenant Woods from the Sixtieth Georgia and John A. Reeves from Company D of the Thirteenth Georgia were interred here. Reeves died of pyemia (septicemia) on July 14 after having his leg amputated.[26]

Weikert filed a damage claim for $1,997.67 and received $1,697.67. His losses included flour, grain crops, fifteen cords of wood, cattle, chickens, two wagons, horse gear, farm equipment, fencing, and damage to the garden, house, barn, and land. The damage to his fields seems to have been Weikert's

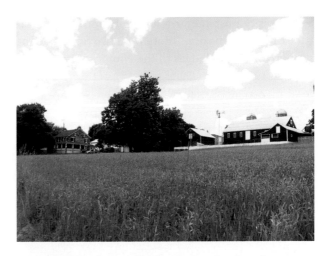

The Weikert farm remains in the Weikert family and is now an egg farm.

biggest complaint. He specifically noted in his claim that the damage done by wagons, horses, and soldiers during the muddy retreat rendered the fields "a disadvantage to farming for several years."[27]

The farm remains in the Weikert family today as an operating egg farm.

14. William Douglass Farm, 2795 Fairfield Road, 39°48.853' N, 77°18.886' W

William Douglass had two farms in the area, both of which served as field hospitals. This one is often referred to erroneously as the David Stewart farm. Stewart did own it, but not until after Douglass died in 1869 and his heirs, David and Martha E. Stewart, inherited the property. It is now a bed and breakfast.

Ambulance trains extended along Fairfield Road as they passed the farm, and the Douglass farm became a temporary hospital for a few men from Hays's Brigade of Early's Division. There were two burials on the property. John F. Hodges of the Ninth Louisiana died on July 4 and was buried at an unknown location on the farm. Horthere Fontenot from the Eighth Louisiana died on July 10 of gangrene. He was buried under an apple tree at the northeast corner of the orchard.[28]

Little is known about this farm. Douglass did file a damage claim for losses of posts and rails, crops, and two cords of wood, but it is not known how much, if anything, he was awarded.

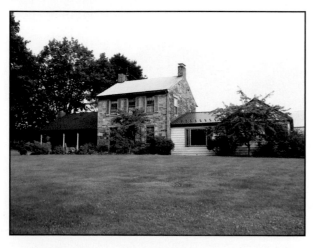

The Douglass farm is often misidentified as the David Stewart farm.

15. John Cunningham Farm, 130 Scott Road, 39°48.117′ N, 77°17.255′ W

Wofford's Brigade of McLaws's Division used the two-hundred-acre farm of John and Margaret Cunningham as their hospital. A few wounded prisoners of war from the Fourth Michigan were also treated here. Most of the wounded came from the Wheatfield on the evening of July 2.

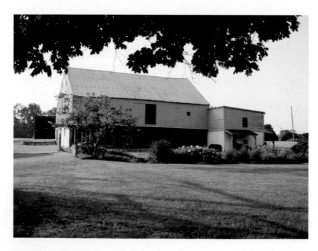

The Douglass farm's barn was pressed into service as a hospital as ambulance trains retreated along Fairfield Road.

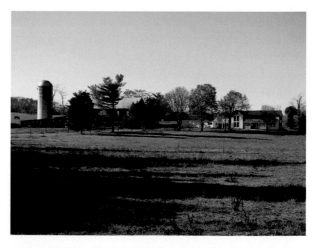

Confederate troops from Wofford's Brigade were treated in Cunningham's barn, while a few Union men were placed outside in the orchard.

Confederate troops were placed in the barn, while the Union prisoners were placed outside in the orchard. Eventually tents were placed in the orchard to provide weather protection for the wounded. A small door to the barn's threshing-room floor was removed and used as an operating table. A Union man who had his leg amputated, Frank Clark from the Fourth Michigan, was said to often return to visit the Cunningham family after the war.

The Cunninghams' domestic worker, known only as Cassie, spent every day for six weeks baking bread for the wounded. The wheat crop for the year had already been trampled by the armies, so she was forced to use the supply of flour from the previous summer. She baked until she exhausted the entire supply, leaving the family with no flour for the coming year. Cassie also served as a nurse, along with Margaret Cunningham, a Mrs. Barnard, and a Mrs. Brain. The latter two women are believed to have come from the Michigan area when they heard of the plight of the Fourth Michigan prisoners.

Erwin James Eldridge (Sixteenth Georgia) was the senior surgeon at Cunningham's farm, assisted by W. D. Bringle (Wofford's Brigade chief surgeon), Robert P. Myers (Sixteenth Georgia), James Broyle Brown (Eighteenth Georgia), Elisha J. Roach (Eighteenth Georgia), and D. H. Ramseur (Eighteenth Georgia).

A makeshift cemetery was set up north of the house in an orchard on a small hill. The graves were dug on the south side of the orchard. There were at least twenty-eight graves, of which sixteen belonged to unknown men. The graves of those who could be identified belonged to men from the Sixteenth and Eighteenth Georgia regiments and Cobb's Legion. John Cunningham diligently cared for the graves for ten years until the bodies could be returned home.

When the Southern army left, a young Confederate soldier remained behind as a deserter. Terrified, the young man was found by Cunningham, sobbing in fear that he would be killed by the Yankees. Cunningham assured him that he would not be killed, and eventually the youth left the Cunningham farm. A few months later, Cunningham got a letter from the young man, who said that Cunningham had been right. Not only had the youth not been killed, he had joined the Union army.[29]

Cunningham filed a claim for $363.50 for losses and damages to livestock, food, wagons and saddles, whips, lines and halters, cow chains, flour, and horse gear. He received an award of $354.00.[30]

16. Lower Marsh Creek Presbyterian Church, 1865 Knoxlyn Road, 39°48.696' N, 77°19.276' W

In the summer of 1740, the Donegal Presbytery began to provide preaching for Presbyterians residing along Marsh Creek. As the congregation grew, they took steps to organize a church. The first house of worship was a log church located at a graveyard on the west bank of Marsh Creek.

In 1790 this site on Knoxlyn Road was chosen for a new church, and this church was constructed. Like the old church, the new building originally had no provision for producing heat in the winter, and it would be several years before this comfort was added. Pews were straight-backed but were considered an improvement over the benches used in the original church, and the pulpit was narrow and deep.[31]

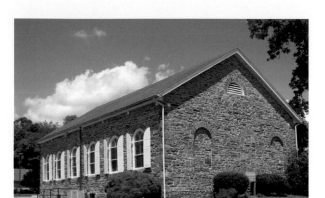

The Lower Marsh Creek Presbyterian church became a hospital while Pickett's Charge was still in progress.

In 1857 the Lower Marsh Creek and Great Cone-wago Presbyterian Churches merged, with Rev. John R. Warner serving as pastor for both. Both were destined to be used as Confederate hospitals. Warner would become an accomplished lecturer and battlefield guide. In fact, his lecture on the battle was so popular that he presented it to the US House of Representatives in the presence of President Abraham Lincoln on May 18, 1864.[32]

On July 3, as Pickett's Charge was still in progress, the Confederate wounded were being brought to the church, as well as other sites along Fairfield Road. Most of the wounded at the Lower Marsh Creek Presbyterian Church were brought from Ewell's Corps in preparation for an eventual retreat southward.

There were an unknown number of burials here, all of them from the First Maryland Battalion and Carpenter's Battery, both from Major General Edward Johnson's Division.

17. William Harner Farm Site, Fairfield Road (?), 39°48.615' N, 77°19.215' W

The William Harner farm does not appear on any period maps, nor is it discussed in great length in any publications. As a result, there is very little known about the farm or its whereabouts. Discussions with licensed battlefield guides and national park rangers place it on Fairfield Road in the general area of the Lower Marsh Creek Presbyterian Church, the David Stewart farm, and the Henry Wintrode farm. The location shown is a "best guess" placement.

The farm was occupied by William (age forty-seven) and Elizabeth (age thirty-three) Harner and their six children, and students of the battle believe it was probably an aid station or short-term hospital. Harner's damage claim confirmed the barn's use as a hospital. There are no known burials on the property.

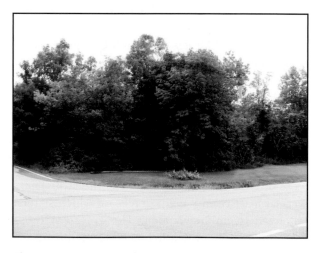

The Harner farm is thought to be in the vicinity of the Fairfield Road–Weikert Road intersection.

Harner's damage claim said the rebels camped on the farm and damaged his land and crops. Unfortunately, the claim offers no further clues about the farm. Harner was awarded $649.00 against his claim of $811.25 for losses of three horses, two bulls, cows and heifers, sheep, lambs, grains, harness, poultry, hay, and fencing, as well as damages to the barn, which Harner specified was the hospital.[33]

18. David Stewart Farm, 3340 Fairfield Road, 39°48.212' N, 77°19.915' W

Now Granite Hill Campground, the property was a 197-acre farm owned by thirty-seven-year-old David Stewart, who lived here with his wife, Martha, and their two children. A farmhand and a domestic worker also lived on the farm during the battle.

A written history of the campground provided by the current owners indicates that Stewart's grand-

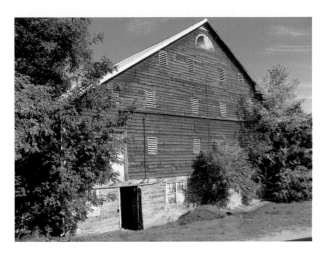

Twelve Confederates were buried under a row of trees near the Stewart barn.

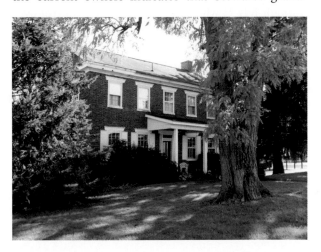

The Stewart farm was used by the Confederates for four weeks.

father was the original property owner. Also named David Stewart, he purchased the property in the 1730s. Stewart (the grandson) sold the farm to Felix Drais in 1865, a Union soldier with the Twelfth US Infantry who had been wounded in the area of Plum Run. It remained a working farm until 1964.

There were thirteen known burials on the farm. Twelve graves were located under a row of trees east of the barn, while the grave location of the thirteenth man was not identified. Of the thirteen burials, only five were identified. Griffin M. Bender of the Second Louisiana suffered a flesh wound of the hip but died either July 6 or 12, probably from infection. Robert Gillespie was listed as being from Virginia, although nobody by this name appears on a list of Virginia casualties at Gettysburg. The remains may have been those of Richard Gillespie of Phillips's Georgia Legion. If so, he probably died in the retreat after being treated at Cunningham's farm as part of Wofford's Brigade. Philip Oldner of the Fourth Chesapeake, Maryland, Battery had been wounded in the knee joint and died on July 20. Knee wounds were generally not considered mortal, so he may also have been a victim of infection. John Sullivan of the First Maryland Battalion received a gunshot flesh wound of the thigh and died of his wound and jaundice either July 28 or August 1. The final identified burial was that of Joseph Cooley (Carpenter's Virginia Battery), who suffered a severe flesh wound of the thigh on July 2 and died on July 4 or 7 of mortification (gangrene).[34]

The present owner of the property described a confirmed death of a fifteen-year-old Georgia soldier who had been shot in his eye. Placed in the barn, he lived several agonizing days before dying. He was buried in the orchard (behind the current woodshop next to the house) and was likely one of the unidentified mentioned earlier.

Surgeon George T. Stevens of the Seventy-Seventh New York treated many Confederate soldiers who had been left behind during the retreat. He wrote of a Southern boy who may have been the one the present campground owner referred to, although some believe this boy may have been at the Harner farm along Fairfield Road. Stevens wrote, "At one of those barns some of our soldiers stopped, and as they passed among the gray-clad sufferers who were lying in rows upon the barn floors, one, a boy apparently not more than sixteen years of age . . . looked more like a delicate girl than a soldier." Stevens went on to say of the same youth, "A piece of linen laid across his face covered a ghastly wound where a ball had passed through his face, and had torn both his eyes from their sockets."[35]

Stewart's damage claim asked for compensation for the loss of forty acres of crops, four thousand rails, farm tools and equipment, bees, sleigh bells, livestock, poultry, bedding, household goods, shingles, bedding, crocks, buckets, whiskey, fly nets, saddle, bridle, harness sets, horse gear, chains, spring wagon, feed trough, spreader, collars, and tallow. He said the rebels used his property for four weeks. His claim for $1,821.08 was reduced to $1,267.83.[36]

19. Henry Wintrode Farm, 260 Weikert Road, 39°48.211' N, 77°19.509' W

Henry Wintrode, described as not yet thirty years old, lived on this farm with his wife, Rebecca, and one child. According to Wintrode's damage claim, a large Confederate wagon train from Ewell's Corps camped on the property the night of July 2, and the house and barn were used as a Confederate hospital from July 2 through July 5, when the Union gained control over the property. The number treated here is unknown, and there were no known burials.

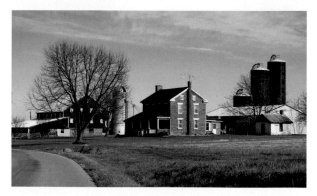

A large Confederate wagon train camped on Wintrode's property, and the house and barn were used to treat the wounded.

In his damage claim, Wintrode claimed losses in the amount of $398.74 for damage to his hay, clover, and wheat. He also noted that many items were stolen or destroyed.[37]

20. Joseph Mickley Farm, Weikert Road, 39°47.884' N, 77°19.757' W

One of twelve children, forty-nine-year-old Joseph Mickley lived on this farm with his second wife, Rebecca (age thirty-nine), and their five children. Mickley's first wife, Harriet, had died at the age of only thirty in 1847. Joseph and Rebecca would have three more children, one of whom, Maria, lived until the age of one hundred, dying in 1965. Joseph and Rebecca's thirteen-year-old son, Amos, would die just three months after the battle.

William Whitehead, surgeon for General Edward Johnson's Division, was in charge of all of Johnson's hospitals, and would certainly have spent some time at the Mickley farm. Rose Quinn Rooney, laundress for Company K of the Fifteenth Louisiana, is believed

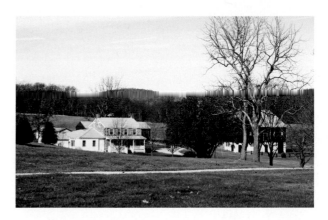

The Mickley house and barn were both used in the treatment of the wounded.

to have served as a nurse at the Mickley farm. There were no known burials on the property.

Mickley's damage claim noted that the house and barn had been used as a hospital, and that he had suffered $425.00 in damage to his house and barn, as well as losses of livestock, grains, fencing, a horse, smoked meat, and flour. His claim was settled for $406.50.[38]

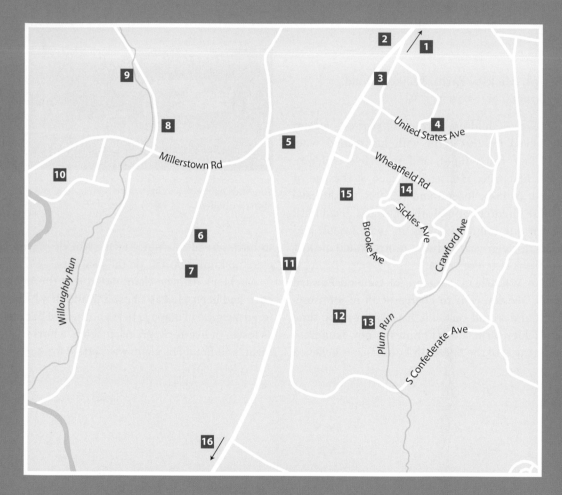

Chapter 7 sites: Emmitsburg Road. (Map by Bill Nelson)

1. Nicholas Codori Farm, 876–998 Emmitsburg Road, 39°48.679' N, 77°14.408' W

One of the most recognizable farms on the battle-field is that of Nicholas Codori. The center of Pickett's Charge on the last day of the battle, it was in a virtual no-man's-land between the two armies. The Army of Northern Virginia had to pass around the house as it moved toward the Union center.

The 273-acre farm was owned by Nicholas Codori, who came to the United States from France in 1828 at the age of nineteen. He purchased the farm in 1854 but was not living in it at the time of the battle. A butcher by trade, he was living in town at 44 York Street (today's Brafferton Inn) and had rented the farm to tenants, believed to be his niece, Catharine Codori Staub, and her husband, John Staub. John was away in the Federal army in Virginia with the 165th Pennsylvania Infantry. It is not known where his family went during the battle.

The house, a two-story brick L-shaped building on a granite foundation, had been built in 1834. The property also had a barn, farm garage, chicken house, wagon shed, and corncrib. During the evening of

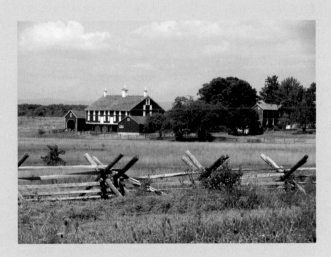

Codori's farm is best known for its highly visible position on the route of Pickett's Charge.

July 2, the 106th Pennsylvania Volunteers charged across the property toward Emmitsburg Road in a gallant assault to retake three guns of Battery B, First Rhode Island Artillery, that had been captured ear-lier in the day. In so doing, the regiment captured 250 Southerners in the immediate vicinity of the house.[1]

The next day the house provided some cover for Garnett's Virginia brigade as it advanced toward the copse of trees during Pickett's Charge, but it also proved to be an obstacle, slowing their progress. Wounded from both sides took shelter in the house until the conclusion of the battle, and Pickett is said to have observed the third day's assault on the Union center from here.

The farm's exposed position prevented its use as a field hospital, but it most likely was used as a temporary aid station. It is known that Confederate general James L. Kemper was carried into the house after he was wounded during the attack. He was given basic treatment and then moved to Bream's Mill.

In June 1872, an effort to return Confederate remains to Southern cities resulted in 325 bodies from Pickett's Division being disinterred just from the Codori farm. Another 225 were removed just two months later.[2] There is no way to determine how many of those buried on the farm were actually treated at Codori's because many were killed instantly during the third day's assault, or died before treatment could be obtained.

Despite the best efforts of those tasked with recovery of the remains, some were missed. In 1886 tenant farmer D. A. Riley plowed up bones near the monument to Colonel G. H. Ward. The skull had a bullet hole through each side, and a thigh bone had another bullet imbedded in the lower end. No positive identification was possible, but a cap box full of percussion caps led to the conclusion that the remains were those of a Southern soldier.

In 1868 Codori was severely injured when he became entangled in his mowing machine. As he was being transported to town for treatment, he was sitting up and giving his customary wave to those he saw, despite his injuries. Unfortunately, his injuries were more severe than they appeared, and he died a short time later.

2.   Peter Rogers Farm Site, Emmitsburg Road, 39°48.501' N, 77°14.645' W

Razed in 1913, nothing remains of the Rogers farm that would give any hint of the ferocity of the fighting in and around the property. During the fighting, Peter Rogers (age fifty-two) had sent his wife, Susan, to safety behind the Round Tops. Peter and Susan's twenty-three-year-old granddaughter, Josephine Miller, remained in the one-story house throughout the battle, spending much of her time in the cellar caring for the wounded.

On the afternoon of July 2, Josephine baked bread and cooked for the soldiers of the First Massachusetts Infantry who were positioned around the house.

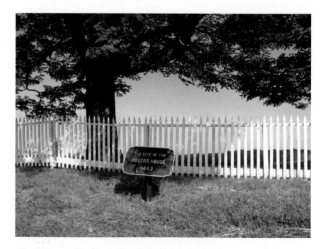

After the battle, the yard around the Rogers house was littered with bodies.

When she had almost run out of supplies to help feed the wounded, six members of the First Massachusetts volunteered to steal three sacks of flour from General Daniel Sickles's nearby commissary stores. Within an hour, the men returned with not only the flour but also raisins, currants, and a whole sheep that was quickly roasted. In the last reunion of the Third Corps, Josephine cooked a meal for Sickles, who presumably never learned of the theft of his supplies years before.

During Pickett's Charge, Confederate troops marched directly across the Rogers farm. Much like the Codori farm, the Rogers farm was situated between the two armies, and the house would be struck nine times by artillery fire. Several Confederates were killed on the farm during the charge, leaving the yard around the house littered with bodies. A rebel sharpshooter was killed on the roof, and another died of exhaustion on the front steps. After the battle, seventeen bodies were removed from the house and cellar, with blue uniforms intermingled with gray. Many of the dead were buried on the farm, and the hastily dug graves yielded their contents on the first day of rain, as body parts soon began to protrude from their shallow confines.

To supplement his income, Rogers spent several days after the battle scouring his fields for lead. He collected more than three hundred pounds and was able to sell it to ammunition manufacturers for thirteen cents a pound.

After the war Rogers filed a damage claim of $158.34. His claim said his carpet had been ruined by bloodstains, a horse had been stolen by a Union cavalryman, his buildings had been damaged by shot and shells, and he had lost bedding, clothing, six panels of garden fence, and corn. He further noted that a bureau had been blasted apart by a projectile from either Cemetery Hill or one of the Round Tops, pinning some of the contents against the log wall; another piece of shell was stuck in a leaf of the table; and a minié ball had struck just above the clock.[3]

In late 1863 Rogers was shot in the abdomen by a former soldier from Maryland in an argument over flowers. The soldier was on his way to the dedication of the new national cemetery. Rogers recovered and lived until 1870, when he died at the age of seventy-five.

In July 1886 the First Massachusetts planned a dedication of their monument near the Rogers house. When the veterans of that regiment learned that both Peter and Susan Rogers had passed away, they also learned that Josephine had married William Slyder a few months after the battle and had moved to Ohio. The veterans insisted that Josephine attend the ceremony and paid her transportation costs both ways, greeting her arrival with three hearty cheers. They also presented her with a gold corps badge in recognition of her care for their wounded, as well as her serving food and baking bread for the regiment. When the veterans learned that the stove she had used to bake the bread was still in the house, they carried it out and placed it next to their new monument for a photo of Josephine standing beside the stove.

3. Daniel H. Klingel Farm, 1024 Emmitsburg Road, 39°48.372' N, 77°14.775' W

Daniel H. Klingel, a boot and shoemaker by trade, lived on this fifteen-acre farm with his wife, Hannah, and two-year-old son, Samuel. The Klingels had purchased the property just three months before the battle from the farm's original owner, Ludwick Essick. The farmhouse is the only war-era building remaining on the farm.

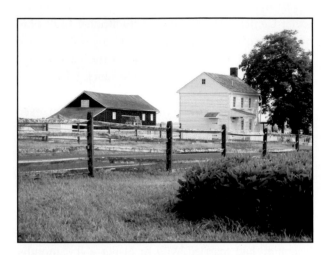

The house is the only remaining building on the Klingel farm that stood during the battle.

After the battle, Daniel's account of activity on his farm was published in the *National Tribune*. In that account, he noted that fourteen to sixteen wounded Confederate soldiers were brought to his house the evening of July 1 and laid on the floor, where Daniel and Hannah gave them water and bathed their wounds through the night.[4]

The next morning, the Klingel family reluctantly left the log house at the insistence of Union officers, going to the foot of Little Round Top. There, Daniel was taken up to the Union signal station on Little Round Top, where he helped identify roads and terrain features for the Union army. He was chased off the hill when it came under fire from a Confederate gun on Warfield Ridge. Rejoining his family, they made their way to a friend's house near Rock Creek, where they remained until the end of the battle.

In their absence from their home, fighting raged around Emmitsburg Road. Men from the Sixteenth Massachusetts entered the house and broke out holes between the logs to shoot through. Confederate brigades from Mississippi and Alabama then focused their attention on the Klingel farm house, driving the Union off and capturing Lieutenant Colonel Frederic Cavada of the 114th Pennsylvania in the orchard. In this portion of the fighting, the house suffered heavy damage, with Lee's army gaining control of the Emmitsburg Road ridge.[5]

The family returned to their house on July 4, encountering Union officers who initially prevented them from entering. Once they eventually got inside, Daniel claimed, nearly everything in the house was taken or destroyed and several dead soldiers were lying on his property. His damage claim describes "damage done to buildings by shot, bullets, glass broken" and "damage done to fruit trees by rifle pits being dug around them." Additional losses alleged were livestock, 3.5 acres of corn, 3.5 acres of oats, 2 acres of timothy grass, a worm fence, a post fence, and boards and pickets. All his shoemaking tools were gone, along with leathers needed to make the shoes. Daniel further claimed that the house was being used as a hospital by the Union army and was "filled with wounded men" when he returned home, and at least one Union soldier was buried at the house. Despite the extensive damage, his $880.00 claim was denied.[6]

4. Abraham Trostle Farm, United States Avenue, 39°48.097' N, 77°14.535' W

Visitors to Gettysburg recognize this farm by its well-known hole in the south gable of the barn, created by the cannon shot that passed through just below the diamond-shaped ventilation openings. The shell is believed to have come from a Confederate battery

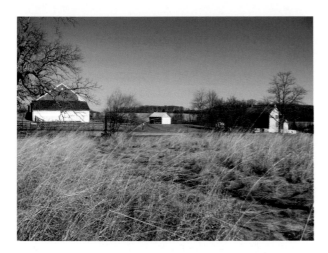

General Daniel Sickles was wounded near the Trostle barn.

firing from a position near Warfield Ridge on the afternoon of July 2. Union general Daniel Sickles, whose headquarters was nearby, was wounded just west of the barn, and the farm is just one of several places credited with being the site of his leg amputation.

At the time of the battle, the 134-acre farm was owned by Peter Trostle but leased to his son, forty-two-year-old Abraham, who had been admitted to an asylum and was not present during the battle. The farm was occupied by Abraham's wife, Catherine, and their nine children.

The two-story house was new, having been built on a granite foundation in 1860, and the farm contained a large bank barn that had been constructed in 1850, an attached wagon shed, a corncrib, and an apple orchard.[7] The family stayed in the home until the fighting forced them to leave. They remained out of the house for several days, and as late as July 6 a witness said that the house was deserted, with the dinner table still containing evidence that the family had left in the middle of a meal.[8]

On the afternoon of July 2, the Ninth Massachusetts Battery was nearly wiped out by the Twenty-First Mississippi on the property. The men from Massachusetts had never been in combat, and they had been involved in a fighting retreat when they realized that Sickles's infantry had withdrawn and the battery had no support. Taking their stand at the Trostle farm, they were soon overrun despite firing double canister, then case shot with the fuses cut short so they would burst at close range. In the chaos, the battery's commander, twenty-two-year-old John Bigelow, was badly wounded. Ignoring orders to retreat and save himself, the battery's bugler, Charles Reed, assisted his wounded captain to the rear, using the heavy smoke as cover. Bigelow survived and Reed was awarded the Medal of Honor for his action.[9] The fighting had been so intense that the battery lost four of their six guns, three officers, six sergeants, nineteen enlisted men, and eighty-eight horses.

A field hospital was quickly set up to accommodate the heavy casualties from both sides, using the house and outbuildings. Surgeon Thomas Sim, medical director for the Third Corps, initially treated General Sickles at Trostle's, then accompanied him to Daniel Sheaffer's and remained with him. The farm remained in Confederate hands until the evening of July 3. After the evacuation of the Confederate army, the farm remained a hospital for several days. There were thirteen from the Confederate First Corps found buried here. The number of Union burials is unknown.[10]

Annie Etheridge was one of the nurses at the Trostle farm. She had earned the Kearny Cross for bravery at Chancellorsville, only one of two women to receive the honor, and continued her actions at Gettysburg.

On July 2, Etheridge was seen walking among bursting shells, retreating from the Peach Orchard with her regiment, and riding her horse back amid falling shrapnel. Periodically she would dismount to tend to a wounded man or help a limping soldier back to the rear. The next day she would move to the Third Corps hospitals behind the Round Tops, where she continued to help with the wounded.

Catherine Trostle filed a damage claim for $3,153.50, noting that there were sixteen dead horses near the house and one hundred more dead horses across the farm. She had lost eighty-two acres of crops and grain, hay, vegetables, a hog, three cows, a heifer, a bull, one sheep, fifty chickens, two hives of bees, flour,

family clothing, hams and shoulders, a saddle, 6,400 fence rails, beds and bedding, stored meat and potatoes, and household and personal items. She further claimed that her livestock and poultry had all been driven off in the fighting, roads had been cut through her fields, her farming equipment had been broken and scattered, and the rebels had set her house on fire. The Compensation Law of July 4, 1864, provided reimbursement only for civilian property damaged or destroyed by Union forces, not those victimized by Confederates or as a result of battle. As a result, she received no compensation for her losses.[11]

In 1899 she sold the farm to the Gettysburg Military Park Commission for $4,500.

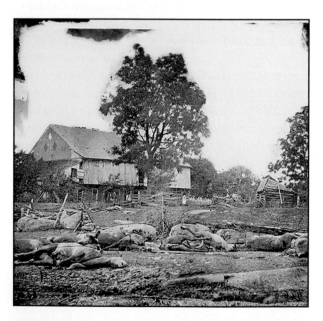

The carcasses of more than one hundred horses littered the Trostle farm after the battle. (Courtesy of Library of Congress, Reproduction Number LC-DIG-cwpb-00905)

5. James Warfield Farm, Millerstown Road, 39°48.100' N, 77°15.318' W

This house, built in 1850, has seen many additions over the years since the battle, but underneath the revisions the original stone walls remain. Confederate artillery deployed near the house drew enemy fire from batteries on Little Round Top and Cemetery Ridge, making its use as a hospital unlikely. However, it did serve to shelter a number of injured who would have received some level of emergency care before being moved to hospitals behind the lines, so it is included here.

The thirteen-acre farm was owned by forty-two-year-old James Warfield, who occupied the property with his four daughters. His wife, Eliza, had died not long before. Warfield operated a highly regarded blacksmith shop on the farm, with at least one customer declaring him "one of the best blacksmiths in the county." The family of free blacks feared being captured and sent into slavery, causing them to flee before the fighting began.

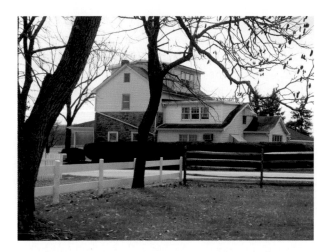

Widower James Warfield and his four daughters evacuated their home during the fighting. The original home is largely hidden by the additions.

There were at least twenty burials on the property. Fourteen were unidentified and disinterred from the garden. Another six were found on the right side of the blacksmith shop.[12]

When Warfield and his daughters returned after the fighting, they found the farm devastated. All his blacksmith tools and equipment, including his heaviest anvils, were gone, depriving him of his ability to earn a living. He also lost fifty bushels of wheat and sixty bushels of corn worth over $500, and fences worth $50. The orchards, gardens, and buildings were all badly damaged, and two head of cattle and three hogs were missing. Abraham Flenner, who saw Warfield's home following the battle, testified on Warfield's behalf that the house, barn, smith shop, and garden orchard had been severely damaged, with the house, shop, and barn plundered of almost everything of value. Warfield eventually received $410 for his losses.[13] The

dejected Warfield put his ravaged property up for sale in 1864 but found no buyer. He moved to Cashtown in 1871 and died in 1875 at the age of fifty-four.

6. John Biesecker Farm (Eisenhower Farm No. 1), 243 Eisenhower Road, 39°47.635' N, 77°15.799' W

John Biesecker purchased his 189-acre farm from Daniel Baumgardner on October 29, 1851. He and his wife, Christiana, both in their midfifties, moved onto the farm with their five children and lived there until returning to their previous home nine years later. At that time, they leased the property to Adam Bollinger and his wife. Although the Bieseckers still owned the property, it was the Bollingers who occupied the farm at the time of the battle. However, they had to leave during the fighting.

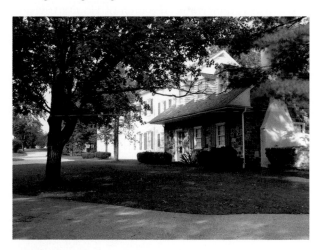

The Biesecker farm eventually became a part of former president Dwight D. Eisenhower's farm after the president retired to Gettysburg.

The two predominant structures on the property were the original farmhouse and the nineteenth-century wooden barn, which covered an area of approximately fifty by one hundred feet. It had three cupolas on the roof and was always painted red. The existing barn is a replacement for the original.

The farm was used as a campsite for Confederate troops and supply trains, with the inevitable damage caused by artillery, trampling, and looting. The house and the double log barn served as an aid station for the wounded, although the farm was too close to the fighting to be a major field hospital.[14]

On the afternoon of July 2, the brigades of Confederate generals Joseph Kershaw and Paul Semmes crossed Biesecker's fields on their way to what today is known as Confederate Avenue. Biesecker's fences posed no obstacle, as the Southern troops simply tore them down. The wheat crop, now ready for harvest, was crushed underfoot. The men of Hood's Division soon followed, and the destruction was repeated. Union artillery fire, largely ineffective, nonetheless tore angry gouges in Biesecker's fields.[15]

When Bollinger returned to the farm after the Confederate retreat, he found little left. Hungry troops had consumed his cows, his crops had been flattened beneath thousands of marching feet, the wheels of artillery trains had torn deep ruts across his fields, and his fences and fence posts had been torn down and used for firewood. Twenty burials dotted the property. The contents of his house and barn had been looted. He filed a claim with the State of Pennsylvania for $441.82 but he received nothing.

After eleven years with no compensation, Bollinger filed a federal claim, with the amount now totaling $1,707.30. His claim was ultimately rejected with the explanation that the damage had not resulted in any advantage to the Union army or any of its soldiers.[16]

After the war, ownership of the farm changed hands several times until it was purchased in 1921 by Alan Redding. Redding held ownership until 1950, when he sold the property to General Dwight David Eisenhower and his wife, Mamie. Eisenhower used it as a weekend retreat during his presidency, moving there permanently in 1960. While he was president, major renovations to the farm were undertaken, requiring much of the original house to be torn down because of severe structural deficiencies.

During the renovations, the remains of a Civil War soldier were discovered when a flower bed was being created near the old pump, southeast of the farmhouse. Mamie directed that the remains be allowed to rest in peace, and the flower bed was relocated.

7. William Douglass Farm (Eisenhower Farm No. 2), 243 Eisenhower Farm Road, 39°47.499' N, 77°15.838' W

William Douglass owned at least two farms, one of which is often referred to as the David Stewart farm, and this one. This second farm eventually became part of the Eisenhower National Historical Site and was referred to as Eisenhower Farm No. 2. The barn on the Douglass farm was said to have been a field hospital.

Douglass obtained the farm in 1841 at a public sale following the death of the previous owner, William McGaughey. The property consisted of a 150-acre farm, a two-story stone house, a double log barn, an orchard, a shed, a bark mill, a courier's shop, and a tannery, plus twenty acres of meadowland and a "due proportion of woodland," a kitchen well, and three springs.

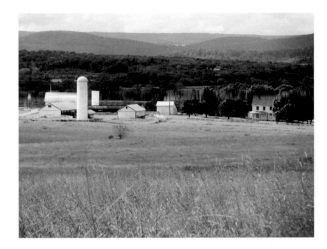

Confederate cavalry occupied the Douglass farm and set up defensive breastworks along the southern and eastern borders of the farm.

During the battle, the property was occupied by Confederate cavalry. Defensive breastworks were constructed along the south and east boundaries of the farm, which was used as an aid station and hospital, as well as a campsite for Confederate units and supply trains.[17] There were fourteen burials shown on the Elliot map, a map of the battlefield drawn by S. G. Elliott after the war in 1864. It also located burials.[18]

Douglass died in 1869 and the farm passed to his heirs, David and Martha E. Stewart, who sold it the next year. After a series of owners, the farm was acquired by President Dwight Eisenhower and his partner, W. Alton Jones, in 1954 from the then owners, Earl and Nellie Brandon. The purchase was not only to expand the farm's program of raising purebred Angus but also to eliminate the possibility of commercial development on the land adjacent to the farm

Eisenhower already owned, which became referred to as Eisenhower Farm No. 1 with this purchase. The Douglass property was now known as Eisenhower Farm No. 2.[19] When Jones died in 1962, the Farm No. 2 property was transferred to the National Park Service. It is now the location of the cattle barns.

8. Samuel Pitzer's Farm and Schoolhouse, Black Horse Tavern Road, 39°48.172' N, 77°15.883' W

Samuel Pitzer's two-hundred-acre farm served as a temporary hospital for Confederate general John B. Hood's Division. The wounded were treated in the farmhouse, the barn, and the schoolhouse Pitzer had built on the southwest corner of his property.

The earliest known owner of the property was John Murphy. A 1767 survey of Murphy's holdings indicated that the farm consisted of 183 acres and a

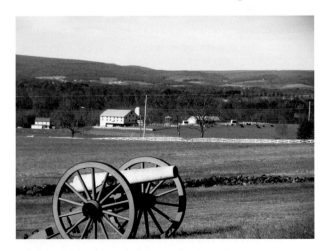

The Pitzer farm, a temporary Confederate hospital, has been acquired by the federal government as Eisenhower Farm No. 3.

one-story log house. The property changed hands at
least four times, including one sheriff's sale, until it
was purchased in 1832 by Emmanuel Pitzer, Samuel's
father. Emmanuel built the stone house on the farm
before selling it to Samuel in 1836.

In the early 1860s, John Flaharty was renting a log
house and barn on a twenty-acre piece of the Pitzer
farm. This tract was carved out of the southeastern
corner of the Pitzer holdings and was separated from
the main farm by the Millerstown Road. The property
became known as the Flaharty Tract, and it eventually
became part of Eisenhower Farm No. 1 when the former president returned to Gettysburg.[20]

In the mid-1850s, Samuel built a small schoolhouse
on the southwest corner of the farm. That portion of the
farm was the site of Kershaw's Brigade's ambulance depot
during the fighting. Dr. T. W. Salmond (Second South
Carolina) served at both the farmhouse and the school
with the brigade's ambulance depot before returning to
the Black Horse Tavern, his earlier assignment.

The marker for Longstreet's headquarters, which
sits near the observation tower on West Confederate Avenue, states, "These headquarters were located
at a school-house 900 yards westerly," giving rise to
the belief that the Longstreet headquarters were in
Pitzer's Schoolhouse. The National Park Service, however, has studied this extensively and has been unable
to confirm that it was Pitzer's Schoolhouse that is
referred to on the marker.[21]

In 1857, Pitzer's Schoolhouse was sold to the local
public school system. The school continued to operate
until it burned down in 1902. A replacement school
was built across Millerstown Road about ten years
later, operating until 1955, when it was sold to John
Eisenhower, the president's son. John lived there with

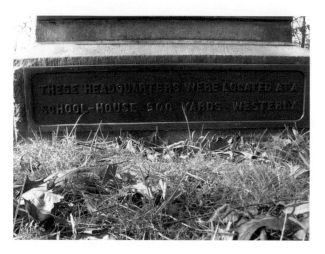

The base of the Longstreet headquarters marker indicates that
the headquarters may have been in Pitzer's Schoolhouse. That
has not been confirmed by the National Park Service.

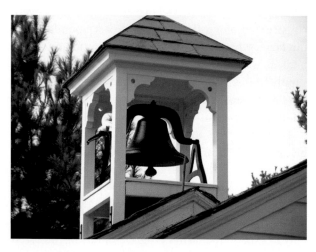

Some sources believe the bell on top of the guesthouse on the
Eisenhower farm came from Pitzer's Schoolhouse.

his family until 1963. The bell from a school has been placed atop the guesthouse on the Eisenhower farm. Some sources indicate that this bell is from Pitzer's Schoolhouse, while other sources say it is not. There is no disputing that the bell is on the guesthouse roof. The only question is where it came from.[22]

Pitzer had the misfortune of being taken captive by the Confederate army and taken to Virginia. He returned by the end of the war, only to discover that some $5,000 worth of gold and silver coins were stolen by troops on his farm.

There were believed to be twelve Confederate graves on the farm, plus several more in the immediate vicinity of Pitzer's, the S. A. Felix farm, and the John Socks farm. Those listed as being on the farm include Thomas M. Bankston of the Sixteenth Mississippi (buried in Pitzer's orchard, near George Culp's), John M. Stricker of the Twenty-First Mississippi (in woods along the road by Pitzer's Schoolhouse), Lieutenant J. M. Daniel of the Seventh South Carolina (on the road near Pitzer's Schoolhouse in a field near the fence, under a wild cherry tree), and nine more near the schoolhouse. Those nine were William Davis of the Forty-Eighth Georgia; J. W. Baley and S. W. Stewart from the Twenty-Second Georgia; and Sergeant Benjamin F. Gregory, T. W. Chapman, James Hodges, C. D. Aaron, Donald H. Montcrief, and Council Wheeler, all of the Third Georgia.[23]

After the war Pitzer filed a claim in which he said that the Confederates held the house for four days and that he had incurred losses or damages to bedding, tablecloths, clothing, farm implements, a buggy, harnesses, a carriage, foodstuffs, poultry, livestock, books, buckets, dishes, a watch, bees, and a rifle. His claim for $2,434.16 was reduced to $1,934.16. There is no request in his claim for reimbursement of the gold and silver coins.[24]

Samuel Pitzer continued to work this farm during the years after the Civil War, still living in the original stone farmhouse built by his father, Emmanuel. During this time, Samuel made additions to the farm, including the construction of a bank barn and a stone smokehouse. In 1875, he sold the farm to his son John, who continued to work the farm for eight more years. John then sold the property to William and Martha Martin in 1883. After a series of owners, the farm came under the ownership of the federal government as Eisenhower Farm No. 3.

9. S. A. Felix Farm Site, Black Horse Tavern Road, 39°48.345' N, 77°16.045' W

Beyond its location on period maps, very little is known about this farm. At least one map identifies it as that of William Felix, rather than S. A. Felix. If that map is accurate, the farm could have been occupied by William and his wife, Sarah. It is also possible that Sarah is the "S. A." in S. A. Felix, as Sarah's middle initial was A. Sarah is also shown in one source as having purchased the farm in September 1864 from Levi D. Maus, so it is likely that she and William were tenants on the Maus farm at the time of the battle.[25] Maus's farm was listed as being only 2.4 acres, so it may be more accurate to refer to this property as the S. A. Felix home. The "farm" has been described as a possible Confederate hospital. It is more likely that it would have been a temporary aid station.

What is known is that there was at least one burial on the property, that of J. W. Price of the Seventeenth Mississippi. The description of the burial location puts it on the road from Plank's to Pitzer's, near a log house on Willoughby's Run. That description fits the

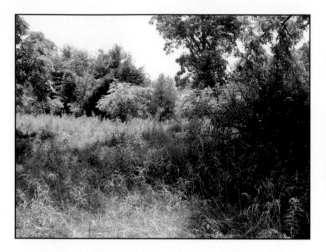

Described as a possible aid station, the Felix farm no longer exists. Period maps indicate its presence in this area.

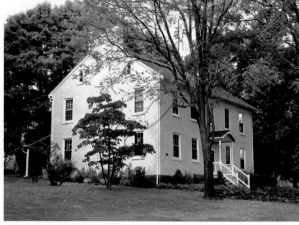

At least two burials, and possibly as many as eight, were found on the Socks farm.

Felix farm location. There were twenty-one Confederate graves in the area bounded by the farms of Felix, Pitzer, and John Socks. I have already shown that twelve of those were on or adjacent to Pitzer's, leaving just nine to locate. Of those nine, only Price's burial location description appears to match the Felix farm.

All physical evidence of the Felix farm is gone.

10. John Socks (Sachs) Farm and Mill, Waterworks Road, 39°47.864′ N, 77°16.445′ W

Owned by John Socks (sometimes spelled Sachs), the property was said to have been occupied by Hood's Division and used as a hospital for two days or more. The mill, gone now, sat near the house, on the banks of Marsh Creek.

The area that formed a triangle from Pitzer's to Felix's to the Socks farm contained twenty-one Con-

federate graves. Twelve of those were on or adjacent to Pitzer's, and one was on the Felix farm, leaving just eight to locate. Two of those appear to have been on or very near the Socks property. J. C. Rife (Eleventh Alabama) was shown as having been buried south of Pitzer's and west of Socks's near a dry watercourse. W. E. Ramsay of the First North Carolina Artillery was buried near the Socks barn.

The remaining six burials of the twenty-one were along roads in the area but not at any particular farm. Four of those were William P. Ray of the Bath Artillery; J. N. (or J. M.) Dance and C. Hammon, both of the First South Carolina; and Corporal Joseph T. Lantz of Taylor's Virginia Battery. The remaining two are unknowns.[26]

Socks filed a damage claim for $3,061.50 and received $2,439.00 for losses of livestock, horses, grain crops, a wagon, harness, a buggy, lumber, poultry, rails, fencing, flour, fish, beef, and lard. He said the lumber that was taken was used for coffins.[27]

11. Philip Snyder Farm, Emmitsburg Road, 39°47.363' N, 77°13.207' W

This eighty-acre farm was occupied by Philip Snyder, a sixty-one-year-old widower, and two of his seven children at the time of the battle. Another son, Adam, was with the Union army but not at Gettysburg. There is nothing specific that states that the farm served as a hospital, but its location as the starting point for General John B. Hood's assault on July 2 makes it likely that it was at least a field aid station. Also, there were six burials on the farm that were later disinterred. One of those was John F. Stephens of Company C, Ninth Georgia Infantry, who was buried east of the house.[28]

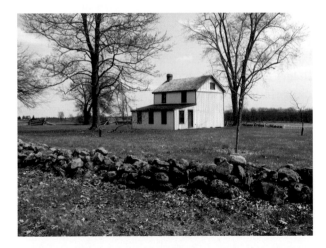

A probable headquarters for the officers of both McLaws's and Hood's Divisions, the Snyder farm was likely at least an aid station for the Confederates as well.

Snyder was born in Bavaria in 1801 and came to the United States in 1832 with his wife, Maria. They moved into this new two-story log home on a granite foundation that had been built just one year earlier. Most of the interior was replaced or reconstructed in the 1970s, but the original log construction remains. The Snyders must have initially been tenants because they did not purchase the farm until August 27, 1838, as part of a larger tract that was offered at a public sale. The house is all that remains.

The National Park Service notes that it was likely used as a headquarters for the officers of McLaws's and Hood's Divisions.[29]

Snyder's claim for $500 in damages was denied on the grounds that the damage was done by the Confederate army and could not have been controlled by the US government. Snyder made an unsuccessful attempt to convince the government that the damage had been done by Union troops.[30]

12. Michael Bushman Farm, 30 S. Confederate Avenue, 39°47.367' N, 77°15.103' W

The Bushman farm is a landmark on the battlefield and is one of the areas that Lieutenant General John Bell Hood's Texas Brigade passed through as they moved to attack Little Round Top and Devil's Den on July 2. The stone house and a smokehouse were built by Samuel Bushman in 1808. In 1829 Sophia Hammer took ownership, and five years later her daughter Amelia married Michael Bushman, a minister in the German Baptist Brethren church and the great-nephew of Samuel Bushman. When Sophia died, Michael and Amelia inherited the farm.

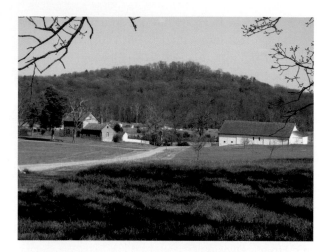

Confederate general John Bell Hood probably suffered his severe arm injury in Bushman's orchard.

The springhouse and the double log barn were built in 1838. In 1860, Michael added the brick portion of the house to the original stone portion built by Samuel.

In the early stages of the fighting on July 2, the house was used by the Second US Sharpshooters until they were driven out in the Confederate advance on Little Round Top and Houck's Ridge. The house then became an obstacle for the Southerners as they moved across the farm under artillery fire.

In this advance, Hood received what would prove to be a serious arm wound in the Bushman orchard. Contrary to popular belief, however, his wound did not render his arm permanently useless. Dr. John Thompson Darby, who treated Hood, kept a detailed account of Hood's progress. He noted following surgery that the healing process was rapidly taking place, and that Hood was able to use the injured arm

to hold a crutch just a few months after his leg amputation at Chickamauga. Darby specifically pointed out that Hood's elbow flexion and extension were perfect, that the wrist could be fully flexed, and that Hood could open and close his fingers. Darby further stated that Hood's thumb was essentially unaffected, with "considerable pronation and supination" existent, and he predicted that the arm would continue to get stronger.[31]

The lane leading to the farm was an old road that connected the Marsh Creek settlement with the Taneytown Road in the eighteenth century. Much of its route was enclosed on both sides by stone and wooden fencing. On July 3 it was used as cover by Union cavalry to harass and attempt to outflank the Confederate infantry.[32]

Michael Bushman was living in town during the Battle of Gettysburg, and when he returned to the farm he found his fences torn down and trenches dug across his land. His house and barn had been used to house and treat the wounded before their being moved to field hospitals west of Seminary Ridge. Many household items had been looted or destroyed, and there were eight Confederate soldiers buried behind his barn.[33] Only one of the bodies was identified, recorded in Dr. J. W. C. O'Neal's journal as J. Ware of the Fifteenth Georgia.

Bushman would file a claim for $717.50 for damages and losses of real estate, wheat and vegetable crops, and bees. His claim would be reduced by more than half, and he was only awarded $317.50.[34]

Amelia died in 1875. Michael then married Louisa Rupp but died in 1893. The farm was sold to the Gettysburg Battlefield Memorial Association in 1894 and transferred to the National Park Service in 1933.

13. John Slyder Farm, 1492 Emmitsburg Road (Slyder Lane), 39°47.331' N, 77°14.802' W

In 1849 John Slyder moved from Maryland to the Gettysburg area, where he purchased this seventy-five-acre property and built a house and barn. In addition to farming, Slyder was a blacksmith and carpenter, and he also established a blacksmith and carpenter shop on the property, as well as a hog pen, privy, chicken house, two-story frame kitchen, smokehouse, and woodshed. The farm also contained an orchard of peach and pear trees, thirty acres of timber, and eighteen acres of meadow. Slyder and his wife, Catherine, lived on the farm with three of their five children: John (twenty), Hannah (seventeen), and Jacob Isaiah (nine).[35]

On the morning of July 2, the family was warned by Union soldiers that they should leave. It was a warning that Slyder and his family were wise to heed. Before the day was over, all four of Hood's brigades would cross the farm on their way to fight at Devil's Den and Little Round Top, driving off the men of Union general Daniel E. Sickles's Third Corps in the process. The

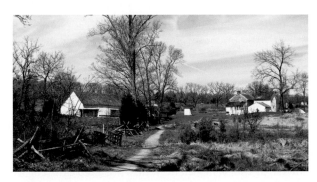

The Slyder farm was the scene of heavy fighting, and the farm's buildings became hospitals for both sides.

buildings on the farm would become a field hospital, treating the wounded of both sides.

From their position behind a stone wall near the house, the Second US Sharpshooters slowed the rebel advance, leading a Confederate officer to later remark that they ran into a "hornet's nest" of sharpshooters. Taking the comment as a badge of honor, two companies of Vermont sharpshooters made sure to include a hornet's nest on their monument along the lane to the farm.

On July 3 the farm witnessed the ill-fated charge of Union brigadier-general Elon Farnsworth, which accomplished nothing and resulted in Farnsworth's death. Of some 300 men he took into the assault, 65 were killed or wounded, with another 120 taken captive. Many of the wounded were treated in the Slyder house or barn.[36]

The Slyders returned after the battle to find their farm devastated, with personal possessions looted or spoiled, crops trampled, fruit taken from the orchard, and the garden dug up. The losses left them with few means of feeding themselves for the rest of the year. John filed a claim for nine acres of crops, destruction of land and fences, three head of cattle, two boxes of bees and honey, a mattock, saddler and shoemaker tools, buggy cushions and shafts, ten quilts and comforters, two rifles, a copper kettle, bedding and carpets, looking glasses, furniture, clothing, ham, bacon, one ton of hay, and thirty bushels of corn. His loss of $619.50 was not reimbursed.[37] Nearly bankrupt, he sold the farm and moved his family to Ohio.

An unknown number of Union bodies, and at least five Confederate bodies, were buried on the farm, including four Confederate officers. Those men were Second Lieutenant Farquhard M. Crimmon of the Twentieth Georgia (buried behind the barn), Second Lieutenant James M. Turnbow of the Fourth Alabama (buried near the barn), and Captain Benjamin L. Hancock of the Second Georgia and Colonel John Augustus Jones of the Twentieth Georgia (both buried under a cherry tree). Jones had been struck in the head by a piece of shrapnel that had ricocheted off a rock on July 2. On December 10, 1866, while being transported home to Georgia, his remains were lost at sea during a storm off the coast of Maryland. A memorial to him was erected adjacent to his wife's grave at the Linwood Cemetery in Columbus, Georgia.[38]

In September 1900 a complete skeleton was unearthed by a work crew building a fence near the house. It was immediately obvious that the remains were those of a Civil War soldier, based on items found with the bones. It was determined that the skeleton probably had been a soldier from the Second US Sharpshooters.

In the 1993 movie *Gettysburg*, the house was used as a substitute for the Thompson house to depict General Robert E. Lee's headquarters.

14. Thirty-Second Massachusetts Temporary Aid Station, Sickles Road Near the Loop, 39°47.832' N, 77°14.695' W

Although many regiments established mobile temporary aid stations as close to the fighting as was practical, this front-line aid station is the only one on the battlefield whose location has been marked. It was set up by Surgeon Zabdiel Boylston Adams, who wanted it close to the front lines. Adams, whose physician father had been an early advocate for the benefits of vaccination, was said to have treated the wounded of both sides for two days and three nights without sleep, finally collapsing from exhaustion and suffering from temporary blindness.

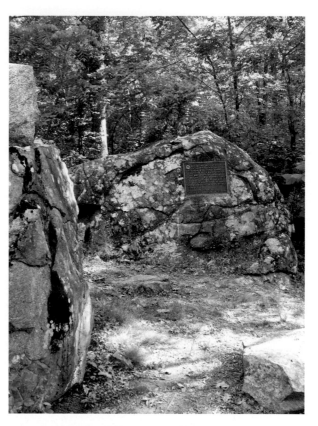

The Thirty-Second Massachusetts aid station is an excellent example of the placement of an aid station as close to the action as prudent.

The large boulder containing the marker was used to shelter the wounded, as well as the attendants, from bullets and bursting shells. A low, flat rock was used as the treatment table. Later in the day, Adams moved his aid station to the northeast corner of the Wheatfield, following the regiment as it moved with the fighting. He reportedly treated about sixty wounded men at the two aid stations.[39]

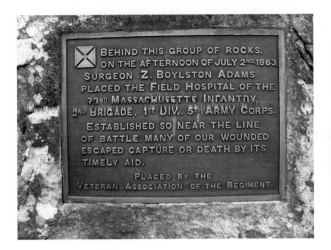

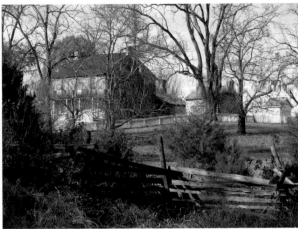

The boulder on which this plaque is placed also served as a means of protection for the wounded during their treatment.

Rose's buildings housed hundreds of wounded, many of whom were beyond treatment.

The wounded from this aid station eventually were taken to the field hospital at the Jacob Weikert farm on Taneytown Road.

15. George Rose Farm, Emmitsburg Road, 39°47.815' N, 77°14.953' W

In 1790 Jacob Sherfig and his wife, Catherine, moved onto this property and reared eleven children. Jacob died in 1842 and the farm passed through a number of owners before being sold to George Rose. Family lore says the house and barn were built with nearly six hundred wagonloads of stones from the farm. During the battle, the 230-acre farm was occupied by the family of John Rose, George's brother.[40]

The house was built in 1811 and during the battle was used to shelter the many Confederate wounded from Kershaw's and Semmes's brigades. The barn was built

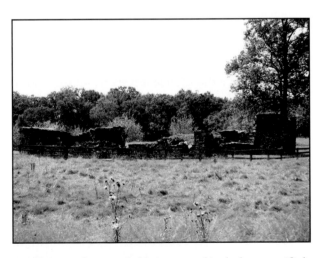

In addition to the wounded being treated in the barn, terrified men used it as a shelter from the Union artillery. The ruins of the stone walls are all that remain.

in 1812. Many of those who took shelter there would say they would always remember the sound of the canister and shrapnel clattering against the barn's stone walls. After the fighting on July 2, the barn was also used as a hospital to shelter Confederate wounded until they could be removed to a field hospital behind Seminary Ridge.[41]

A lightning strike in 1910 ignited a fire, causing extensive damage to the barn, and in 1935 a windstorm tore the roof from the barn. The building deteriorated rapidly from that point until it was acquired by the National Park Service in the mid-1950s. Only a portion of the barn's stone walls have survived the years of decay. They have been stabilized to prevent future deterioration. Other farm buildings, however, still remain.

The names of the beleaguered doctors who labored here went largely unrecorded, although Surgeon James B. Clifton of Semmes's Brigade is known to have treated men in the barn. Dr. Simon Baruch, Third South Carolina Battalion, also briefly assisted here until Dr. John Syng Dorsey Cullen, medical director for Longstreet's Corps, moved him to the Black Horse Tavern on July 2.

Several thousand casualties occurred on the farm on July 2 alone, although not all were treated here. Rose claimed that there were 1,500 burials on his property, but while there were certainly hundreds of graves documented, the total number is believed to be lower than that. Semmes was mortally wounded, and many from his brigade were killed on the Rose property. Semmes, however, was not buried here. He had been moved to the John Crawford farm before his death.

The famed Wheatfield is part of Rose's farm and is one of the bloodiest parts of the entire Gettysburg battlefield. More than 50 were buried there, and more than 175 buried behind the barn. Another 33 burials, mostly from the Eighth South Carolina Volunteers, were found north of the barn. Other nearby graves

contained the remains of men from the Fifty-Third Georgia, while another 100 or so, including ten officers, were placed in Rose's vegetable garden.[42] Several burials occurred in the yard, and another officer, believed to be Lieutenant Colonel Francis Kearse of the Fiftieth Georgia, was buried just a few feet from the kitchen door. Several additional dead were found in the stream when the battle ended, while others lay in Rose's well and spring, rendering the water unusable.[43] Witnesses claimed that there were so many casualties that their bodies created dams when nearby streams flooded in the rainy days after the battle.

John Rose, George Rose, and former tenant Francis Ogden, who retained a financial interest in two fields of wheat on the Rose farm, all filed damage claims. Ogden claimed the loss of nine sheep, and he said that "two fields of wheat were fought over and entirely destroyed by the Union and rebel armies on July 2d and 3d 1863." His claim for $526 was rejected.

John Rose filed one state claim and two federal claims and won awards from both, although it is unclear whether he received any payment because the records reveal contradictory information. His state claim was for $750 for losses of oats, corn, a cow and heifer, farming utensils, clothing, carpet, furniture, beds and bedding, hams and shoulders, dried beef, flour, china, tableware, and mirrors. Rose was awarded $600 but he said he never received payment. His first federal claim was for $2,152.93 for the same items on his state claim, with only a few variations. He also revalued the items on the claim. Most of the claim was denied, for various reasons. His award was for $50 for the loss of corn and oats only. His second federal claim, for $750, was denied.

George Rose's state claim was similar to his brother's, asking for reimbursement for damages to flooring boards, weather boarding, wheat, oats, corn, grass, fencing, the house and barn, and land. He asked for $3,306 but was awarded only $1,606. The amount of the award really did not matter, though, because he never received any payment. Six years after filing his state claim, Rose filed a federal claim, with the amount revised to reflect current values. He added fifty peach trees, house repairs, timber, and a cow and bull. He also was more specific in the claim for damage to his land, stating that it was caused by roads, rifle pits, and breast-works. His total claim for $9,299 was disallowed.[44]

16. Cornelius Houghtelin Farm, 2264 Emmitsburg Road, 39°46.467' N, 77°15.598' W

Today the Battlefield Bed and Breakfast, this farm belonged to Cornelius and Anna Houghtelin. Cornelius had been vice president of the Gettysburg Anti-slavery Society and was active in the Underground Railroad. The farm is also sometimes referred

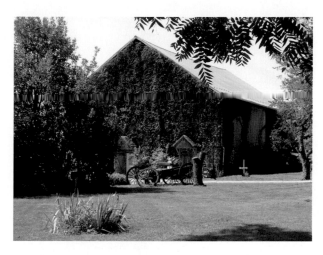

Houghtelin's barn became a small aid station on the last day of the battle.

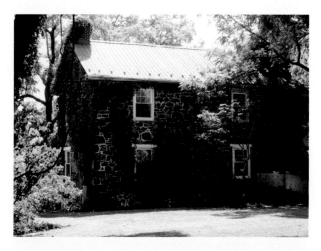

The Houghtelin house served as the headquarters for General Wesley Merritt.

to as the Heagy or Hagey farm. The Houghtelins had two sons in the Union army, but neither fought at Gettysburg. They also had two daughters.

Built in 1809 as a single-family fieldstone farmhouse with a wooden summer kitchen and barn, the house served as General Wesley Merritt's headquarters, with a cavalry camp set up on the property. An artillery position was set up at the farm's entrance, and the barn was pressed into service as a small field hospital or aid station.

During the battle, Cornelius was captured by Confederate forces. He was released and sent home when he was recognized as a Mason by a Confederate fellow Mason.

The farm witnessed fighting by the Sixth Pennsylvania Cavalry (Rush's Lancers), fighting dismounted, on July 3. The Lancers suffered three killed, seven wounded, and two missing. Most of the wounded were among those treated at the Houghtelin farm.

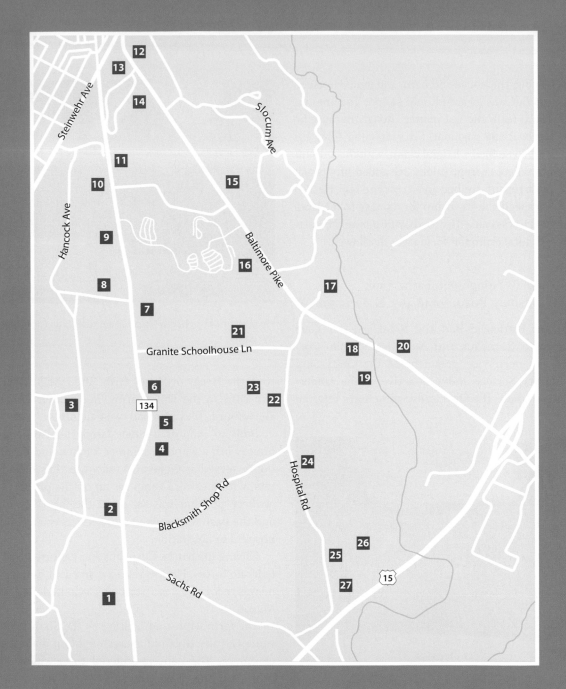

Chapter 8 sites: Taneytown Road/Baltimore Pike, west of US Route 15. (Map by Bill Nelson)

1. Jacob Weikert Farm, 1051 Taneytown Road,
    39°47.262' N, 77°13.822' W

This 102-acre farm was heavily used as a campsite and hospital by the Union's Third and Fifth Corps, and to a lesser degree by the Second Corps, from July 1 to 5. The farm was occupied at the time of the battle by sixty-six-year-old Jacob and Sarah Weikert (age sixty-one) and their thirteen children. Also on the farm at the time of the battle were Hettie Shriver, her daughters, and Matilda "Tillie" Pierce, a neighbor of the Shrivers on Baltimore Street. The Weikerts had purchased their farm in 1840 from John Hoke. Parts of the house date to the 1700s, although most of the house was built around 1825.

Jacob Weikert, his family, the Shrivers, and Tillie Pierce went to the cellar during the fighting. Numbering twenty in all, they found the space cramped but serviceable. A well-known story associated with the farm relates to the family's retreat to the cellar. As they moved to their place of safety, Jacob Weikert took the hand crank for the well along with him, fearing that the soldiers would use so much water that his well would run dry. Obviously, the soldiers took

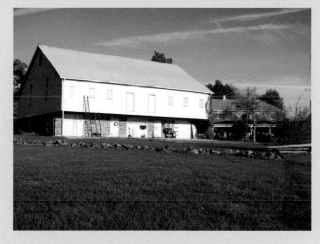

Nearly one thousand wounded were treated at Weikert's farm before artillery fire forced it to close.

issue with Weikert's action, and First Lieutenant Ziba B. Graham of the Sixteenth Michigan threatened to shoot Weikert if he did not relinquish the crank. Graham must have been very convincing, because the crank quickly appeared, allowing the wounded from both sides to have all the water they needed.[1]

As the battle raged, a steady stream of wounded flowed into the eight-room house, its carriage house, and the barn. Nearly one thousand eventually were treated at Weikert's, including Confederates from McLaws's Division. When the buildings filled up, tents were used to provide weather protection for the wounded. Amputated limbs were piled in the field across the road, reaching the height of the fence. Many of the more seriously wounded developed pyemia, known today as septicemia. This condition, common to most of the hospitals, was nearly always fatal, and soon the farm was dotted with the graves of men from both sides. Across Taneytown Road, one hundred were hastily buried in the field. Even those otherwise healthy individuals helping the wounded found themselves getting nauseated from the odor of blood, perspiration, and anesthesia that permeated the air in the house and barn. Bloodstains still mar the dining-room floor of the Weikert house.

Fifteen-year-old Tillie Pierce carried food and water daily for the wounded soldiers and helped care for the wounded. Mrs. Shriver and her daughters baked bread, while Mrs. Weikert gathered all her linen and muslin and tore it into bandages.

One of the nurses at Weikert's was Mary "French Mary" Tepe, a vivandière attached to the 114th Pennsylvania Infantry.[2] Tepe's photograph and details about her are located in Chapter 1.

Brigadier General Stephen Weed, Colonel Patrick O'Rorke (140th New York), and Lieutenant Charles Hazlett (Battery D, Fifth US Artillery) were all brought to the Weikert house.[3] The latter two had been killed almost instantly on Little Round Top. Some accounts also state that Weed was killed instantly, but Tillie Pierce insisted that Weed was alive when he arrived at Weikert's. She said she sat and talked with him in the house basement, promising to return in the morning. When she did, however, she learned he had died. The bodies of Weed, O'Rorke, and Hazlett were placed on the front porch following their deaths.

Hazlett was temporarily buried in the garden, near the road. Later, his body was disinterred and taken to his hometown of Zanesville, Ohio, for reburial in Woodlawn Cemetery. The bodies of Weed and O'Rorke were moved to the Lewis Bushman farm on July 3 when the Weikert farm was abandoned as a hospital after Confederate artillery began to hit too close to the farm. Not long after, O'Rorke's widow came to Gettysburg and had the body removed to Rochester, New York, for reburial. Weed's body was eventually reburied on Long Island.

The farm was selected as a hospital by Dr. Clinton Wagner from the Second Division, Fifth Corps. Surgeon Joseph Thomas (118th Pennsylvania), Assistant Surgeon John S. Billings (US Volunteers), Dr. Cyrus Bacon Jr. (US Regulars), Dr. Edward Breneman (US Regulars), Dr. Benjamin Howard (US Volunteers), Surgeon Ira Russell (US Volunteers, who stayed with Weed), and Surgeon Edward T. Whittingham (US Regulars) also assisted the wounded on the Weikert farm. Billings noted that there were eleven surgeons there, in addition to himself, so there obviously were some who are not on this list. Interestingly, Billings made a point of mentioning that eight of the twelve, including himself, became ill while at the Weikert farm.

Weikert filed three claims, for $186.00, $1,277.00, and $2,756.00, for damages to thirty-nine acres of crops, 3,500 rails, timber, breastworks thrown up and entrenchments dug on his property, fields trampled by marching troops and cavalry, artillery, and wagons that drove across the property, bed clothing, linens, underclothing, kitchen furniture, tin and tableware, and personal property. He received $45.00.[4]

The farm today is much smaller than it was in 1863, only about 13.5 acres.

2. Leonard Bricker Farm, Taneytown Road, 39°47.570' N, 77°13.862' W

Also a hospital or aid station for the Third and Fifth Corps, the small farm of seventy-four-year-old Leonard Bricker and his wife, eighty-year-old Catherine, filled quickly with wounded. As more wounded arrived, especially from the Eighty-Third Pennsylvania in the Little Round Top fighting on July 2, they had to be directed to the nearby farms of Jacob Weikert, Michael Fiscel, and Lewis Bushman.

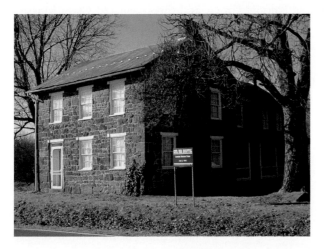

This small farm quickly received more wounded than it had room for on July 2.

There were at least seven Union burials around the house, including that of Lieutenant Eugene L. Dunham of the Forty-Fourth New York, who was buried near the garden fence. Another man from the Forty-Fourth New York who was buried with Dunham was Captain Lucious S. Larrabee, who was killed on Little Round Top on July 2. Larrabee had told a companion that he had a premonition that he would be killed in the battle. When Larrabee's premonition proved accurate, the friend took Larrabee's body to the nearby Bricker farm for burial.

Bricker filed a claim for $982.00 to cover his loss of straw and bandages. There is no record of any award.[5]

Bricker died in 1870 at the age of eighty-one and is buried in Evergreen Cemetery in Gettysburg.

3. George Weikert Farm, 365 United States Avenue, 39°48.114' N, 77°14.096' W

George Weikert moved to the Gettysburg area in 1838 and purchased this property in 1851 from Henry Bishop. He lived here with his wife, Ann, and four of their six children. The two oldest sons lived nearby. The house and barn on the property were built in 1798 and were probably used for shelter and concealment by Union skirmishers engaged with Confederate skirmishers close to the nearby Trostle buildings. Also on the property were a carriage house, corncrib, and summer kitchen. After the battle, the house was used for hospital purposes.[6]

The family left before the fighting began, and twelve-year-old Elizabeth recalled later that when the family returned, they found that their home was in use as a hospital. Six men had died in the parlor alone, and there were burials around the yard and surrounding area, with the Weikerts' carpet being used to line a mass

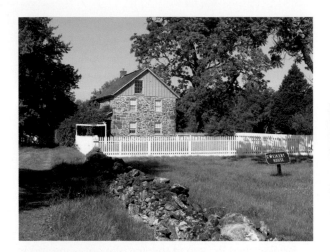

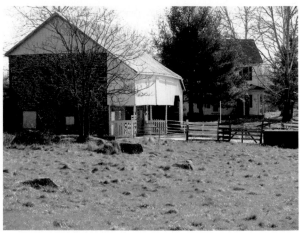

When the Weikert family returned home after the battle, Mrs. Weikert calmly opened the windows and tossed amputated body parts into the yard.

Nearly five hundred wounded were treated in and around the Patterson barn.

grave. At several windows were piles of amputated limbs. Elizabeth said her mother simply opened the windows and tossed the body parts out into the yard.[7]

The New Jersey Brigade had held this ground during the battle, and after the war the surviving members purchased the farm and placed their monument across what is now Sedgwick Avenue, southeast of the house. The land, known as Weikert Hill, later became part of the battlefield park.[8]

Weikert filed a damage claim for $1,156.00 for damage to his hay, crops, fencing, and land. No record of payment has been found.[9]

4. Sarah Patterson Farm, 630 Taneytown Road, 39°48.011' N, 77°13.663' W

Sarah Patterson, thirty-two years old at the time of battle, lived here with seventy-six-year-old Julia A.

Patterson, probably her mother. Also on the farm were eighty-four-year-old Elizabeth Epply, twelve-year-old Samuel Grove, and three-year-old Clara Musser. Sarah was the sister of William Patterson, whose nearby farm also served as a hospital. The barn was built circa 1830. The east wing of the house is likely original, but the rest of the house is most likely postwar. The farm is one of several where General Daniel Sickles's leg was said to have been amputated.

The farm served as a temporary hospital for Gibbon's Division of the Second Corps (but troops from other divisions of the Second Corps and Third Corps were also treated here, as were a number of wounded Confederates). An estimated five hundred wounded were treated inside and outside the barn, including in the orchard. Many of the wounded were out in the open with no shelter because tents had not yet arrived from Westminster, after General George

Meade's orders to keep supply wagons in the rear to allow better access for ambulances and wagons carrying ammunition.

With Confederate artillery fire making it impractical to remain on the farm, the wounded here were relocated July 2 to a position along Rock Creek after the Second Corps' medical director, Dr. A. N. Dougherty, instructed Captain Thomas Livermore (chief of ambulances) to find a more sheltered location for a general field hospital capable of caring for all the wounded of the corps.[10]

Dr. Justin Dwinell, who was surgeon in charge of the Second Corps field hospitals, was here most of the first day. He was assisted by a number of unnamed regimental surgeons.

S. G. Elliott's burial map showed fifty-four Union and three Confederate graves on the Patterson property.[11]

5. Jacob Swisher Farm, 597 Taneytown Road, 39°48.086' N, 77°13.747' W

This small farm served as a temporary aid station for the Union Third Division, Second Corps, until the Second Corps general field hospital was established.

Family records indicate that Jacob Swisher was married to Eve Elizabeth Bender of York County, Pennsylvania. They had seven children: Sarah, Abraham, Samuel, Jacob, Nancy, Mary (Polly), and Elizabeth.

Somewhat vague records indicate that Jacob Swisher had died in April at the age of eighty-five, just ten weeks before the battle, and the farm is believed to have been in the process of being sold to John Musser at the time of the fighting.

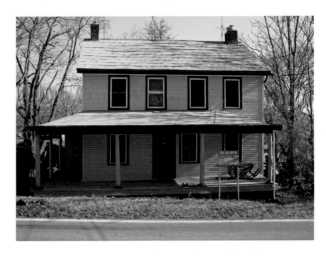

At least sixteen burials took place on the Swisher farm.

There were at least sixteen Union burials on the fifty-nine-acre farm. Two of these came from the Sixth New York Cavalry, and a third man was believed to have been Private Bartlett Brown from the 111th New York Infantry. Brown was killed on July 3 when he was shot in the chest. When he was reinterred in the national cemetery, he was mistakenly buried in the New Hampshire section, rather than that set aside for New York soldiers.

6. Michael Frey Farm, Taneytown Road, 39°48.215' N, 77°13.788' W

This farm of Michael and Sarah Frey was used from July 2 to July 4 as a temporary field hospital for the Union Third Corps and as a staging area for the ambulances of the Second Corps. General Robert O. Tyler of the US Artillery Reserves had his headquarters in the immediate area, possibly on the farm itself. The

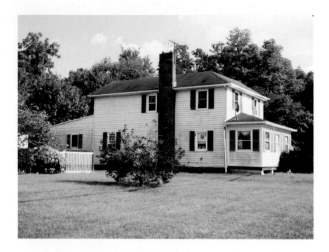

The barn, no longer standing, stood across Taneytown Road from the Frey house and held as many as three hundred wounded.

barn, which sat across Taneytown Road from the house, was said to be filled with as many as three hundred wounded. The barn is gone now, and the house has been replaced with a more modern one.

There were several Union burials on the farm, but no Confederate ones. One of those buried here was First Lieutenant Joshua Garsed of the Twenty-Third Pennsylvania, which was better known as Birney's Zouaves. Garsed was not treated at Frey's, however. He had been struck by a solid shot between the right shoulder and neck on Culp's Hill late in the afternoon of July 3. His brother Frank said the impact tore him to pieces, killing him instantly.

His body was brought to the Frey farm and buried in a shallow grave behind the house. Regimental chaplain James Shinn notified the family, and Garsed's father and brother made the trek from Philadelphia to Gettysburg, arriving on July 11. There, the

body was disinterred and Mr. Garsed positively identified his son.

A casket was brought to the farm and Garsed was taken to Dr. William Burnell's tent on East Cemetery Hill for disinfecting. The task accomplished, Mr. Garsed clipped a lock of hair from the young lieutenant and placed it in his pocket. A clean casket was purchased and the body was removed to the Adams Express office. From there, the remains were shipped home at a cost of fifteen dollars.

While in Gettysburg, Garsed's father and brother visited the site where Joshua had been killed. Frank Garsed placed a piece of iron engraved with his brother's initials as a memorial. The family visited the site each year for the next twenty years.

Joshua's sword and watch were also sent home but were lost. They remained missing until 2003 when they were discovered in an attic in Philadelphia, along with photos and letters. Also included in the articles that were found was a gold ring belonging to Joshua's mother. Inside the ring was the lock of Joshua's hair that his father had taken before he had been shipped home for burial.[12]

7. William Patterson Farm, Taneytown Road, 39°48.372′ N, 77°13.811′ W

William Patterson, forty years old, and his wife, Lydia, lived on this seventy-five-acre farm along Taneytown Road. Patterson was the brother of Sarah Patterson, who lived a short distance away and whose farm also served as a temporary hospital. William Patterson's house and barn were utilized by the First Division, Second Corps, for housing and treatment of their wounded. The barn, which was located across the

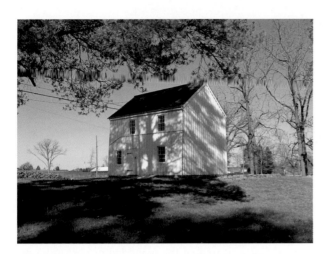

William Patterson's house, built in 1798, is the oldest log plank house on the battlefield.

he moved to the Aaron Sheely farm on the Baltimore Pike.

William, Lydia, and their children left the farm during the fighting. While they were gone, a shell from a Confederate signal gun being used to launch Pickett's Charge on July 3 struck the barn, tearing off the arm of the young black servant of a New York officer. Several other artillery shells also landed on the farm. Patterson's claim for $1,300.00 to cover his damages was denied.

There were ten Union burials on the William Patterson farm, along with twenty-four Confederate ones.[15]

8. Jacob Hummelbaugh Farm, 45 Pleasonton Ave, 39°48.474′ N, 77°13.894′ W

road from the house, is gone, but the original house remains. The wounded were relocated on July 2 because of Confederate artillery fire, to a more protected site along Rock Creek.

The house was built by Samuel Patterson around 1798, making it the oldest log plank house on the battlefield.[13] The original house was a one-and-a-half-story log home; it was later raised to two stories. Alterations to the house were made in 1825, 1930, and 1982. General Alfred Pleasonton used the house as his headquarters late in the battle, according to the Library of Congress.[14] Other sources place his headquarters at the Jacob Hummelbaugh farm, which was likely after the battle ended. He may have moved from one to the other at some point, using either or both of them over the three days of the battle. Provost Marshal General Marsena Patrick also briefly set up a headquarters here before

One of the first hospitals set up by the medical officers of the Second Corps, the Hummelbaugh farm is best known for having treated Confederate general William Barksdale before he died. Barksdale had been mortally wounded in the legs and chest on July 2 while leading his Mississippi troops in an advance that one (Union) observer called the "grandest charge that was ever seen by mortal man." Barksdale had been found lying against his dead horse by troops from the Fourteenth Vermont, who brought him here. He died that night and was buried beside the house. His remains were disinterred in January 1867 and taken for reburial in Greenwood Cemetery in Jackson, Mississippi.

Jacob Hummelbaugh, forty-five years old, was a widower. His wife, Sarah, had died in 1853 at the age of forty. His only son was in the 138th Pennsylvania Infantry and was assigned to the Harpers Ferry garrison at the time of the fighting in Gettysburg. He would

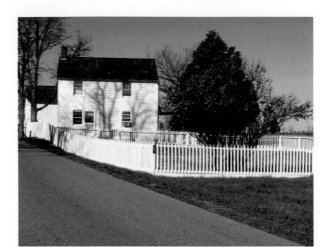

Confederate general William Barksdale was treated here before he died.

be badly wounded at the Battle of the Wilderness in 1864 but would survive his wounds and live until 1888.

The house was built in 1840, and the farm also included a stable, carriage house, chicken house, and smokehouse. A water pump stood in the front yard. All the buildings except for the house are postwar.

The house reputedly was used by General Alfred Pleasonton as his field headquarters.[16] Both the house and barn were used as a hospital. There were about fifteen Union men buried here. Barksdale's was the lone Confederate burial.[17]

Dr. Alfred T. Hamilton (148th Pennsylvania Infantry) was the only surgeon at this position on July 2 and 3. He said Hummelbaugh had fled in a hurry, leaving a partly eaten meal on the kitchen table. He also noted that there were so many wounded around the property that the house, barn, and surrounding grounds were completely filled.

Hummelbaugh filed a damage claim for a bay horse, wheat, corn, grass, hay, potatoes, rails and posts, vegetables, chickens, three feather beds, carpets, bedding, tin buckets, knives, and forks, as well as damage to his house. His claim stated that all were taken by the US Eleventh Corps.[18]

9. Peter Frey Farm, Taneytown Road, 39°48.673' N, 77°13.876' W

The buildings of the Peter Frey farm provided cover for Union troops during the battle, as well as shelter for the wounded being treated there. Established for the Union's Second Corps, it treated the wounded of both sides on July 2 and 3. Its location so close to major action during the battle made it one of the busiest of all the forward aid stations and hospitals. The stone house was there during the battle, having been built in 1850. The two-story bank barn, however, is a replacement that was constructed in 1890, probably on the foundation of the original barn. The property also included a summer kitchen and wagon shed. The farm was sold in 1865 to Basil Biggs, a free black.[19] The farm is believed to have been occupied by a tenant farmer named Brown during the battle.

Surgeon Francis Wafer (108th New York Infantry) indicated that most of the doctors there only stayed on the farm for a short time, providing what would be referred to today as basic first aid in preparation for moving the wounded to a larger hospital in the rear.[20] Fighting on the farm, which included such well-known battlefield landmarks as the Angle and the Copse of Trees, made it difficult to retrieve the wounded, let alone spend much time treating them.

There were 122 Federal burials on Frey's property and at least one Confederate, Second Sergeant William

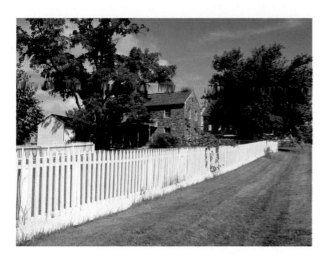

Despite suffering heavy damage during Pickett's Charge, the Frey farm became one of the busiest hospitals on the battlefield.

S. Jinkins of the Seventh North Carolina. Lieutenant Abner Small of the Sixteenth Maine was with Jinkins when he died. Small said Jinkins's last words were, "I'm cold. So cold. Won't you cover me up?"[21]

Frey's damage claim asked for $1,063.97 for his losses. He said his house had been damaged, including the roof being torn off in several places. He also noted that all his outbuildings had suffered damage and his fences and orchard were destroyed. Most of this damage occurred during the artillery barrage before Pickett's Charge.[22]

10. Lydia Leister Farm, Taneytown Road, 39°48.870' N, 77°13.926' W

This small farm was used as the headquarters of Union general George Meade on July 2 and 3. Meade and his staff were forced to evacuate during the artillery

duel that preceded Pickett's Charge because of Confederate shells overshooting the Federal positions on Cemetery Ridge. The property served as a temporary hospital and ambulance collecting area during the fighting, and the barn was also used as a signal station. As with most of the hospitals and aid stations, the wounded from both sides were taken care of here.

A central gathering area for Confederate prisoners of war is believed to have been located in the area immediately around the Leister farm. They were guarded by the Second Pennsylvania Cavalry, under Colonel Richard B. Price.

The night of July 2, Meade called his famous council of war. Twelve generals met in Lydia Leister's small parlor: Major General John Newton (First Corps), Major General Winfield Scott Hancock (Second Corps), Brigadier General John Gibbon (Second Corps), Major General David Birney (Third Corps),

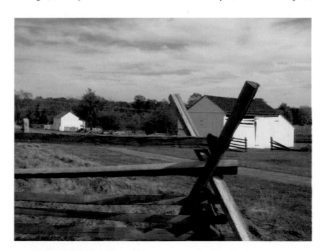

Widow Lydia Leister's farm served as General George Meade's headquarters and was the site of the famous council of war on the night of July 2.

Major General Dan Butterfield (Meade's chief of staff), General George Sykes (Fifth Corps), General John Sedgwick (Sixth Corps), General Oliver O. Howard (Eleventh Corps), Major General Henry Slocum (Twelfth Corps), General Alpheus Williams (Twelfth Corps), Brigadier General Seth Williams (adjutant general, Army of the Potomac), and General Gouverneur Warren (chief engineer). Warren fell asleep in a corner but apparently awoke in time to offer his opinion on the next day's action. The vote was unanimous to remain in position and fight.

Lydia Leister was the fifty-two-year-old widow of James Leister, who had died in 1859. She had purchased the nine-acre farm in 1861 from Henry Bishop. The farm had a log barn and several small outbuildings, an orchard, a pasture, and several tillable fields. A spring supplied her with water. Leister fenced off a small garden, put up sturdy fences to protect her fields planted with wheat and oats, and pastured a cow and a horse.

Two of her six children still lived with her. Her two oldest daughters had married and moved away, her youngest son was living with and working for another family, and her oldest son was serving in the Union army but Leister was not sure where, nor did she remember the ages of any of her children. The family was forced to flee the premises for a safer location along the Baltimore Pike on July 1.

Leister later said she lost "a heap" because of the battle. When she and her children returned on July 5, she found seventeen dead horses on the property, several of which had been burned in her peach orchard, ruining several of the trees. Other orchard trees had been broken, and her wheat crop was destroyed. Her barn siding had been removed for firewood and grave markers. Two tons of hay were gone, as were her horse and cow.

Her house did not fare any better. The porch pillars had been knocked down, and there were holes in her roof and the east side of the farmhouse. One artillery round had entered the garret, while another had destroyed a bedstead. Most of her furniture lay outside in the yard. Bedding and clothing were missing, probably torn for use as bandages, and her food stores were gone.

The dead horses on her property had contaminated her spring, forcing her to have a new well dug. She received no payment for her losses, so over a two-year period the resourceful widow gathered and sold the bones of the dead horses for fifty cents for each one hundred pounds. Leister lived on the farm until 1888, when she sold it for $3,000 to the Gettysburg Battlefield Memorial Association.[23]

A visitor to the farm four months after the battle claimed that the stench was still intolerable. He said that bones and skulls still littered the area and the ground remained strewn with knapsacks, haversacks, canteens, pieces of uniforms, blankets, and bedrolls.

In May 1882 the remains of a Union soldier were plowed up on Leister's property. Efforts to identify the unfortunate man were unsuccessful, and he was reinterred as an unknown in the national cemetery.

11. Catherine Guinn Farm, Taneytown Road, 39°48.935' N, 77°13.921' W

Although all the original buildings on this farm are long gone, they served as a temporary aid station and hospital for Brigadier General Alexander Hays's Division of the Union Second Corps during the battle. The

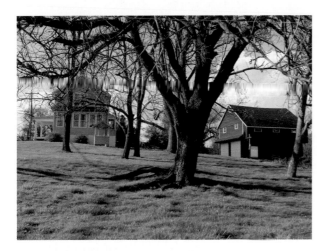

Now an office for park rangers, Catherine Guinn's farm became a hospital during the fighting. The current buildings are all replacements.

current house is believed to be sitting approximately where the original barn stood. Today the house serves as a park ranger office, and part of the original farm is used for overflow parking for the adjacent national cemetery.

The original two-story log house was built in 1776 by William Guinn and was occupied by seventy-two-year-old Catherine "Katie" Guinn during the battle. The family moved into the house on July 4, 1776, with William immediately leaving to fight the British in the Revolutionary War.

During the 1863 battle, the house was struck by thirteen shot and shell, with one striking a bureau near where Katie Guinn was sitting. Described as feisty, she was known to use her broom to chase away any soldier she found on her property.

The farm has also been referred to as the Wright farm, and there were several burials from the Eighth

Ohio, 111th New York, and 125th New York along the east side of the house. H. M. McAbee (Fourth Ohio) was the physician in attendance during the battle.

Guinn's damage claim of $700.00 was not accepted.

12. Catherine Snyder House Site, Baltimore Pike, 39°48.928' N, 77°13.919' W

Catherine Snyder's home sat in what is now the parking lot for the 1863 Inn of Gettysburg. Catherine (thirty-nine years old) was a widow with ten children ranging in age from four to twenty-two. Her husband, Conrad, had died in 1860 at the age of fifty-four. The two oldest sons were not living with the family at the time of the battle. Both were in the Union army and both were captured. One was sent to Libby Prison, the other to Andersonville. Both survived and eventually made it home to Gettysburg.[24]

The Snyders were the proprietors of the Wagon Hotel, which sat across the street from their home.

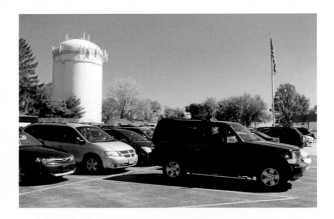

Catherine Snyder's home served as a hospital during the battle. Its site is now a hotel parking lot.

The hotel, which was situated at the intersection of Baltimore Pike and Steinwehr Avenue, is long gone and the site now contains a convenience store.

The two-and-a-half-story Wagon Hotel had been built in 1821 by John Espy to accommodate wagoners and teamsters. Conrad Snyder had purchased the hotel in 1837, sometimes operating it himself, other times leasing it out. When he died, ownership fell to Catherine and her son-in-law, David Blumbaugh, who operated it from 1862 to 1865. During the battle, Union soldiers took over the hotel, shooting from the windows and through holes they bored in the roof.

During the fighting, the children were sent to stay with relatives for their safety. On the first day of fighting, Confederate prisoners were being marched past the Snyder home. One of the prisoners, weakened by exhaustion and the effect of his wounds, could go no

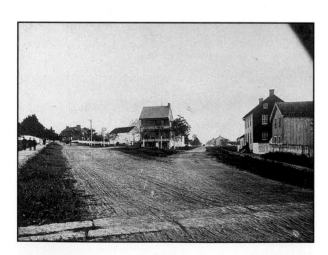

Catherine Snyder was the proprietor of the Wagon Hotel, which sat across the street from her home. The site is now occupied by a convenience store. (Courtesy of Library of Congress, Reproduction Number LC-DIG-ppmsca-35053)

farther and collapsed in front of the house. Mrs. Snyder told the Union guards to bring the man inside and put him in the bed in the spare room. The wounded man protested, saying he did not want to get the bed dirty. Mrs. Snyder insisted, and the man was made as comfortable as possible. Not long after, his arm was amputated.

Damage claims were filed by Blumbaugh, asking for payment to cover damage to the hotel, as well as the loss of linens, bedclothes, and silverware. The same claim also asked to be reimbursed for the loss of thirty-eight gallons of whiskey, five gallons of brandy, eight gallons of gin, four gallons of applejack, twelve gallons of wine, eighteen gallons of cherry brandy, seventeen gallons of ginger brandy, and two gallons of bitters. Catherine Snyder's son William also filed a claim for two lost mares.

After the war, the new hotel owners changed the name to the Battlefield Hotel as a means of attracting more visitors. The hotel was razed in the late 1800s and replaced by a newer one.

13. John Myers House, 777 Baltimore Pike, 39°49.345' N, 77°13.840' W

At the time of the battle, this property of Captain John Myers on Baltimore Street consisted of two acres, a large brick house, a stable, a well, a garden, and an orchard. Myers (age seventy-nine) lived here with Mary E. (fifty), David Plank (fourteen), and Anna M. Plank (ten).[25] Union general Oliver O. Howard set up his headquarters here during the battle.

On the evening of July 1, Elizabeth Thorn, wife of the caretaker at Evergreen Cemetery, said she set out for Myers's house to retrieve some meat, four hams,

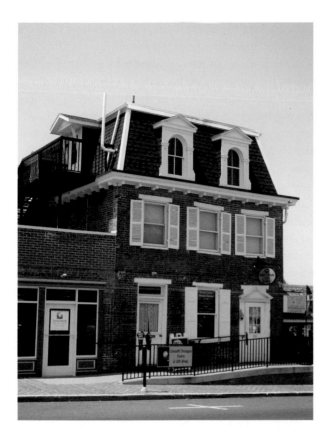

The John Myers home became the site of the National Soldiers' Orphan Homestead.

and a shoulder that she had kept there. She said that when she arrived, the house was filled with wounded men. Six of them showed no signs of life. Badly shaken, she immediately returned to her home, leaving the meat behind.[26]

When the battle was over, the gruesome task of burying the dead began in earnest. Dead soldiers lay in every part of the town. One of them was found lying on Stratton Street, near today's fire station. He had no identification but was clutching an ambrotype of three children. Dr. J. Francis Bourns was intrigued. Who were these children? Who was this soldier?

Haunted by the image, he had copies of the photo made and circulated. The *Philadelphia Inquirer* wrote a story about the unidentified soldier, which other newspapers reprinted. Eventually Philinda Humiston in Portville, New York, read the story and thought it sounded as if the photo may be of her children. She had not heard from her husband, Amos Humiston, a soldier in the 154th New York, in some time. Fearing the worst, she obtained a copy of the photo, confirming that she was now a widow.

With so many children losing their fathers in the war, it was quickly recognized that many of them could no longer be properly cared for. The National Association of Philadelphia was founded with the mission of establishing an orphanage to care for them. Gettysburg was selected as the location for such a facility, and in 1866 the John Myers house was purchased as the home of what would be called the National Soldiers' Orphan Homestead. Much of the funding had come from the sale of copies of the famous photo. It was only fitting that Philinda Humiston be selected as the matron, and her three children, by now known as the Children of the Battlefield, would become the first residents. Not long after the orphanage opened, it was visited by Ulysses S. Grant, commanding general of the US Army.

When Philinda remarried in 1869, she and the children left the orphanage. The Homestead would exist for eleven years, closing under the shadow of a scandal when the new matron was convicted of cruelty to the children and forced to leave town.

In 1957 television personality Cliff Arquette, whose television persona was known as Charlie Weaver, purchased the building and used it to house his Soldiers' National Museum. The museum closed in November 2014 and the building was refurbished.

14. Evergreen Cemetery Gatehouse, 799 Baltimore Street, 39°49.252' N, 77°13.753' W

With all the local church cemeteries closing in on their capacities, the Ever Green Cemetery Association of Gettysburg was established in November 1853. The cemetery opened in 1854 with the burial of Mary M. Beitler in October.

Caretakers Elizabeth and Peter Thorn, both born in Germany, lived in the three rooms in the north side of the gatehouse arch with their three sons, ranging in age from two to seven. Elizabeth's parents, John and Catherine Musser, lived in the three rooms south of the

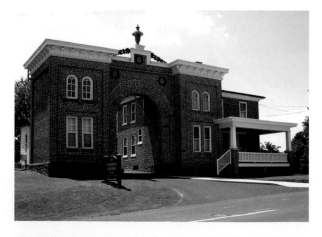

The gatehouse also served as the home of Elizabeth and Peter Thorn and became a hospital during the battle.

arch. At the time of the battle, Peter was near Harpers Ferry serving with the 138th Pennsylvania; Elizabeth was six months pregnant. She and her father maintained the cemetery in the absence of her husband.

On July 1 Elizabeth spent the early part of the day baking bread and giving it to hungry soldiers heading toward the fighting. She and her family also distributed water from their well for the soldiers as they passed. When the battle sounds drew closer, everyone went to the cellar except Elizabeth, who escorted Union officers around the area. She also provided meals to Union generals Howard, Sickles, and Slocum.

As the battle grew in intensity, the irony of three cemetery signs could not be overlooked. The first prohibited destruction of any shrubs, trees, and stones. The second warned, "Driving, riding, or shooting on these grounds strictly prohibited. Any person violating this ordinance will be punished by fine and imprisonment." The third threatened ominously, "All persons using firearms in these grounds will be prosecuted with the utmost vigor of the law." As General Howard and a staff member read the signs during the fighting, a shell smashed the second one. Nonplussed, Howard turned to his aide and said, "Well, that ordinance seems to have just been rescinded."[27]

That night Elizabeth and sixteen others huddled in the cellar. As dawn broke, a messenger came and told them that Howard said they were no longer safe and that everyone must leave immediately and go as far as they could go in ten minutes. As shells burst around them, Elizabeth, her sons, and her parents hurried to relative George Musser's farm on the Baltimore Pike. There Elizabeth and her father shared their concerns about their home and decided to return to check on their hogs.

As they prepared to leave, one of the wounded beckoned to Elizabeth. Showing her a picture of his three sons, he asked Elizabeth if she would allow her three boys to sleep next to him. Elizabeth obliged, and the sight of her sons brought a smile to the man's face. He, no doubt, dreamed of home that night.

Elizabeth and her father, John, cautiously made their way home, the groans of the wounded reaching their ears before they arrived at the gatehouse. John immediately went to the hog pen but the hogs were gone, the pen having been used for firewood, along with the old stable and all other available wood. Inside the gatehouse, wounded men from the Eleventh Corps lay in the cellar. Gathering a shawl and a quilt, Elizabeth and her father quickly left, vowing to move the family farther out the Baltimore Pike to get farther away from the battle.

Three hours after departing the Musser farm to return home, the family was on the road again, this time stopping at White Church before proceeding to the Henry Beitler farm, where they remained for three nights. Along the way they were joined by neighbor Margaret McKnight. While there, Elizabeth, her mother, and Margaret helped treat the many wounded on the property. They also received word of Jennie Wade's death. President Lincoln would deliver his famous Gettysburg Address a few months later in Evergreen Cemetery, just a few yards from Wade's grave.

The family returned home on July 7, only to find all their windows broken, the pump broken, and everything in the cellar gone except for three bloody featherbeds, on which six legs had been amputated. They also found sixteen soldiers' graves, as well as that of an African American civilian beside the pump shed. In the cemetery they saw that gravestones had been toppled and the ground torn up from artillery fire. Fences had been thrown down to facilitate artillery movement. Fifteen dead horses lay in front of the house and another nineteen in the field.[28]

Over the next several days, friends who came to assist quickly became ill from the stench and could not stay, leaving the burials of the dead to Elizabeth and her father. Together they buried 105 soldiers, 2 of them Confederates. About 50 of the 105 were eventually reinterred in the national cemetery. The rest remain in Evergreen, including the two Confederates, who are not buried beneath their markers. Townspeople did not want enemy soldiers buried in Evergreen, so the rebels were placed elsewhere in the cemetery and the location was left unmarked. Elizabeth noted that, for all the extra work of burying the soldiers, they never received any extra pay from the cemetery or from any other source, only their monthly salary of $13.00.[29]

Less than three months after burying 105 dead soldiers in the heat of summer, Elizabeth gave birth to a daughter. Unfortunately, that daughter would die at the age of thirteen. Peter Thorn survived the war and filed two damage claims, one for $405.00 and one for $355.00 for the loss of two tons of hay and four bushels of corn, as well as general damages to his property. He received $41.50.[30]

In 2002 a statue honoring Elizabeth was dedicated just inside the cemetery entrance. Titled the Civil War Women's Memorial, it shows Elizabeth taking a brief rest from burying the dead soldiers, and it honors all the women of Gettysburg for their efforts during and immediately after the battle.

15. Henry Spangler Farm, 1118 Baltimore Pike,
     39°48.869' N, 77°13.407' W

Sometimes referred to as the Abraham Spangler farm,
this property actually was occupied by his thirty-two-
year-old son, Henry, and his family during the battle.
The family included Henry's wife, Sarah, and their
three children.

Abraham had purchased the 230-acre property
in 1827 but was living on another farm he owned
along Chambersburg Road. To confuse matters just a
bit more, Henry owned a farm just off Emmitsburg
Road that was being farmed by tenant Jacob Ecken-
rode. That farm was not used as a hospital, and Henry
would not live on that property until after the war.

The log home on the Baltimore Pike farm was built
in 1744, with the stone addition constructed in 1819.
The barn, which, along with the other outbuildings,
no longer remains, was used as a hospital for the
Union Second Division, Twelfth Corps. As with most
hospitals, however, it also treated Northern soldiers
from other divisions, as well as some Confederates.
The wounded were moved to the Twelfth Corps hospital at the George Bushman farm on July 4.

Most of the wounded here were from the Culp's Hill
fighting. The worst cases were put in the barn so they
would have some protection from the weather. Others were placed outside on the grass. Known doctors
here included Surgeon Isaac H. Stearns (Twenty-Second Massachusetts), William Altman (Twenty-Eighth
Pennsylvania), and Cornelius M. Campbell (150th
New York).

There were seventy-eight Union burials on the
farm, with twenty-five of them from the 137th New
York, and as many as fifteen Confederate.[31]

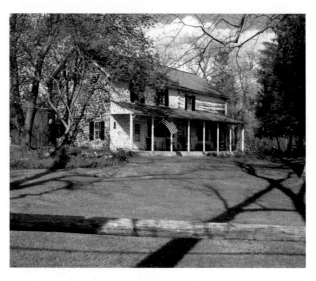

Most of those treated here had been wounded in the Culp's
Hill fighting. Owned by Abraham Spangler, the farm was
occupied by Spangler's son Henry during the battle.

Henry filed a damage claim of $1,714.11 for dam-
ages to his real estate, plus another $195.12 for loss of
personal items, for a total claim of $1,909.23.[32]

16. Nathaniel Lightner Farm, 1251 Baltimore
     Pike, 39°48.624' N, 77°13.200' W

Nathaniel Lightner (age thirty-nine) purchased this
twenty-six-acre farm in the late 1850s and lived here
with his wife, Catherine (also age thirty-nine), and
six of their seven children. An eighth child would be
born in 1869. The family had already experienced the
tragedy of war a week before the battle actually began,
when George Sandoe was killed near the Lightner
property. He was on patrol with Lightner's son, also
named Nathaniel. Both were with the Twenty-First

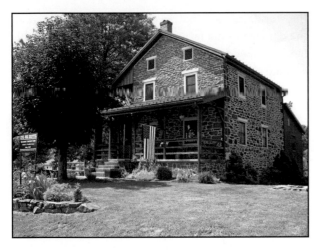

The Lightner family had to live in the farm's carpenter shop for six weeks because the house was filled with wounded.

Pennsylvania Cavalry. They got into a skirmish with a party from the Thirty-Fifth Virginia Cavalry and Sandoe was killed, making him the first man to die from enemy action at Gettysburg. Lightner was able to get away safely, possibly to his family's home.

On the sultry morning of July 1, Lightner and neighbor John Tawney were mowing Lightner's meadow. The two decided a drink was in order, and Lightner was dispatched to go into town and buy a jug of whiskey. When he saw what was happening in town, he scurried back home.

The atmosphere had changed dramatically since he had left Tawney. Surgeons had moved his dining-room table outside, where they were in the process of amputating a man's leg. The pile of limbs under the apple tree provided mute evidence that this was only the latest of several such surgeries. Inside the house the floor was covered with wounded. His terrified family had taken refuge in the stable.

Lightner asked a surgeon what he should do, considering the situation. The surgeon advised him to leave. When Lightner asked whether he could go inside the house to gather some clothing, the surgeon told him he could if he could find anything. Lightner soon realized what the surgeon meant when he went inside the house and saw that clothing, linens, bedclothes, and anything else that could be torn into bandages had been taken for that purpose.

Lightner and his family departed with only the clothing they were wearing, wending their way through oncoming troops and wagons until they reached the home of an unnamed relative, probably Isaac Lightner. Late that night he left his family and worked his way to his friend Tawney's, where he spent the night. At daybreak the two of them walked to the Signal Corps headquarters, where they could look down on Lightner's farm. Lightner saw wagon trains in his wheat field and orchard, while a drove of beef cattle was being herded in the meadow. Realizing that there was nothing he could do, he returned to his family and moved them still farther out Baltimore Pike. He then returned to the Signal Corps headquarters, where he spent the rest of the day.

He was finally able to get to his house on July 3, where he discovered all his fencing gone, all his poultry and livestock missing, and the family dog nowhere to be found. The army's mules had eaten the orchard of four-year-old trees down to the core. His house was still filled with wounded, and a weary-looking General Henry Slocum was seated in front of the barn, in which he had made his headquarters. A number of wounded prisoners had also been brought to the farm.

A week later he returned with his family and lived in the carpenter shop for six weeks. They moved into the house when the wounded were moved out about mid-August, but it was in such poor condition that they could not stand to stay there. The smell of blood and medicine permeated every surface. Opening windows to clear the air only made it worse, with the stench from the yard and meadow wafting in. Huge biting bottle flies covered the walls.

A few days after the family returned to the farm, a man from New York stopped by and told Lightner's children he would buy any relics they found, although newspapers had published warnings against picking up government property found on the battlefield. Anyone found with "battle souvenirs" would be required to help bury the dead or, if they had a team, haul gathered weapons to a central location. Most farmers in the area, however, reasoned that it was worth the risk, considering most of them had lost everything and were desperate for ways to rebuild their farms. Lightner was no different, and he and his children began gathering what they could find around the farm.

Meanwhile, Quartermaster General Montgomery Meigs sent Captain Henry B. Blood of the Quartermaster Corps and Captain William Smith of General Halleck's staff to Gettysburg to gather all property left on the battlefield by both sides, including any material picked up by civilians. The Twenty-First Pennsylvania Cavalry, in which Lightner's son served, was ordered to search all area farms and confiscate any property that belonged to the government. Some was found at Lightner's.

Blood had Lightner arrested and the confiscated items taken to the Washington Arsenal. After several days Lightner's neighbors were able to get him released, but Lightner told anyone who would listen that he considered Blood to be the meanest man in the world. He said that, even when he considered all the damage to his farm and the hardships he and his family had endured, the thing that angered him most was the way he had been treated by Blood.

Early in the spring of 1864, Lightner was able to obtain a stocked farm on shares, and he moved from his Baltimore Pike farm. Speaking of his old farm, he said he "gave it to an old Dutchman, who did not seem to mind the smells and filth."[33]

Nine years later he returned and tore all the woodwork and plaster out and made the house new from the cellar to the garret. The family moved back, but Catherine, who had never been well since they had tried to live in the home immediately after the battle, died a few years later.

Nothing remains on the farm now except the house. The farm had been used as a hospital from July 1 to August 12, 1863, by the Sixth and Twelfth Corps, plus some of the First and Eleventh Corps. Colonel William Colvill (First Minnesota) had been treated here before being moved to James Pierce's house in town. Colvill claimed that he was aware of at least thirty amputations that had been performed at Lightner's. Despite all this, Lightner's claim for nearly $1,500.00 in damages was rejected.

Lightner lived until November 14, 1911, when he died at age eighty-seven after receiving internal injuries when he was struck by a wind-damaged tree that he had been removing.

17. James McAllister Farm and Mill Site, Baltimore Pike, 39°48.552' N, 77°12.844' W

James McAllister purchased this 295-acre property in 1822, which included not only a farm but also a gristmill that ground barley, oats, and wheat. The seventy-seven-year-old McAllister lived here with his wife, Agnes, and their seven children, ranging in age from sixteen to thirty-four. Their son Samuel ran the mill. Another son, James Alexander McAllister, was with the Union army. He was destined to be killed at Vicksburg at about the same time his family was coping with the fighting in Gettysburg.

McAllister was a staunch abolitionist and the site served as an important stop on the Underground Railroad, becoming one of the earliest networks through which runaway slaves passed. Slaves were hidden in the mill's cog pit in a room concealed by the water wheel. The door to the secret room was so massive that it had to be opened by a pulley system. Using streams and secondary roads at night to avoid bounty hunters who heavily patrolled this area, runaway slaves were conducted over one of two routes to freedom. The first took the runaways to Carlisle and Harrisburg, then either east to Philadelphia or north to New York, and finally to Canada. The second route went due east to York, Lancaster, Chester, and Philadelphia.[34]

On July 4, 1836, the farm was the site of a major gathering of abolitionists that led to the formation of the Adams County Anti-slavery Society.

In July 1863 the McAllister house became a hospital for wounded soldiers from Slocum's Twelfth Corps. The wounded from the First Division of the Union Second Corps moved here from Granite Schoolhouse after artillery fire forced them to relocate. Bloodstains remain on the dining-room floor. On July 4, as Confederate prisoners were being transported down Baltimore Pike on their way to Westminster, Maryland, the most severely wounded among them were removed from the march at a checkpoint at the foot of Powers Hill. A small hospital was set up near the mill on July 4 to treat those deemed unfit to make the trek

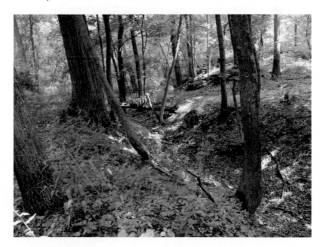

The mill's cog pit sat here and hid slaves in a secret room whose door could only be opened with an elaborate pulley system.

The remains of the old mill race that provided water to operate the mill wheel.

to Westminster. Agnes and her two daughters, Mary and Martha, treated the wounded at both hospitals under the direction of Dr. William Warren Porter of the Fifty-Seventh New York.

The first Union soldier killed in action at Gettysburg, George Sandoe of the Twenty-First Pennsylvania Cavalry, was killed on McAllister's property. The elderly McAllister reprimanded the rebel soldiers who had killed him, and made them bury the young man. He would be listed among the thirty-five burials on the farm, which also included at least three Confederates.

McAllister put in a claim for $1,200.00 in damages, which appears to have been rejected. He died in 1872, and after the family left, the mill sank into disrepair. Eventually the property was used as the town dump until it closed in the 1950s. As if to humiliate the property even more, it then became a construction waste site and an automobile junkyard, an ignominious fate for such a historical piece of land. Finally, in 2011 the federal government recognized McAllister's Mill as one of several properties having a verifiable connection to the Underground Railroad, restoring some dignity to the old mill site. A marker was erected in 2012 in recognition.

Nothing remains at this site today. It is now private property, accessible only by authorized tours conducted by Historic Gettysburg Adams County.

18. George Musser Farm, Baltimore Pike, 39°48.297' N, 77°12.754' W

Seventy-year-old George Musser and his wife, Elizabeth, lived on this small, eighteen-acre farm during the battle, and on July 2, Crawford's Division of the

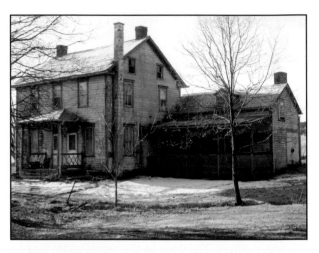

The Musser farmhouse served as an aid station. Amputated limbs are believed to remain somewhere on the property.

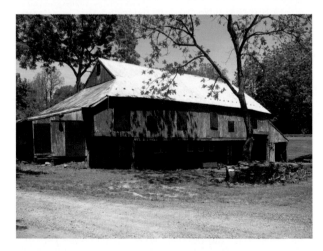

The Musser barn also was used as a hospital.

Union Fifth Corps bivouacked in the Musser fields. Both the house and barn are believed to be original to the property.

The farm was used as a hospital during the battle, primarily as an aid station for wounded Confederate prisoners passing on Baltimore Pike as they were being taken to Westminster, Maryland.

Several amputations were performed in the house, with the removed limbs tossed onto the porch until they could be buried somewhere on the farm, where they presumably remain.

According to an oft-repeated account of the Musser farm, Elizabeth Thorn, caretaker for the Evergreen Cemetery, arrived at the farm with her parents and three young sons during the fighting. Thorn was six months pregnant at the time and had been told to leave her home for her own safety by General O. O. Howard. She and her family would move farther out Baltimore Pike a day later. It was here that Thorn allowed her boys to sleep next to a wounded Confederate soldier who had asked for her permission. He said they reminded him of his own three sons at home.

The Mussers' son George was serving in the Eighty-Seventh Pennsylvania Volunteers and had been captured at Carter's Woods near Winchester, Virginia, just two weeks before the fighting began in Gettysburg, a fact that the elder George and Elizabeth Musser probably were not aware of when their house and barn were being used as a hospital. Young George would eventually be paroled and discharged on a surgeon's certificate. He was able to return home but died just a year later.

19. Isaac M. Diehl Farm Site, 1575 Baltimore Pike, 39°48.281' N, 77°12.745' W

This 150-acre farm abutted that of George Musser and is now a stone quarry. Nothing of the farm remains today, but during the battle it was owned and

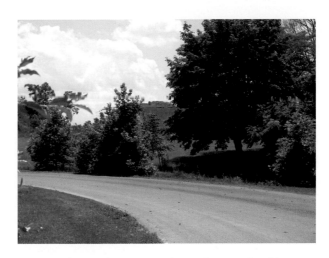

The Diehl farm no longer exists, having been replaced by a quarry, which is visible in the background.

occupied by thirty-one-year-old Isaac Diehl; his wife, Elizabeth Catherine; and their five children. The farm had a two-story stone house, a stone and log barn, an orchard, and a small stone quarry that was likely the beginning of the major quarry operation that stands on the property today. The house and barn were used as a hospital for about five weeks.

William Cable Meredith, age eighteen, was buried behind the barn. He was serving with the Eighteenth Virginia and had been wounded in the ankle and abdomen. It is uncertain whether he had been treated at Diehl's. His records only note that he died in an unknown field hospital. It was likely that it was either Diehl's or George Musser's. Meredith is the only burial recorded on the farm. He was disinterred in 1872 and reburied in Hollywood Cemetery in Richmond.[35]

Diehl claimed losses of $2,274.20 for livestock, flour, grain, houseware, food, stone fencing, thirty-five panels of post and rail fence, and 6,270 rails. His award was reduced to $1,574.20.[36]

20. G. Flemming Hoke Toll House, 1630 Baltimore Pike, 39°48.273' N, 77°12.591' W

This stone house served as a tollhouse for the Gettysburg-Petersburg Turnpike. As on today's toll roads, fees were imposed for those transporting animals or goods to the markets in Baltimore. G. Flemming Hoke was the gatekeeper for this particular tollhouse, giving rise to its unofficial name: Hoke's Gate.

Much like the farms of George Musser, Isaac Diehl, James McAllister, and others along Baltimore Pike, Hoke's tollhouse was used to treat wounded Confederate prisoners who were being transported along that route. It also treated a number of Federal soldiers, most notably Brigadier General Samuel Zook.

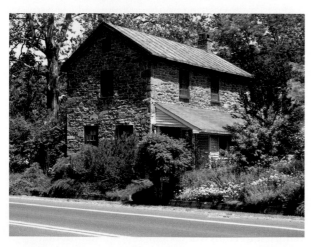

The tollhouse was used to treat wounded from both sides, including the mortally wounded Brigadier General Samuel Zook.

Zook had been shot through the abdomen in the Wheatfield on July 2 and was brought to Hoke's that evening. The house was already filled with wounded. Zook, despite being in severe pain, asked that a blanket be placed under him to avoid getting the bed bloody. It really did not matter, as witnesses said that the floor was already streaming with blood. Surgeon Charles Squire Wood from the Sixty-Sixth New York pronounced Zook's wound mortal.

The next day, with fears growing that Lee's army could break through the Union line, Zook was moved from Hoke's, and he died later that afternoon. Surgeon William Warren Porter (Fifty-Seventh New York) stayed with Zook until he died.

More than twenty burials were recorded in Hoke's yard.

21. Granite Schoolhouse Site, Granite Schoolhouse Lane, 39°48.290' N, 77°13.356' W

This schoolhouse served as the headquarters for Union general Winfield Scott Hancock's First Division of the Second Corps. As such, it treated Hancock's wounded, and may have also been an aid station for the Artillery Reserve. When Hancock was wounded, he received his initial treatment here. The wounded were relocated to McAllister's Mill when artillery fire made the area unsafe on July 2.

Some historians believe that this is where Meade came when overfire from cannons preceding Pickett's Charge forced him to relocate his headquarters from the Lydia Leister farm.

Dr. H. B. Buck from the US Artillery Reserve treated the wounded here, as did Dr. William Warren Porter of the Fifty-Seventh New York until he accompanied

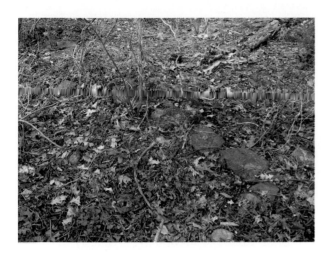

Remains of the old schoolhouse foundation, which was a hospital until artillery made the area unsafe.

General Samuel Zook's mortally wounded body to Hoke's tollhouse for treatment.

In 1920 the George Rosensteel family purchased the school and had it razed. Rosensteel used many of the stones from the school to construct an addition, with living quarters, to their tourist stand on the Taneytown Road across from the west gate entrance to the national cemetery. That home, the Rosensteel's National Civil War Museum, eventually became the National Park Service visitor center for the Gettysburg National Military Park. It was torn down in 2008 when the new visitor center was constructed.

Portions of the old foundation for the school remain but are difficult to locate. Those wishing to do so should look for the marker for Lieutenant Edward Heatons's Batteries B and L, Second US Artillery. This marker is surrounded by a stone wall and sits on the right side of Granite Schoolhouse Lane when driving from Taneytown Road toward Hospital Road. The foundation for the schoolhouse is across Granite Schoolhouse Lane from this marker, on the opposite side of the small stone wall running along the north side of the road.

The foundation is likely to be covered with leaves, and there are many rocks and stones in the area that are not part of the foundation, so it is difficult to locate. The easiest way to find it is to locate a corner where the stones form a ninety-degree angle.

22. Eleventh Corps Hospital Tablet, Hospital Road, 39°48.065' N, 77°13.097' W

Often referred to as the German Corps because of its high concentration of German troops and officers, the Eleventh Corps suffered significantly on July 1. When the right flank collapsed, it led to a chaotic retreat of Union forces through the town to the safety of Cemetery Hill, and the corps lost many captured on the way. On the second day, it regained some stature when it participated in a successful defense of East Cemetery Hill. At Gettysburg the corps suffered 368 killed, 1,922 wounded, and 1,511 captured or missing, for a total of 3,801, out of fewer than 9,000 engaged.

This marker sits at the entrance to the George Spangler farm. Its inscription reads,

Army of the Potomac
Medical Department
Field Hospitals
Eleventh Corps

The Division Field Hospitals of the Eleventh Corps were established July 1st at the Spangler House two

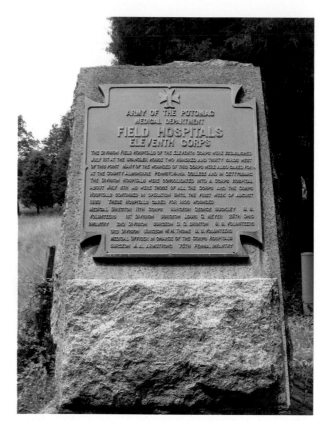

Eleventh Corps Hospital Tablet on Hospital Road, at the entrance to the George Spangler farm. Confederate General Lewis Armistead died here.

hundred and thirty yards west of this point. Many of the wounded of this Corps were also cared for at the County Almshouse, Pennsylvania College, and in Gettysburg. The Division Hospitals were consolidated into a Corps Hospital about July 6th as were those of all the Corps and the Corps Hospitals continued in operation until the first week of August 1863. These hospitals cared for 1400 wounded.

Medical Director 11th Corps, Surgeon George Suckley, U.S. Volunteers
1st Division, Surgeon Louis G. Meyer, 25th Ohio Infantry
2nd Division, Surgeon D.G. Brinton, U.S. Volunteers
3rd Division, Surgeon W.H. Thome, U.S. Volunteers
Medical Officer in charge of the Corps Hospitals, Surgeon J.A. Armstrong, 75th Penna. Infantry

23. George Spangler Farm, 488 Blacksmith Shop Road, 39°48.069′ N, 77°13.095′ W

This 156-acre farm belonged to George Spangler and served as the primary hospital for the Eleventh Corps. After a major refurbishment, it looks very similar to the way it looked in 1863. George Spangler was forty-eight years old and lived here with his wife, Elizabeth (forty-five). The couple had four children: Harriet (twenty-one), Daniel (twenty), Sabina (nineteen), and Beniah (fifteen). Beniah would live to age

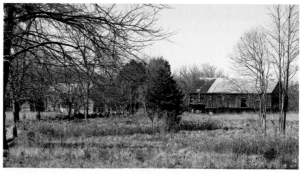

The Spangler farm was in near ruins until a major restoration was undertaken in 2012–2013.

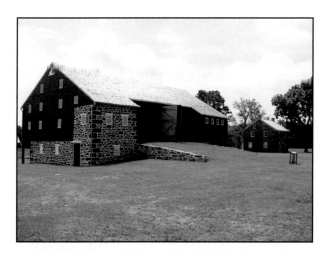

Spangler house and barn shown after restoration.

eighty-four and was extremely proud of having been in the crowd to hear Lincoln's Gettysburg Address. The family lived in one of the six rooms in the house, with the wounded of the Eleventh Corps taking up the other five.

Spangler had purchased the property in 1848, and it proved to be an ideal site for a hospital during the battle. It was easily accessible from both Baltimore Pike and Taneytown Road, it had multiple water sources, and the size of the barn guaranteed the availability of planks and doors that could be used for operating tables. The open layout provided ample space to place patients and for the surgeons to work. Still, the throng of wounded caused the hospital to run out of space and supplies. The farm was used as a hospital for five weeks.

Contributing to the overcrowding was the presence of batteries from the Reserve Artillery and ammunition train that used the farm as a gathering area, known as an artillery park. At one time this park held 114 cannon with limbers and caissons, 2,376 officers and men, and 1,500 horses, plus ambulances, wagons to haul reserve ammunition, and forges to repair equipment.

More than two thousand wounded were treated here, including about one hundred Confederates. The barn, outbuildings, yard, and surrounding fields were used, with hundreds of tents set up to provide protection from the weather. Still, many were forced to lie in the open air, and when heavy rains hit on July 4, those lying in the barnyard were forced to endure the mud and manure as it soaked into their bandages. Every inch of space inside the barn held a wounded man, with men propped up in stalls and cribs to make room for more. Confederate wounded were isolated in the wagon shed, which no longer exists.

Four crude operating tables were set up outside with tarps or blankets stretched on poles to keep the rain off. All four tables were filled night and day, with surgeons working virtually nonstop from July 1 to July 5. They worked with their sleeves rolled up, their arms and aprons covered in blood. Standing in pools of blood, they were surrounded by heaps of amputated limbs.

Three Union colonels were treated here, but undoubtedly the best-known patient was Confederate general Lewis Armistead. Armistead had dropped out of West Point after he broke a plate over the head of fellow cadet Jubal Early, who also became a general in Lee's army, though some historians speculate that the primary reason that Armistead resigned from the academy was academic difficulties. During Pickett's Charge, Brigadier General Armistead had been wounded in the lower leg and (depending on

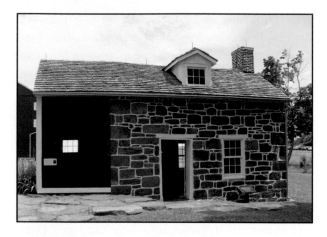

Confederate general Lewis Armistead died in the kitchen of the Spangler farm.

the source) in either the forearm or the pectoral area of the chest. Union captain Henry Bingham assisted Armistead after he was taken from the Angle and was lying with other wounded behind Cemetery Ridge. Armistead was brought to the summer kitchen on the Spangler farm, where Dr. Daniel Brinton and another doctor dressed both wounds, neither of which was considered serious. However, Armistead died a few days later, surprising Brinton, who determined that the death was not caused directly by the wounds but more likely by secondary fever and prostration. The reference to secondary fever probably meant that he had developed an infection. A more likely explanation for his death, however, would be a blood clot that ultimately resulted in a pulmonary embolism. He was buried behind the barn and later reinterred in Old Saint Paul's Cemetery in Baltimore.

The dead were quickly carried outside to allow more wounded to be brought in. Burials took place in four long trenches that had been dug in the field south of the house. There were at least 20 Confederate and 185 Union burials on the farm.[37] Rev. William R. Keifer of the 153rd Ohio provided spiritual comfort and officiated funerals. One of those buried here was George Nixon, great-grandfather of President Richard Nixon.

Most of the Union dead were eventually reinterred at the Gettysburg National Cemetery. While it is not known exactly where all of the Confederate soldiers were reinterred, most would have been removed with the rest of the Southern troops in 1872.

The Eleventh Corps medical director was Surgeon George Suckley (US Volunteers), and the officer in charge of the hospital was Surgeon J. A. Armstrong (Seventy-Fifth Pennsylvania). Other doctors here included Daniel Brinton (US Volunteers), Robert Hubbard (Seventeenth Connecticut), Louis G. Meyer (Twenty-Fifth Ohio), W. H. Thome (US Volunteers), Jacob Y. Cartwell (Eighty-Second Ohio), W. S. Moore (Sixty-First Ohio), John P. Kohler (153rd Pennsylvania), and B. van Benst (US Volunteers). Moore was badly wounded on July 3 and died on July 6, the only doctor to be killed at Gettysburg.

Assisting the surgeons were several regimental stewards, including Reuben Ruch, a hospital steward with the 153rd Pennsylvania Infantry. Further assistance came from relatives of many of the wounded, who rushed to Gettysburg upon hearing of the wounding of their loved ones.

On July 3 the farm came under fire from artillery during the cannonade before Pickett's Charge. Many of these shells landed near the barn, killing several horses. The wounded lying in the barn reported that they lay on the floor and watched the shells exploding just outside the barn door, some saying within twenty feet.

Spangler claimed losses of $3,000.00 but received only $375.00 in compensation.[38]

24. Bushman Tenant House, Baladerry Inn, 10 Hospital Road, 39°47.866' N, 77°13.042' W

The oldest section of the Baladerry Inn was constructed in 1812 as a farmhouse, with the rest of the structure completed in 1830. It served as a tenant house on the George Bushman farm at the time of the battle and is believed to have handled some of the overflow of wounded from the Bushman hospital.

The main hall was used to treat both civilians and wounded soldiers. Amputations were carried out in this portion of the house. Seven Confederate burials were said to have taken place on the part of the property now occupied by the tennis courts. There were no Union

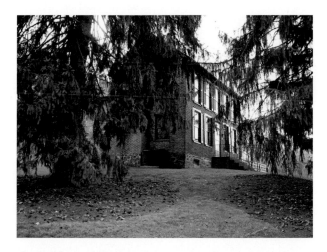

The Baladerry Inn, a tenant house on the George Bushman farm, probably treated wounded who could not be accommodated on the main farm.

burials recorded on the farm, so it is possible that the house was used to isolate the Confederate wounded from the Union men being treated at Bushman's.

A second possibility stems from the fact that the two divisions of the Twelfth Corps initially may have had separate hospitals that were near one another, situated "around and north of the Bushman farmhouse."[39] This description fits the location of the inn, so it is possible that the tenant house served as the hospital, at least for a while, for one of the divisions of the Twelfth Corps.

The house was converted into a bed and breakfast in 1992.

25. Twelfth Corps Hospital Tablet, Hospital Road, 39°47.447' N, 77°12.895' W

The two divisions of the Twelfth Corps fought principally on the right flank of the Union army at Culp's Hill. The corps suffered a loss of 204 men killed, 812 wounded, and 66 either captured or missing, for a total casualty count of 1,082. Most of these casualties took place while the corps was positioned in the vicinity of Culp's Hill.

The inscription on the tablet reads,

Army of the Potomac
Medical Department
Field Hospitals
Twelfth Corps

The Division Field Hospitals of the Twelfth Corps were located July 2nd at the Bushman House one hundred and sixty yards east. These hospitals cared for about 1200 wounded and were in operation until about August 5th, 1863.

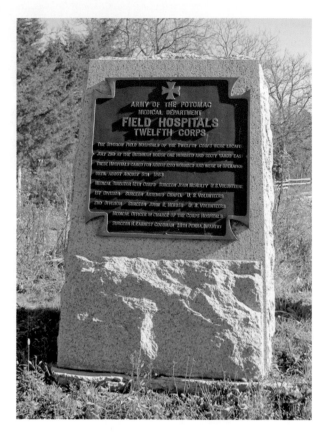

Twelfth Corps Hospital Tablet at the entrance to the George Bushman Farm. The hospital was forced to relocate here from Powers Hill on July 2, 1863, when it came under heavy artillery fire.

Medical Director, 12th Corps Surgeon, John
McNulty, U.S. Volunteers
1st Division Surgeon, Artemus Chapel, U.S. Volunteers
2nd Division Surgeon John E. Herbst, U.S. Volunteers
Medical Officer in charge of 12th Corps Hospitals,
Surgeon H. Ernest Goodman, 28th Pennsylvania
Infantry

26. George Bushman Farm, Hospital Road, 39°49.433' N, 77°12.805' W

At the time of the battle, this farm extended across what is now US Route 15 and served as the hospital for Major General Henry Slocum's Twelfth Corps. George Bushman, fifty-three years old, lived here with his wife, Anna. The couple had three children, but it is not known whether they were on the farm during the battle. However, their granddaughter Sadie, nine years old, was known to be there, having been sent from town to get away from the fighting. She assisted in helping the wounded.

The oldest part of the house was built around 1800 and was used during the battle as a dining place for the surgeons and attendants. The women of the family prepared and served the food.

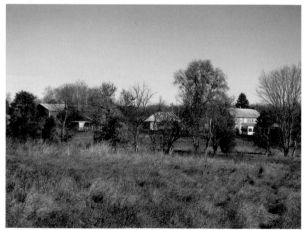

The Bushman farm hospital treated Lewis Powell, who was destined to become one of the Lincoln assassination conspirators.

The Twelfth Corps hospital had initially been behind Powers Hill before artillery fire forced it to relocate to Bushman's. Here, the wounded were housed in the barn until it was full, then in two rows of tents that ran north and south. Tents on the west side held wounded from the Second Division, while those on the east held those from the First Division. Tents were available almost immediately because the corps had its own wagons and ambulances, enabling Slocum to ignore Meade's order to send supply wagons to the rear. Nearly 1,200 Union men were treated here, along with 125 Confederates.

One of those wounded Confederates, with the colorful name of Captain Decimus et Ultimus Barziza (Fourth Texas), wrote that as he was being brought to Bushman's, he saw that every shelter in the neighborhood was crammed, including haylofts. At Bushman's he noted that the dead were laid out in rows, on their backs, until dragged away and thrown into a pit for burial.[40]

Perhaps the best-known Confederate prisoner to be treated at Bushman's was Lewis Powell. A private in the Second Florida Infantry, Powell had been wounded in the wrist near the Peach Orchard on July 2. He would eventually gain notoriety for his role in the Lincoln assassination plot, when he stabbed Secretary of State William Seward several times. Powell would be hanged for his part in the conspiracy.

Burials were mostly east of the house, with one section for Union dead and another for Confederates. There were fifty-two Union burials on the farm, and Dr. John W. C. O'Neal recorded the names of another forty-one Confederates buried on the property.[41]

Surgeon H. Ernest Goodman (Twenty-Eighth Pennsylvania) was in charge of the hospital here. He was assisted by as many as a dozen additional doctors, including John E. Herbst and Artemus Chapel (both from the US Volunteers), W. C. Bennett (Fifth Connecticut), Amos Fifield (Seventh Ohio), James L. Dunn (109th Pennsylvania), John H. Love (Thirteenth New Jersey), William Tibbals (Fifth Ohio), W. H. Twiford (Twenty-Seventh Indiana), Patrick H. Flood (107th New York), J. Alfred Ball (Fiftieth Ohio), Surgeon William C. Rogers (Forty-Sixth Pennsylvania), and H. C. May (145th New York). May's wife joined her husband in Gettysburg to serve as a volunteer nurse on the Bushman farm.

Surgeon George Burke (Forty-Sixth Pennsylvania), Surgeon Evelyn Lyman Bissell (Fifth Connecticut), Dr. James A. Freeman (Thirteenth New Jersey), Dr. C. H. Lord (107th New York), and Assistant Surgeon Robert T. Paine (Twenty-Eighth New York) all served as records, food, and shelter officers.

Lieutenant James E. Crocker had been the valedictorian of the Pennsylvania College in 1850. He was now in the Ninth Virginia Infantry and had been wounded at Pickett's Charge. He had been mistakenly reported killed back in Virginia. He was brought to Bushman's for treatment.

When he felt strong enough, he obtained a pass and went into town, meeting old classmates and professors. One of the friends he met was Henry Louis Baugher, son of the president of Crocker's alma mater and a staunch abolitionist. Political viewpoints were put aside as the old friends reminisced. Then, young Baugher invited his former classmate to dinner with his family, including President Baugher, the abolitionist. By all accounts the evening went well, no arguments over abolition or slavery arose, and Crocker returned to Bushman's saying he thoroughly enjoyed his time with the Baugher family. Crocker would be sent to a prisoners-of-war camp a few weeks later and was paroled in February 1865.[42]

The farm was used as a hospital from July 2 through August 5. Only the house remains from the original farm.

27. Second Corps Hospital Tablet, Hospital Road, 39°47.358' N, 77°12.876' W

The Second Corps encountered the heaviest fighting it had ever experienced on July 2, when it fought in the Wheatfield, and July 3 in the repulse of Pickett's Charge. The loss in the corps was 796 killed, 3,186 wounded, and 368 missing, a total of 4,350 out of fewer than 10,500 engaged. Generals Hancock and Gibbon were seriously wounded, while four brigade commanders were killed: General Samuel K. Zook and Colonels Edward E. Cross, George L. Willard, and Eliakim Sherrill.

The inscription on the tablet reads,

Army of the Potomac
Medical Department
Field Hospitals
Second Corps

The Division Hospitals of the Second Corps were located July 2nd at the Granite School House but were soon removed to near Rock Creek west of the creek and six hundred yards southeast of the Bushman House. They remained there until closed August 7th, 1863. These Hospitals cared for 2200 Union and 952 Confederate wounded.

Medical Director 2nd Corps Surgeon, A.N. Dougherty, U.S. Volunteers

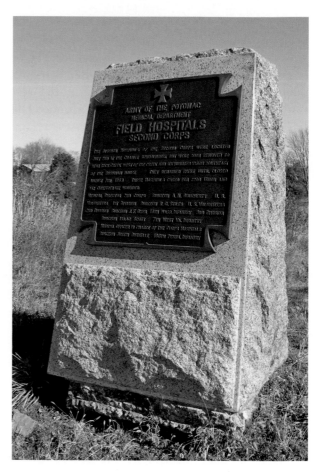

Second Corps Hospital Tablet, marking the location of the hospital after moving from the Granite School House on the second day of fighting.

1st Division Surgeon, R.C. Stiles, U.S. Volunteers
2nd Division Surgeon, J.F. Dyer, 10th Massachusetts Infantry
3rd Division Surgeon, Isaac Scott, 7th West Va. Infantry

Medical Officer in charge of the Corps Hospitals, Surgeon Justin Dwinell, 106th Pennsylvania.

Other doctors who served in unspecified Second Corps hospitals included Surgeon John Akin (Seventy-First Pennsylvania), Assistant Surgeon J. D. Benton (111th New York), Surgeon Frederick F. Burmeister (Sixty-Ninth Pennsylvania), Surgeon William J. Burn (Forty-Second Massachusetts), Surgeon W. J. Burr (Forty-Seventh New York), Assistant Surgeon W. P. Bush (Sixty-First New York), Assistant Surgeon Theodore O. Cornish (Fifteenth Massachusetts), Surgeon U. Q. Davis (148th Pennsylvania), Surgeon Ebenezer Day (Thirty-Ninth New York, surgeon in charge, Third Division, Second Corps), Surgeon Nathan Hayward (Twentieth Massachusetts), Bushrod W. James (civilian doctor), Assistant Surgeon A. Stokes Jones (Seventy-Second Pennsylvania), Surgeon Charles T. Kelsey (surgeon in charge, Second Corps), Assistant Surgeon Henry C. Levensaller (Nineteenth Maine), Surgeon H. M. McAbee (Fourth Ohio), Assistant Surgeon J. W. McCullough (First Delaware), Surgeon W. S. Cooper (125th New York), Surgeon William Child (Fifth New Hampshire), Surgeon Philip Plunkett (Second Delaware), Assistant Surgeon Charles Swart (Sixty-Third New York), and Surgeon J. Wilson Wishart (140th Pennsylvania).

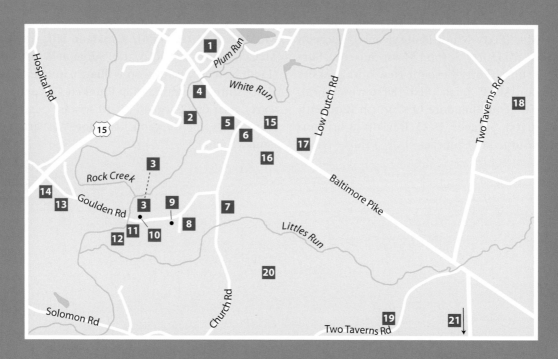

Chapter 9 sites: Baltimore Pike, east of US 15. (Map by Bill Nelson)

1. Adam Wert Farm, White Road, 39°47.906' N, 77°11.713' W

War of 1812 veteran Adam Wert was a medical doctor and educator, teaching both German and English. He served as the burgess of Gettysburg and was instrumental in the creation of the Adams County Anti-slavery Society.

Adam lived with his wife, Catherine, and his son J. Howard, and the Wert family had been involved in the antislavery movement for three generations. The farm was an integral part of the Underground Railroad, and many escaped slaves had been hidden on the property.

During the battle, the house became a refuge for wounded soldiers, as well as civilians seeking safety. Out of necessity, Catherine soon became a nurse, assisting her husband as he treated the wounded. Known to her neighbors as Aunt Katie, Catherine also helped with the wounded at the nearby Jacob Schwartz farm. While the family was trying to make the wounded men comfortable and find places for visitors to sleep, Union officers regularly came into the farmhouse to consult a large map of Adams County that Adam had affixed to his wall. The entire scene had to be chaotic.

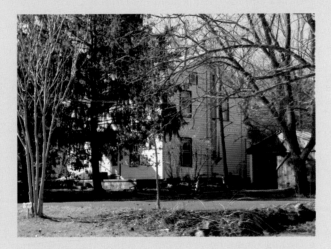

The Wert farm was a stop on the Underground Railroad that became a hospital during the battle.

Meanwhile, the adventurous teenage J. Howard explored the battlefield during and after the fighting. Fortunately for historians, he left well-documented stories of scenes from the battlefield in the days immediately after the battle. He became so fascinated with what he saw and wrote about that he joined the 209th Pennsylvania Volunteer Infantry a year after the battle.

Returning from the army, J. Howard was accepted to study at Pennsylvania College, where he joined an unsanctioned fraternity known as Beta Delta. Far from innocent, the Beta Deltas, or BDs, as they became known, had earned a reputation for their late-night parties and bad behavior. The name Beta Delta had not been chosen without considerable thought, and it was soon a poorly kept secret that BD actually stood for Black Ducks, a secret society that often hid slaves as part of the Underground Railroad. Young J. Howard and his friends fashioned hiding places in the rocks on Culp's Hill where runaways were taken until they could be moved northward.[1]

The barn is now gone, and the house is not original to the farm.

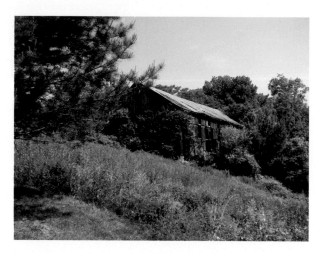

The Sheely farm was the headquarters for General Marsena Patrick and a prisoner-of-war depot, in addition to treating wounded.

2. Aaron Sheely Farm, Baltimore Pike, 39°47.515' N, 77°11.961' W

The Aaron Sheely farm was not a hospital in the true sense of the word. However, it was taken over as a prisoner-of-war depot and the headquarters for General Marsena Patrick, the provost marshal general for the Union army. As such, Patrick was responsible for guarding Union deserters and Confederate prisoners, many of whom were wounded. A map made by the US Christian Commission shortly after the battle shows a hospital on the Sheely farm, and there is evidence that the farm may have taken in patients from nearby hospitals. The farm briefly hosted several thousand Confederate prisoners, from which they were sent south on the Baltimore Pike to Westminster, Maryland.

Shortly after the battle, Dr. Bushrod W. James of Philadelphia arrived with a load of medical supplies. He would spend several days here and at Jacob Schwartz's farm treating the wounded. The less seriously wounded were moved to division hospitals over time, but those who were unable to be moved stayed at Sheely's for several weeks. Representatives from the Christian Commission provided assistance in the treatment of the wounded.

Sheely claimed a loss of four horses at $150 each from Stuart's raid of October 1862, and further claimed the loss of a mare, a wagon bed, a spring wagon, two horse gears, a chain, a wagon saddle, three bridles and halters, and a string of bells, all lost during the battle or in the time the farm was used by Patrick. The two claims came to $843.00, with Sheely being awarded $817.75.[2]

The house no longer stands, and the barn is in very poor condition and is not expected to survive much longer.

3. Jacob Schwartz Farm, White Church Road,
39°47.266' N, 77°12.159' W

The sprawling three-hundred-acre farm of Jacob Schwartz, often incorrectly referred to as the Moses Schwartz farm, held two separate hospitals serving the Union's Second, Third, Fifth, and Sixth Corps. The two are shown interconnected by a broken line on the map at the beginning of this chapter. Moses was Jacob's brother and was the previous owner of the farm, but he sold it to Jacob about five years before the battle. Jacob was the owner at the time of the battle.

The farm buildings and the fields immediately surrounding them treated some 2,300 Union men, mostly from the Second Corps, and 1,000 Confederate wounded. Most of the Southern wounded resulted from Pickett's Charge on July 3.

The farm contained a two-story brick house, a brick-and-wood barn, a wagon shed, a corncrib, a

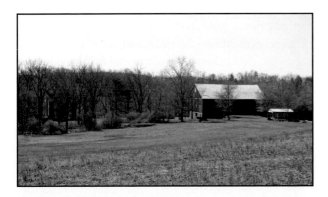

The Second Corps hospital utilized the Schwartz farm buildings and the immediate surrounding area. The area in the foreground became a cemetery for Union dead.

carriage house, and a smokehouse. The barn was built in 1817 and remains, but the current house is not original. The barn was completely filled with wounded, most of them Confederates, and nearly all of whom had lost at least one limb. Several had lost more than one, and many had to be fed like infants. The blood of the wounded flowed so freely that it ran through the floorboards of the threshing floor and dripped on those below.

While neighbors felt that the barn should have been used for Union men and the Confederates should have been the ones to be placed outside, the reasoning was sound for keeping the Southerners inside: as prisoners of war, they would be easier to guard if confined, and escape would be more difficult, although most were in no condition to try.

An amputation table, made from removed barn doors, was set up beside the barn, and as the arms and legs piled up they were taken away by the wagonload to trenches used specifically for them. One of those who had a leg amputated was a soldier named Charles N. Drake, of the Twelfth New Hampshire Infantry. During the night, scavenging hogs chewed on his amputated limb. He said he felt the pain as much as if the leg were still there.[3]

Initially at the Granite Schoolhouse, the Second Corps had relocated its hospital several times, first to the area around the Lewis Bushman farm, then to a spot along Rock Creek on the George Bushman farm, just south of today's US Route 15. This last site seemed to be perfect, with Rock Creek providing a good source of water and the wooded terrain providing ample shade and protection from the heat. The First and Second Divisions sat along the north side of Rock Creek, with the Third Division setting up across the creek on the south side. Unfortunately, the site proved to be anything but ideal.

On July 4 and 5, heavy rains caused Rock Creek to overflow. The water spread out on the lower side of the stream to a depth of about two feet. Those who were mobile desperately tried to assist the incapacitated but were unsuccessful in relocating all the wounded to higher ground, and at least twenty of the Confederate wounded drowned. The death toll would have been even higher had not heroic attendants dragged many patients, screaming in pain, to elevated areas.

In addition to the drownings, more than four hundred men died here of their wounds, of which nearly half were Confederates. Burials took place in four makeshift cemeteries on the farm. The field northeast of the barn and house was used for Union fatalities. To the southwest, between the Schwartz farm buildings and the Lewis Bushman farm, a second field was used for burials from both sides, as was the third cemetery, located on Red Hill above Rock Creek. The fourth cemetery, also used for both Union and Confederate burials, was located along a lane through a cornfield, off what is now Sachs Road.

Only seventeen medical officers were present on a regular basis to treat the more than three thousand wounded, although some civilian doctors did come in from time to time. Five days after the fighting had ceased, nurse Cornelia Hancock wrote a letter to her sister saying, "There is a great want of surgeons here; there are hundreds of brave fellows who have not had their wounds dressed since the battle."[4] She did not exaggerate. A Union officer who had been wounded three times had to wait six days to receive medical attention, except for what minimal help could be provided by friends.

Doctors here included Surgeon A. N. Dougherty (US Volunteers and Second Corps medical director), Surgeon Justin Dwinell (108th Pennsylvania, who was in charge of the hospital), Acting Assistant Surgeon William Hays (US Volunteers), Surgeon Thaddeus Hildreth (Third Maine), Surgeon Jonas W. Lyman (Fifty-Seventh Pennsylvania), Surgeon H. B. Fowler (Twelfth New Hampshire), Surgeon William Warren Porter (Fifty-Seventh New York), Surgeon Pierre D. Peltier (126th New York), Assistant Surgeon Isaac Scott (Seventh West Virginia), Assistant Surgeon W. W. Sharp (140th Pennsylvania), Surgeon Martin Rizer (Seventy-Second Pennsylvania), and Surgeon Fred Wolf (Thirty-Ninth New York). A civilian volunteer, Dr. Bushrod James, arrived from Philadelphia with an abundant supply of badly needed medical supplies and worked until exhaustion. He eventually came down with what was referred to as violent cholera morbus, a gastrointestinal disease, and was forced to return home.

Most civilian doctors, however, were not as conscientious as James, at least in Justin Dwinell's eyes. Dwinell never hesitated to voice his distrust of the skill and dedication of civilian volunteer and contract surgeons, citing them as too "unreliable." He also complained of the hundreds of able-bodied skulkers who invaded these safe areas and who "consume the food and occupy the shelter provided for the wounded."[5]

Hancock was a nurse here, and her letters home are used extensively by historians. A Quaker from New Jersey, she gained the respect of her patients almost immediately despite her lack of medical experience. She had been turned down by Dorothea Dix as a volunteer nurse because she was too young and attractive. Undaunted, she was accepted as a volunteer by the Second Corps. After Gettysburg she volunteered at the Wilderness, Fredericksburg, Port Royal, White House Landing, City Point, and Petersburg and was one of the first Union nurses to arrive in Richmond after its capture. After the war, she opened a school for freed slaves and helped children orphaned after the Johnstown Flood.

Other nurses here, in addition to Mrs. Schwartz and Hancock, included Mrs. Emily Bliss Thatcher Souder of Philadelphia, Jane Boswell Moore, Charlotte McKay, and Clarissa F. Jones, the last of whom attended the fiftieth reunion of the battle and spent time with some of the men she had treated. Catherine Wert, who lived on the nearby Adam Wert farm, also was here, spending much of her time treating wounded Confederates. She was known locally as Aunt Katy, and her patients became especially fond of her for her kindness.

Helen Gilson (age twenty-eight) was another volunteer nurse who was highly thought of for her compassion. Turned down by Dix, probably because of her age and attractive appearance, she was mentioned by both the US Christian Commission and the US Sanitary Commission in their formal reports for the respect the wounded accorded her. Although all the nurses tended to wounds and fed the men, she went beyond the normal expectations. The wounded said she sang to them to calm their fears, read to them, wrote letters for them, and sat with many dying men until they breathed their last. She even was called on to settle arguments. Her calm demeanor also led to her assisting with amputations and conducting religious services.

This hospital was utilized until August 8, 1863, when the last of the wounded here were moved to the Camp Letterman General Hospital.

About a third of a mile southwest, just south of the junction of Rock Creek and White Run, sat the hospital for the Third Corps (39°46.961' N, 77°12.293' W), still on the Jacob Schwartz farm. This hospital also served wounded from the Fifth and Sixth Corps, along with hundreds of wounded Confederate prisoners.

Levi Baker of the Ninth Massachusetts Battery said that the operating table here was simply a barn door placed across two barrels, with amputated legs piled at one end, arms at the other.[6]

Under Surgeon Thaddeus Hildreth (Third Maine Infantry), this camp handled about 2,600 Union wounded and 259 Confederate. It closed its operations on August 8. Other doctors known to have treated wounded here were James T. Calhoun (acting as Third Corps medical director), William Hays (US Volunteers), Surgeon Jonas W. Lyman (Fifty-Seventh Pennsylvania), H. B. Fowler (Twelfth New Hampshire),

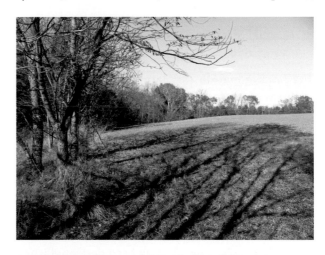

A second hospital was established in these fields on the Schwartz farm to serve the Third Corps, as well as wounded from the Fifth and Sixth Corps.

William Watson (105th Pennsylvania), and Bushrod James, a civilian contractor with the US Christian Commission, previously mentioned. The Third Corps medical director, Thomas Sim, would ordinarily have been present but had left to accompany General Daniel Sickles, who had lost a leg, to Washington.

The medical staff was shorthanded the entire time. Watson said he was assigned with seven other doctors to provide treatment for 813 wounded and 100 captured Confederates, who were "in a most distressing condition." He indicated, "The mortality among the wounded is fearful—caused principally by Gangrene, Erysipelas, Tetanus and Secondary Hemorrhage. Our secondary operations have been very unfavorable. Most of the cases die." (Erysipelas is a serious infection of the skin.) Watson said that he performed fourteen operations without a break, and that by July 7 he had performed more than fifty amputations.[7]

4. Daniel Sheaffer Farm, 2159 Baltimore Pike, 39°47.676' N, 77°11.764' W

The brick home on this farm was built in 1791 by Nicholas Mark and was owned by sixty-one-year-old Daniel Sheaffer, who lived here with his wife, Lydia, and several children. Sheaffer had purchased the farm in 1845. Under the advisement of Federal officers, he left with his family during the battle.

In 1863 the farm consisted of about sixty-nine acres, although it is smaller today. The original barn was a double log structure (now gone), and Sheaffer operated a small sawmill located on White Run, although it is also gone, having been destroyed when White Run overflowed its banks years later. The wounded were treated in the house, barn, and out-

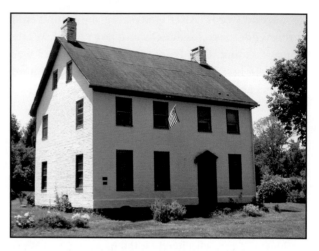

The Sheaffer farm included a small sawmill that provided lumber to be built into coffins during the battle.

buildings.[8] Lumber from the sawmill was purportedly used to make coffins for Union dead.

Sheaffer's farm was the site of a hospital for soldiers from the Union's Third and Twelfth Corps. Amputations were performed in the barnyard, and the house still contains bloodstains on the floors, as well as holes drilled into the floors to allow the blood to drain to the cellar.

The Sheaffer farm is one of many locations that claim to be the site of the amputation of General Daniel Sickles's leg. Of all the field hospitals that make this claim, the Sheaffer farm arguably presents the best case.

Mrs. Sheaffer noted in her damage claim that Sickles had his leg amputated here on July 2 and stayed overnight, and the National Register of Historic Places agrees that there is evidence to support that claim. Also, neighbor J. Howard Wert, who provided documented information about the battlefield and the environs, insisted that the leg was amputated here. Sickles himself did not provide much information to resolve the controversy, saying only that the leg was removed by Dr. James T. Calhoun at "the field hospital on Baltimore Pike."

Wherever the leg was amputated, the flamboyant Sickles ordered that it be preserved and the shattered bones donated to the Army Medical Museum in Washington. He made a point to visit his bones each time he went to Washington.

Sickles received the Medal of Honor for conspicuous gallantry on the field. He also served as a congressman after the war and was instrumental in gaining national park recognition for the battlefield, introducing the bill to Congress that was approved in 1895 to establish the Gettysburg National Military Park.

As so many citizens did, Sheaffer collected a great deal of material left on the battlefield. When authorities inspected the farm, they found three hundred shirts and drawers, fifty blankets, twenty-eight guns, and artillery harnesses, all concealed in a well and in four large sinks that had been filled with water. The guns had been hidden under piles of boards at the sawmill, along a fence, and in the garret of the house.

5. White Church (a.k.a. Mark's German Reformed Church), 5 White Church Road at Baltimore Pike, 39°47.517' N, 77°11.525' W

Founded in 1789, the church served as a hospital for the Union First Corps and a medical headquarters for its First Division. The church was named for Nicholas Mark, who donated the land for the church. In 1863, the building was constructed of hewn logs, with weatherboard on the outside and plastered walls on

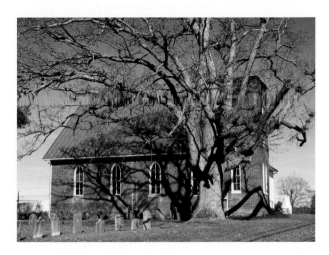

The church's central location along Baltimore Pike made it a logical site for a hospital, medical supply depot, and prisoner-of-war holding area.

the inside. It had no steeple, and locally it was called the White Church. The current brick church stands on the site of the original church.

The area around the church also served a number of additional functions beyond being a hospital. Dr. John Brinton established a temporary medical department supply depot that served the corps hospitals in the surrounding area, and a prisoner holding pen was set up in an open field adjacent to the church. The church and the Isaac Lightner farm, located a short distance farther out the Baltimore Pike, were both supervised by General Marsena Patrick, and the two hospitals combined to serve 1,229 wounded, including several hundred Confederates.

Wounded filled the church, as well as the surrounding yard. An amputating table, made from one of the church's doors, was set up in the front yard. Other tables were pressed into service as beds. Pews were removed and cut up to make bunks, and hay and lumber were brought from the nearby Isaac Lightner farm to use as bedding.

The Philadelphia *Daily Evening Bulletin* reported that the fighting had been so fierce that many of the wounded had their clothing torn from them in the battle. What little clothing they had left was usually so covered with blood and dust that doctors removed it, leaving the men totally naked. The newspaper said that female nurses could not go into certain areas around the church because of this.[9]

George W. Ramsey (Ninety-Fifth New York) was the surgeon in charge. Other doctors here were Andrew J. Ward (First Corps surgeon) and George W. New (Seventh Indiana). Henry Marsh, hospital steward for the Nineteenth Indiana, and Elmina K. Spencer, a civilian volunteer, provided nursing assistance to the wounded.

There were at least two Confederate burials in the church cemetery. One was a soldier from the Second North Carolina named Gates; the other was Private Edgar Hammond from the First Maryland Battalion.[10]

6. First Corps Hospital Tablet, White Church Road, 39°47.333' N, 77°11.983' W

This area is referred to as the Rock Creek/White Run Union Hospital Complex, and it represents the largest cluster of corps hospitals associated with the battle. Nearly ten thousand were treated within the boundaries of the complex.

There were thirteen hospital sites (see individual sites for more information) within this complex: the Jacob Schwartz farm (two sites), the Daniel Sheaffer farm, the John Trostle farm, the Lewis Bushman farm, the Michael Diener farm, the Peter Conover farm, the

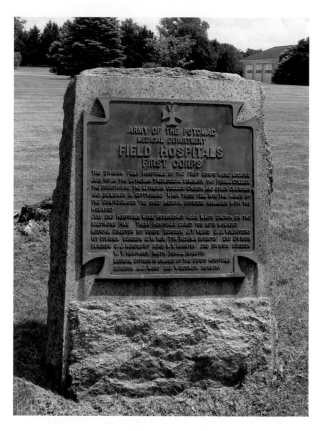

First Corps Hospital Tablet. The corps suffered a casualty rate of 36 percent at Gettysburg.

Isaac Lightner farm, the Henry Beitler farm, Mark's German Reformed Church, the Jane Clapsaddle place, the George Bushman farm, and an unnamed property between the Daniel Sheaffer farm and Mark's Church (once part of the Sheaffer farm). Although the Michael Fiscel farm lies within the boundaries of this complex, it is not considered part of the National Register of Historic Places with the other thirteen because none of the original site remains.[11] The hospitals were placed here because the hilly terrain offered protection, they were distant from the combat area and the artillery zone, and there was an abundance of good water from Rock Creek and White Run.

The first caption on this tablet reads,

**National Register with Medical Department
Field Hospitals
First Corps**

The Division Field Hospitals of the First Corps were located July 1st at the Lutheran Theological Seminary, the Penna. College, the Courthouse, and other churches and buildings in Gettysburg. When these fell into the hands of the Confederates the chief medical officers remained with the wounded.

July 2nd Hospitals were established near White Church on the Baltimore Pike. These Hospitals cared for 2379 wounded.

Medical Director 1st Corps, Surgeon J.T. Heard,
U.S. Volunteers
1st Division, Surgeon G.W. New, 7th Indiana
Infantry
2nd Division, Surgeon C.J. Nordquist, 83rd N.Y.
Infantry
3rd Division Surgeon, W.T. Humphrey, 149th
Penna. Infantry
Medical Officer in charge of the Corps Hospitals,
Surgeon A.J. Ward, 2nd Wisconsin Infantry

Other doctors who served in First Corps hospitals include Surgeon George W. Ramsey (Ninety-Fifth New York), Assistant Surgeon Lucretius Ross (Fourteenth Vermont), Assistant Surgeon George W. Towar

(Twenty-Fourth Michigan), Surgeon A. T. Woodward (surgeon in charge, Third Division, First Corps), Surgeon William B. Chambers (surgeon in charge, Second Division, First Corps), Assistant Surgeon Simon C. Place (147th New York), Surgeon Abram William Preston (Sixth Wisconsin), and Surgeon Charles E. Humphrey (142nd Pennsylvania).

The three divisions of the First Corps had 3,231 casualties out of about 9,000 engaged, or about 36 percent. The First Division placed its men around Mark's German Reformed Church (the White Church), and on the farm of Barbara and Isaac Lightner; the Second Division set up on Peter and Ellen Conover's farm; and the Third Division lay on the Jonathan Young property.

7. Jane Clapsaddle Farm, 307 White Church Road, 39°47.001' N, 77°11.659' W

This small, twenty-two-acre farm was the home of forty-one-year-old Jane Clapsaddle, widow of Jesse, who had died in 1858 at age forty-three. She would later marry her second husband, Civil War veteran Andrew Bender. Clapsaddle lived on this farm with her three children, Amanda (twenty years old), George (seventeen), and Jacob (fifteen). Three other children had died young. Eight months after the fighting at Gettysburg, her son George would enlist in the Twenty-First Pennsylvania Cavalry and be captured at Cold Harbor in June 1864. He would die of typhoid fever seven weeks later at age seventeen. The farm became the hospital for the Second Division, Fifth Corps, after the wounded were moved from the Jacob Weikert farm, located on the Taneytown Road, on July 3.

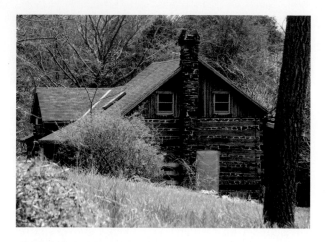

About eight hundred were treated on this small farm owned by Jane Clapsaddle.

The original log house was built in the mid-nineteenth century, and only a small portion remains. It has been incorporated into the newer sections of the house. The wounded were sheltered in the house, barn, and outbuildings until August 2, when they were moved to Camp Letterman. About eight hundred were treated here.

Dr. Augustus M. Clark, medical officer in charge of all the Fifth Corps hospitals, spent some of his time on the Clapsaddle farm.

Jane Clapsaddle died in 1906 and was buried in the White Church cemetery.

8. Michael Fiscel Farm Site, 835 Goulden Road, 39°46.815' N, 77°12.038' W

At the time of the battle, this golf course was the farm of Michael and Matilda Fiscel. In July 1863 it became the hospital for the Union Fifth Corps after the hospital relocated from the Jacob Weikert farm. It also served a handful of wounded from the Third and Sixth Corps. Most of the Fifth Corps wounded arrived from the second day of fighting and were placed in the house and barn, which held the most severely wounded. The current house on the property is not original, and all of the other original buildings are long gone.

Michael was forty-one years old; Matilda was thirty-seven. The couple had eight children living with them at the time of the battle. The farm, although a prominent hospital, was not included in the National Register of Historic Places for the Rock Creek/White Run Union Hospital Complex because nothing remains of the original site and the landscape has been significantly altered in the construction of the golf course.

Some eight hundred wounded were treated here, only a portion of whom could be accommodated in

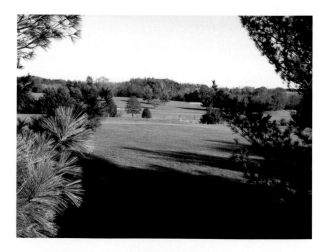

Now a golf course, the Fiscel farm became a hospital for the Union Fifth Corps.

the house and barn. Tents and other shelters arrived to house the others, though overcrowding forced many to lie side by side in the yard with no protection from the weather until they could be moved.

Eleven surgeons were here to treat the wounded, including Surgeon John J. Milhau (Fifth Corps medical director), Augustus M. Clark (medical officer in charge of all the Fifth Corps hospitals), Cyrus Bacon (US Regulars), William H. True (Eighty-Third Pennsylvania), Thaddeus Hildreth (Third Maine Infantry), Jared Free (Eighty-Third Pennsylvania), Dr. Porter (Fifth Corps), Dr. Von Teague (a civilian doctor from Philadelphia), and three others. Treatment took place around the clock, and Bacon reportedly became so exhausted that he fell asleep on the operating table.

There were at least 186 burials on the farm, including 12 Confederate ones. Prominent among the Confederate burials was that of First Lieutenant John Oates of the Fifteenth Alabama, brother of Colonel William Oates, who led the attack against the Twentieth Maine on Little Round Top on July 2. John Oates was wounded seven times in the hips and legs, and he died of pyemia (septicemia) on July 25. Others were from Cobb's Georgia Infantry Legion, the Fourteenth Alabama, the Fifteenth Alabama, the Fifth Texas, and the Sixteenth Georgia. The burials took place east of the barn in a small field overlooking a stream. Witnesses said the graves were so shallow that they often gave off an eerie phosphorescent light at night.

9. Fifth Corps Hospital Tablet, Goulden Road, 39°46.962' N, 77°12.120' W

The Fifth Corps hospital was initially located at the Jacob Weikert farm on Taneytown Road. It was moved on July 3 to the Michael Fiscel farm.

The inscription on the tablet reads,

Army of the Potomac
Medical Department
Field Hospitals
Fifth Corps

The Division Field Hospitals of the Fifth Corps were established July 2nd at the Weikert House and other

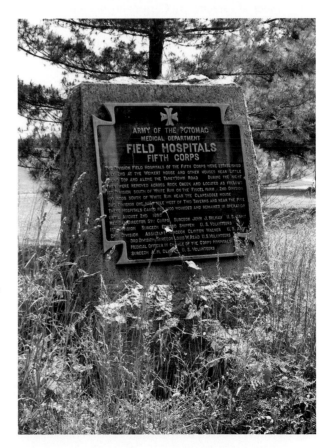

Fifth Corps Hospital Tablet. There were at least 186 burials at this hospital, including twelve Confederates.

houses near Little Round Top and along the Taney-town Road. During the night they were removed across Rock Creek and located as follows: 1st Division south of White Run on the Fiscel Farm. 2nd Division 100 rods south of White Run near the Clapsaddle House. 3rd Division one half mile west of Two Taverns and near the Pike. These Hospitals cared for 1400 wounded and remained in operation until August 2nd 1863.

Medical Director 5th Corps, Surgeon John J. Milhau, U.S. Army
1st Division, Surgeon Edward Shippen, U.S. Volunteers
2nd Division, Assistant Surgeon, Clinton Wagner, U.S. Army
3rd Division, Surgeon Louis W. Read, U.S. Volunteers
Medical Officer in charge of the Corps Hospitals, Surgeon A.M. Clark, U.S. Volunteers

Other doctors who served in Fifth Corps hospitals, in addition to those shown on the plaque, include Dr. Cotton (regiment unknown), Dr. Porter (surgeon, Fifth Corps), Assistant Surgeon Robert A. Everett (Sixteenth Michigan), Jared Free (Eighty-Third Pennsylvania), John Kollock (118th Pennsylvania), Surgeon J. A. E. Reed (155th Pennsylvania), Surgeon Benjamin Roher (Tenth Pennsylvania Reserves), and Assistant Surgeon W. Stockton Wilson (155th Pennsylvania).

10. Third Corps Hospital Tablet, Goulden Road, 39°46.946' N, 77°12.295' W

Although shown on the tablet as the Third Corps medical director, Surgeon Thomas Sim was not present after July 1. He was ordered to accompany corps commander General Daniel Sickles, who had been badly wounded on the Abraham Trostle farm, to Washington.

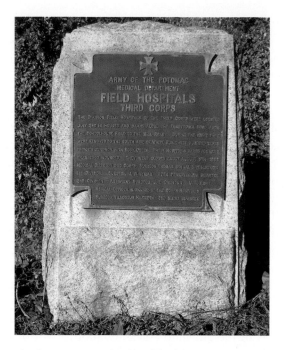

Third Corps Hospital Tablet. The large hospital sat just north of the tablet, with 10 percent of those treated being wounded Confederates.

Under Surgeon Thaddeus Hildreth, the Third Corps hospital handled about 2,500 Union wounded and 259 Confederates, and closed its operation on August 8. One division there reported 813 casualties; of these there were ninety-seven operations performed, with fifty-three being amputations.

The inscription on the tablet reads,

Army of the Potomac
Medical Department
Field Hospitals
Third Corps

The Division Field Hospitals of the Third Corps were located July 2nd in houses and barns along the Taneytown Road from the Schoolhouse Road to the Mill Road. During the night they were removed to the south side of White Run three hundred yards from its junction with Rock Creek. These Hospitals cared for more than 2500 wounded. They were closed about August 6th 1863.

Medical Director 3rd Corps, Surgeon Thomas Sim, U.S. Volunteers
1st Division, Surgeon J.W. Lyman, 57th Pennsylvania Infantry
2nd Division, Assistant Surgeon J.T. Calhoun, U.S. Army
Medical Officer in charge of the Corps Hospitals, Surgeon Thaddeus Hildreth, 3rd Maine Infantry

Doctors who served in the Third Corps hospitals, in addition to those shown on plaque, included Surgeon H. B. Fowler (Twelfth New Hampshire), John H. Love (Thirteenth New Jersey), Assistant Surgeon Albion Cobb (Fourth Maine), Assistant Surgeon Charles W. Hunt (Twelfth New Hampshire), Surgeon Nahum A. Hursam (Seventeenth Maine), Surgeon Robert V. K. Montfort (124th New York), Assistant Surgeon John H. Sanborn (Twelfth New Hampshire), Surgeon John H. Thompson (124th New York), Assistant Surgeon William Wescott (Seventeenth Maine), and Assistant Surgeon Samuel C. Whittier (Eleventh Massachusetts).

11.   Sixth Corps Hospital Tablet, Goulden Road, 39°46.887' N, 77°12.383' W

Used sparingly at Gettysburg, the Sixth Corps could be considered the most fortunate corps to take part in the battle. Its medical director, Charles O'Leary,

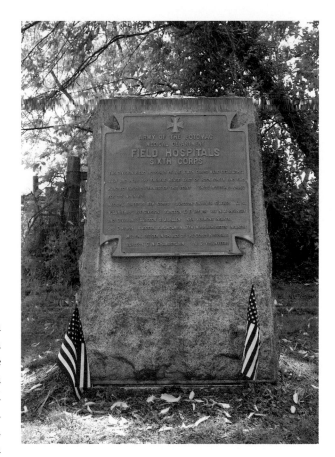

Sixth Corps Hospital Tablet. The corps was used sparingly in the battle and suffered relatively few casualties.

assigned Dr. C. N. Chamberlain to manage the corps hospitals, which treated only about 315 wounded.

The Sixth Corps had undertaken a forced march of thirty-two miles to get to Gettysburg, after covering one hundred miles in the four previous days. Many of the corps's infantrymen were thoroughly exhausted by the time they reached Gettysburg, and being held in reserve was a welcome respite. Since it was not heavily engaged, the corps suffered only twenty-seven killed, 185 wounded, and thirty missing.

The inscription on the tablet, which sits at the entrance to the John Trostle farm, reads,

Army of the Potomac
Medical Department
Field Hospitals
Sixth Corps

The Division Field Hospitals of the Sixth Corps were established July 2nd near the Trostle House east of Rock Creek and two hundred yards southwest of this point. These Hospitals cared for 315 wounded.

Medical Director 6th Corps, Surgeon Charles O'Leary, U.S. Volunteers
1st Division, Surgeon E.F. Taylor, 1st N.J. Infantry
2nd Division, Surgeon S.J. Allen, 4th Vermont Infantry
3rd Division, Surgeon S.A. Holman, 7th Massachusetts Infantry
Medical Officer in charge of the Corps Hospitals, Surgeon C.N. Chamberlain, U.S Volunteers

Other doctors known to have served with the Sixth Corps included Surgeon George T. Stevens (Seventy-Seventh New York), and Surgeon Augustus M. Clark (US Volunteers). All served at the John Trostle farm.

12. John Trostle Farm, White Church Road, 39°46.838' N, 77°12.378' W

Often referred to as the Michael Trostle farm, the farm was actually owned by John Trostle, Michael's son, during the battle. John (thirty-five years old) and

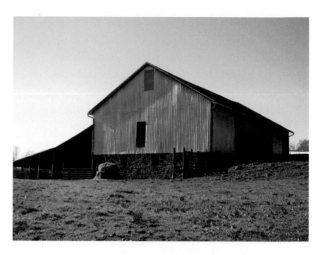

Temperatures inside the barn became so oppressive that the wounded had to be moved outside.

Suzannah (thirty-one) and their two children lived on the sixteen-acre property that became the Sixth Corps field hospital during the battle.

The house is now sided but is thought to be log construction with a stone extension. It is now two stories high but was probably only one story at the time of the battle.

Casualties were relatively light in the Sixth Corps, allowing the farm to also treat overflow from the hospitals of the Second, Third, and Fifth Corps, as well as a few wounded Confederates. The low number of wounded here meant that conditions were good, overcrowding was nonexistent, and all the wounded could be cared for in the house, barn, outbuildings, and a few tents. None of the wounded were exposed to the elements, with one exception: those in the barn eventually were moved outside onto the hill behind the barn when the heat became too oppressive inside.

Only about 315 Union men were treated here, and possibly a dozen Confederates. Still, there were seventy burials on the property, including eleven Southerners. The burials took place north of the barn in an area known as "Walnut Row.

Doctors known to have served at the Trostle farm included Surgeon Charles O'Leary (US Volunteers and medical director for the Sixth Corps), Surgeon C. N. Chamberlain (US Volunteers and medical officer in charge of the Sixth Corps hospitals), Surgeon E. F. Taylor (First New Jersey), Surgeon S. J. Allen (Fourth Vermont), Surgeon Silas A. Holman (Seventh Massachusetts), Surgeon George T. Stevens (Seventy-Seventh New York), Surgeon E. F. Taylor First New Jersey), and Surgeon Augustus M. Clark (US Volunteers). Chamberlain also served as the embalmer at this hospital.

The Sixth Corps hospital closed in early August 1863.

13. Rodkey-Diener (Dener) Farm, 491 Sachs Road, 39°47.083' N, 77°12.850' W

Also known today as the Sachs farm, a house was built on this property in 1857 by John Rodkey. The barn on the farm is believed to predate the house. Rodkey sold the farm to Henry Beitler in 1859, and although Beitler owned the property during the battle, it was occupied by tenant Michael Diener.

The house is two stories tall with three bays, and the house, barn, and surrounding grounds served as an aid station for the Fifth Corps.[12] The property contained fifty-nine acres, and there are bloodstains on the upstairs floors.

There was at least one burial here, a Confederate buried on the south side of the house at the corner

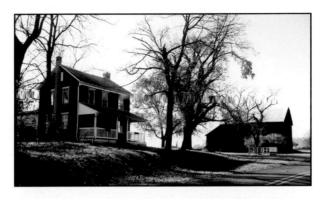

The Rodkey-Diener farm served as a hospital for the Union Fifth Corps.

of the woods. Sometime in the 1940s another set of remains was found on the farm.

In 1951 the farm was purchased by the Sachs family, whose descendants still own the property at the time of this writing.

14. Lewis Bushman Farm, 489 Sachs Road, 39°47.084' N, 77°13.025' W

Lewis Adolphus Bushman (age thirty) lived on this farm with his wife, Caroline (age twenty-nine), and their son George (age two). Their first son, Harry, had died at the age of two just three years before the fighting at Gettysburg. George would live until 1918, when he was murdered by Clarence Collins and Charles Reinecker.[13]

The farm was used by the First Division of the Union Fifth Corps as a field hospital. The current house is a replacement for the original house, which sat several hundred feet to the east of the present structure. The present barn is believed to have been here during the

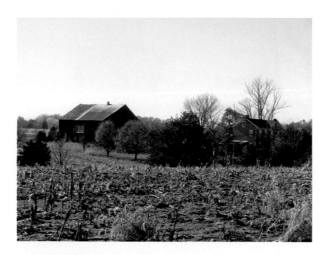

The First Division, Fifth Corps, moved here to the Lewis Bushman farm when artillery fire became too intense to remain at the Jacob Weikert farm.

battle. The Fifth Corps came here when it was forced to leave the Jacob Weikert farm on July 3 when artillery rounds began striking there.

When the move was made from the Weikert farm, the bodies of General Stephen Weed and Colonel Patrick O'Rorke (140th New York) were moved to the Lewis Bushman farm. Here, they were temporarily buried by Sergeant Major James Campbell and Lieutenant William Crennell, both of the 140th Pennsylvania. Crennell had served as an aide to Weed during the battle, and Weed had uttered his famous quote, "By sundown I will be as dead as Julius Caesar," to Crennell when he was mortally wounded on Little Round Top. Weed and O'Rorke were buried behind the Bushman house near an apple tree. Campbell and Crennell marked the spot in the event the families wished to recover the bodies. O'Rorke's widow came to Gettysburg a short time later and did just that,

taking her husband's body to Rochester, New York, for final burial. Weed's body was eventually reburied on Long Island.

Also brought here were two officers who had been mortally wounded, Colonel George Willard of the 125th New York and Colonel Strong Vincent of the Eighty-Third Pennsylvania. Both were destined to die on the Bushman farm.

Caroline Bushman, pregnant at the time of the battle, gave birth to a son two months later. She and Lewis named the baby Strong Vincent Bushman.

Doctors here included James P. Burchfield (Eighty-Third Pennsylvania Volunteers) who took care of Vincent here; Henry C. Dean (140th New York); and Assistant Surgeon Mathias L. Lord (140th New York).

15. Isaac Lightner Farm, 2350 Baltimore Pike, 39°47.464' N, 77°11.369' W

Fifty-three-year-old Isaac Lightner and his wife, Barbara (age fifty-four), lived on this 115-acre farm along Baltimore Pike. Also living with Isaac and Barbara in 1860 were their children Elizabeth (twenty-four), Sarah (twenty-two), David (twenty), Barbara (eighteen), Amanda (sixteen), William (fourteen), and Isaac N. (twelve), although it is not known whether all of them were still there in 1863; the ages shown are what they would have been at the time of the battle. Three white convicts (Jacob Stover, whose occupation was listed as shoemaker; James Shildt; and Henry Craig) and two black prisoners (Jacob Jones and Weldon Singleton) were also shown on the census as living in the home in 1860, with no explanation of why they were there.[14] There is also no explanation for the designations of the white men as convicts and the

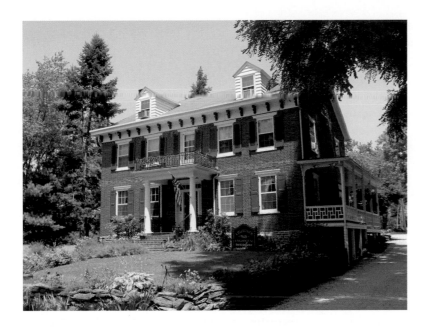

Contrary to the hospital sign at the entrance, the Lightner farm was primarily a First Corps hospital, rather than one for the Eleventh Corps.

black men as prisoners. All five may have been gone from the home before 1863. The family had moved out to the barn during the fighting. When they returned to their house, they found the stench so bad that they could no longer live there.

Lightner had served as the sheriff of Adams County from 1857 to 1860, and their house was new, having been completed less than a year before the battle. The house is still there, as is the original stone beehive oven. The original barn, which sat on the north side of the house and was used to house wounded, was in poor condition and razed around 1970. The barn had sat behind the house and was filled with wounded.

In his damage claim, Lightner said all his buildings were used to treat the wounded from the First Corps, although the sign at the entrance says it was an Eleventh Corps hospital. He said there were many tents set up around the house to allow for more men to be treated. His claim for $1,465.07 was for the loss of hay that had been confiscated and taken to White Church for bedding, shingles and boards that were used for crutches and coffins, and burned fence rails.[15] The farm was used as a hospital until July 20.

One of the wounded was Private John F. Chase of the Fifth Maine Artillery. During the fighting with his battery on Stevens's Knoll, Chase was horribly wounded by shrapnel from an exploding case shot. His forty-eight entry wounds were believed to be mortal and thus were not dressed for three days. It was several more days after that when he was moved from the barn to the house. Chase was eventually relocated to the hospital at the Lutheran Seminary, where he recovered.

Doctors here included Surgeon C. J. Nordquist (Eighty-Third New York) and Surgeon Andrew J. Ward (Second Wisconsin). Barbara Lightner and the adult children served as nurses.

The farm has been reduced to nineteen acres today.

16. Peter Conover Farm, Baltimore Pike, 39°47.198' N, 77°11.268' W

The wounded from General George Stannard's Second Vermont Brigade and General Gabriel Paul's Brigade were probably treated on this farm occupied by Peter and Ellen Conover and their five children. A small number of Confederates were also treated here. Witnesses describe seeing desperate men crawling into the barn while the cattle were still there. When they were discovered, they were moved to a nearby log structure and placed on clean straw.

The farm currently occupies 111 acres, and the four-bay bank barn's cornerstone shows that the structure was built in 1859. The house is postwar.

The surgeon here was Andrew J. Ward, who was in charge of the First Corps hospitals.

There were eleven burials recorded on the property. The names of the seven Federal troops buried here were not recorded, but Dr. John W. C. O'Neal did record the four Confederate names: Jacob McGrady (Thirty-Seventh North Carolina); another North Carolina soldier named Scrabbs; Lieutenant J. P. Mims (Eleventh Mississippi), who was wounded on July 3 and died on July 9; and Robert Wooden (Forty-Seventh North Carolina).[16]

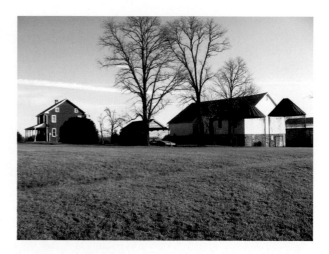

Desperate men, badly wounded, crawled into the Conover barn and took shelter among the cows.

According to an army voucher dated July 4, 1863, Conover sold the government seventy-five gallons of milk and 510 pounds of meat to feed the wounded in the hospital on his farm. He later filed a damage claim for $60.20 to cover his costs, raising the ire of his neighbors who had donated similar items.[17]

17. Henry Beitler Farm, Baltimore Pike, 39°47.307' N, 77°10.453' W

Henry Beitler, twenty-eight years old; his wife, Matilda (twenty-six); and their two small children lived on this twenty-four-acre farm during the battle but were forced to leave for their own safety. They fled to Littlestown, where they stayed with friends, leaving the house vacant. The Beitlers also had two young children who had died in 1860, three-year-old

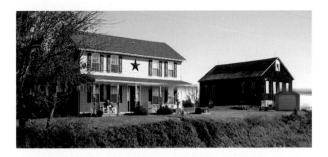

Amputations at Beitler's took place in the wagon shed, with the severed limbs placed in a corncrib before being hauled off in wagons.

John Edward and infant William, who only lived a few weeks.

The farm's farmhouse, barn, barnyard, and outbuildings were used for the wounded. Amputations took place in the wagon shed, with the severed limbs placed in a corncrib before being hauled off in wagons. The farm also served as an encampment for Hall's Fifth Maine Battery on July 1 and 2, and for General Alfred Pleasonton's headquarters on July 2 and 3.[18] There was at least one burial here, a soldier from the Fifth Maine Battery. A small store was said to also operate on the site.

Elizabeth Thorne arrived here on July 3 and said the house was filled with wounded and sick soldiers. It was here that she first learned of the death of Jennie Wade, who became the only civilian to be killed in the battle when she was struck by an errant sniper's shot while baking bread at her sister's house.

Henry Beitler filed a damage claim in the amount of $1,050.15 for loss of wheat, grass, hay, corn, three head of cattle, bees and honey, tools, buggy cushions and shafts, bedding, two broken rifles, clothing, flour, salt, boards, a copper kettle, a looking glass, and furniture, as well as fence and land damage. Unfortunately, he never received any compensation for his losses and died in 1867.[19]

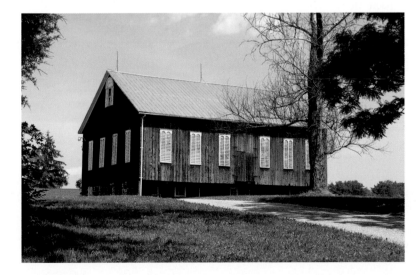

The Beitler barnyard was pressed into service as a hospital when all the farm's buildings became full.

18. Samuel Durboraw Farm, Two Taverns Road, 39°47.713' N, 77°9.635' W

Formerly known as the Baubalitz farm, this property was occupied by Samuel Durboraw, a sixty-three-year-old former state legislator, with his third wife, Mary R., age forty-four, and four of his five living children. (His son Isaac was serving with the Union army.) Durboraw's first wife, Hannah, had died in 1832 at age thirty-two, and his second wife, Mary J., had died in 1849 at age thirty-seven. He also had lost his sixth child, who had died in 1861 at age two.[20]

On July 2 Samuel's son Isaac had been fighting in the Wheatfield with Company K of the First Pennsylvania Reserves as Sergeant Isaac Newton Durboraw. Isaac was able to get away for a few hours and visited his family's farm. When he arrived, he found the house filled with wounded soldiers, one of whom was Brigadier General Solomon Meredith, commander of the famous Iron Brigade. Not wishing to disturb the wounded man lying in his bed, Isaac slept on the floor.

The house is the original wartime structure, while the barn is a replacement of the one that stood here in 1863. At the time, Durboraw's farm was made up of one hundred acres of tillable land.

There were two Confederate burials on the Durboraw property: Chester Farmer of the Fourteenth Virginia, who was identified only by his initials, CHF, when he was buried, and John R. Gibson of the Twenty-Second Georgia, who was wounded in the left shoulder on July 3 and lingered until July 14 or 15. Both these burials are also shown as having taken place on the Jonathan Young farm, an indication of the chaotic record keeping in the heat of war.[21]

19. Jesse Worley Farm, Barlow-Two Taverns Road, 39°46.315' N, 77°10.453' W

Many of the original buildings on the Jesse Worley farm are still in use, and the farm remains in a good state of repair. The owners at the time of the battle were thirty-three-year-old Jesse Worley and his wife,

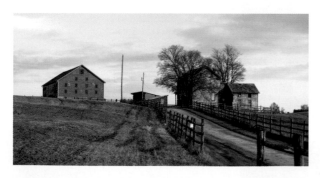

Durboraw's son Isaac Newton Durboraw was serving with the First Pennsylvania Reserves. After fighting on July 2, Isaac was able to visit his home that evening.

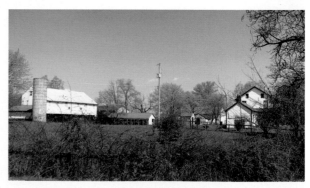

Although the Worley farm was a field hospital for the Union Fifth Corps, more Confederates than Union were buried on it.

Ann, also thirty-three. Their three small children were also living with them on the farm, which served as a field hospital for the Third Division of the Pennsylvania Reserves, Fifth Corps. About 181 wounded from both armies were treated here.

Dr. Alexander Clarke (US Volunteers) served as medical officer in charge of all the corps hospitals, and the medical director of the corps was Surgeon John J. Milhau. Neither of them spent any appreciable time on the Worley farm. However, Dr. W. W. L. Phillips (First New Jersey Cavalry) and Surgeon Louis W. Read (US Volunteers) both remained with the wounded from the time they were brought to the Worley farm on July 2 until they were moved to Camp Letterman.

There were at least six, and possibly seven, known Confederate burials on the Worley farm. William Sensabaugh of the Fifth Texas was shot in the left thigh and had his leg amputated. He survived until July 21, when he was buried but incorrectly identified as William Sensalman. Also from the Fifth Texas was J. J. Galluper, who may actually have been John Goldsticker. He was shot in the left thigh and had the leg amputated on the southwest slope of Little Round Top the night of July 2. Brought to Worley's, he died on July 15. James L. Gould of the Fourth Texas also had a leg amputated after he was captured. He died on July 8. John Booth, Fifth Texas, died on July 10 after being shot in the head and side. A sixth Texan, John Greene of the Fourth Texas, was shot in the right side of his chest on July 2. He died on July 13. A member of the Fifth Texas, William Nelms was shot in the right thigh on July 2 and died on July 9.[22]

Burial records for the Worley farm indicate seventeen Federal burials. Two of the Union soldiers, Private Andrew J. Pettygrew (Fortieth Pennsylvania) and Private John Lusk (Thirtieth Pennsylvania) were

identified. Pettygrew was wounded on July 2 and died from his wounds on July 13 following amputation of his right leg. Lusk had been wounded on July 3 and survived until July 11.[23]

20. Alexander Schwartz Farm, Unnamed Road, 39°46.608' N, 77°11.306' W

Little is known about this farm, including the exact location. The farm was described as being about one mile south-southeast of White Church and about the same distance southwest of Two Taverns. Plotting that information on a modern map leads directly to a farm at this location, although there is no way to plot the location with a high degree of accuracy based on the limited description available. If this is not the site, however, it must be nearby.

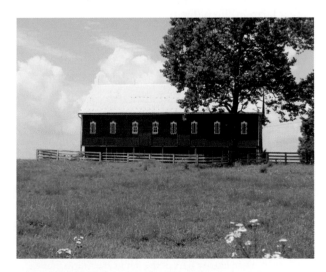

This modern farm may sit on the site of the Alexander Schwartz farm.

Alexander Schwartz purchased the property shortly after Christmas 1862, and he said that his farm became a hospital for about six weeks. It was probably not very large and may have been better called an aid station. Considering the geographic location, it would have served Union troops.

21. James Barr Farm, Krug Road, 39°44.937' N, 77°10.020' W

Another farm whose location is difficult to pinpoint is this farm, often identified as the J. Bair or J. Barr farm. The farm was said to have been two miles south of Two Taverns. Plotting that distance on a modern map of the area, much as was done for the Alexander Schwartz farm, puts it at these GPS coordinates, just east of the intersection of Krug Road with Hoffman Home Road. An 1863 map of Adams County does indicate a farm in the name of J. Barr at this approximate

location, and there was a James Barr on the tax roll at the time, so it is a good guess that this was the site of the farm in question.

Forty-nine-year-old James Barr and his thirty-nine-year-old wife, Elizabeth, lived on 261 acres here, and there were five known Federal burials. It was used primarily by the First Brigade, First Division, First Corps, although there may have been some wounded from the Third Corps treated here as well.

X. Jonathan (Jesse) Young Farm, Baltimore Pike Area, Location Not Identified at Request of Owner

This farm is not shown on the accompanying map, nor is an address or GPS coordinates provided, because the current owner has specifically requested that we refrain from identifying the farm's location.

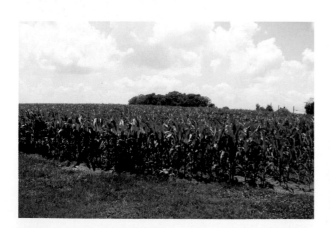

These fields were likely a part of the James Barr farm in 1863.

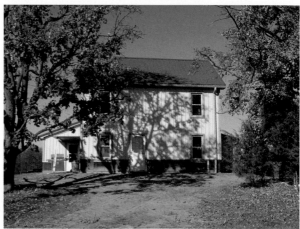

The Union Third Division, First Corps, established a hospital on the Young farm, where a large meteorite would be found in 1887.

The Union's Third Division, First Corps, set up on the Jonathan Young property. The original farmhouse, which dated back to the pre-1800s, is gone, although the remains of the foundation can still be found on the property. The house that currently sits on the farm is the one that sat here during the battle. The farm totaled 124 acres in 1863.

Chester M. Farmer (Fourteenth Virginia) had been wounded in the left shoulder on July 3 in Pickett's Charge. He died on July 10 and was buried in a grave marked only as CHF. John R. Gibson (Twenty-Second Georgia) was wounded the same day as Farmer and died on either July 14 or 15. Their exact burial sites are no longer known, as they are also shown as being buried on the Samuel Durboraw farm.

In 1887 Jacob Snyder discovered what would become known as the Mount Joy meteorite as he dug a hole to plant an apple tree nearby. Weighing 874 pounds, it was one of the largest meteorites ever found in North America; it is now on display in the Vienna Museum of Natural History, Austria.

Nearly 1,300 men were cared for on this farm. It is not known how many died, although the regimental history of the 151st Pennsylvania notes that at least one of their members, forty-four-year-old Private Jacob Zimmerman, was buried here.[24] Records kept by the current owner of the property indicate that there were seven Federal burials here. The current owner also has records showing that at least one horse drowned in the farm's pond, which is still in use.

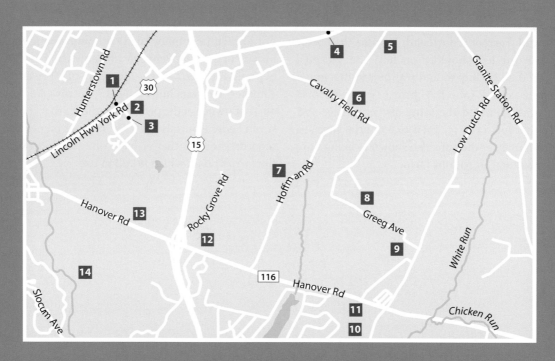

Chapter 10 sites: York Road/Hanover Road area. (Map by Bill Nelson)

1. US Sanitary Commission Lodge Site, 1060 York Road, 39°50.443' N, 77°12.498' W

Created at the beginning of the war to provide services to soldiers that were not provided by the government, the US Sanitary Commission played a very active role at Gettysburg, providing medical supplies and services, meals, and various other things to make the life of a soldier somewhat more bearable. A precursor to today's American Red Cross, its functions were much the same.

Trains full of wounded men began leaving Gettysburg twice a day, bound for the general hospital facilities of larger cities. The number of wounded requiring transport soon overwhelmed the ability to move them, and the Sanitary Commission stepped in to establish facilities to provide some relief for those left behind. Two relief lodges were erected, one at the railroad station and one at this site. Patients discharged from Camp Letterman General Hospital on the south side of the York Road were brought to the lodge, where they were prepared for transportation by rail to permanent hospitals in Philadelphia, New York, and Alexandria, Virginia.

This lodge consisted of two large tents capable of holding seventy-five men each, plus a field kitchen. A Dr. Hooper was placed in charge. The lodge provided

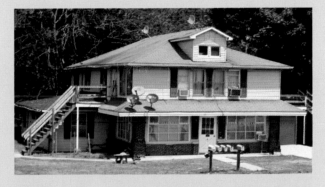

The US Sanitary Commission established a relief lodge on this site, preparing wounded for transport to larger general hospitals.

the essentials patients needed while awaiting transportation, such as food, beds, and medical treatment. A government surgeon remained on hand to oversee treatment and the moving of the wounded into the trains for transport. Once the cars were loaded, Sanitary Commission workers passed from car to car, providing soup, fresh bread, coffee, milk punch, and brandy.

For those who had to stay behind, dressings were changed, and basins of water, soap, and towels were made available for the comfort of those wishing to use them. Most of the men took advantage of the offer, as well as the provisions of new socks, shirts, drawers, and dressing gowns.

2. Army of the Potomac Medical Department Tablet, York Road, 39°50.489' N, 77°12.351' W

Situated along the York Road border of Camp Letterman, this marker serves to note the locations of the

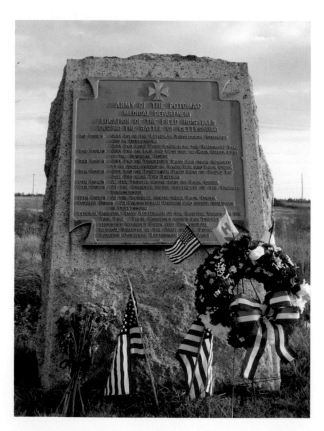

Army of the Potomac Medical Department Tablet showing he general location of each of the individual corps hospitals.

various Union Corps field hospitals at Gettysburg. The inscription reads:

Army of the Potomac
Medical Department
Location of the Field Hospitals
During the Battle of Gettysburg

1st Corps: July 1st at the Lutheran Theological Seminary and in Gettysburg
July 2nd near White Church on Baltimore Pike
2nd Corps: July 2nd on east and west side of Rock Creek east of the Bushman House
3rd Corps: July 2nd on Taneytown Road and soon removed to an angle formed by White Run and Rock Creek
5th Corps: July 2nd on Taneytown Road west of Round Top
July 3rd near Two Taverns
6th Corps: At the Trostle House east of Rock Creek
11th Corps: At the Spangler House southeast of the Granite Schoolhouse
12th Corps: At the Bushman House near Rock Creek
Cavalry Corps: At Presbyterian Church and other buildings in Gettysburg
General Hospital Camp Letterman at the Hospital Woods on the York Pike. These hospitals cared for twenty thousand wounded Union and Confederate.
Medical director of the Army of the Potomac, Surgeon Jonathan Letterman, U.S. Army.

3. Camp Letterman Site, York Road, 39°50.367' N, 77°12.360' W

As the battle expanded from McPherson Ridge into town and then into the surrounding countryside, hospitals began to spring up throughout the area. Some were official division or corps hospitals, but many were less official, often set up in the barns or cellars of homes and farms spread over a large expanse. These hospitals, while necessary and credited with saving countless lives, also presented a logistical nightmare for those responsible for knowing where the hospitals were located so supplies could be provided. Many men went for days with no treatment beyond what a farmer and his family could extend from their own meager provisions. Medical knowledge at many of these outlying aid stations and field hospitals was virtually nonexistent.

The need for a central system became acutely apparent when Dr. Jonathan Letterman, medical director for the Army of the Potomac, left Gettysburg a few days after the battle, placing responsibility for

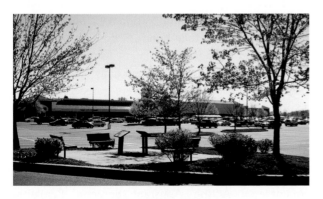

A shopping center now sits where Camp Letterman once treated as many as 1,700 wounded per week.

the treatment of more than twenty thousand wounded in the hands of only 106 surgeons. The addition of a few more doctors did little to relieve the problem. Surgeon Henry Janes (US Volunteers) was placed in charge of all the field hospitals and unwittingly revealed, through no fault of his own, the extent of the problem when he wrote that he had been placed in command of "some 60 different hospitals."[1] In truth, unbeknownst to Janes, there were three times that many if he were to include every site where wounded soldiers were being treated.

Letterman had conceived the idea of a general hospital on the battlefield. Such a hospital would have to meet strict criteria to be effective, however, criteria that were deemed impractical by many. The ideal property would sit on high ground, for good drainage. There would need to be shade for the comfort of the wounded, as well as good air movement. A reliable source of pure water was essential, and it should be near a railroad to facilitate the transportation of men and supplies. Good ambulance access was obviously vital. Surprisingly, despite the devastation throughout the Gettysburg area, a site that met these criteria was found.

That site was the farm of George Wolf, a popular picnic spot before the war that locals referred to as Wolf's Woods. An inspection of the site revealed that it had already been used as a field hospital, with as many as seventeen Confederate burials on the property.[2]

Under the command of Dr. C. N. Chamberlain (US Volunteers), the camp consolidated the services of all the Union hospitals in the Gettysburg area with the exception of three: the Lutheran Theological Seminary, the Adams Express office, and the Public School

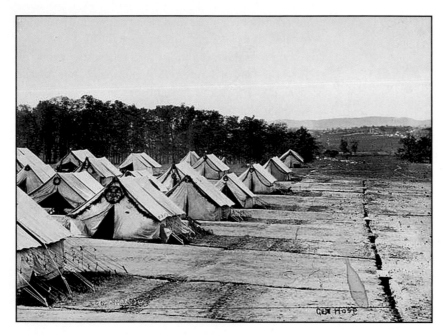

Some four hundred tents, each containing up to twelve wounded, made up the treatment area of Camp Letterman. (Courtesy of Library of Congress, Reproduction Number LC-DIG-ppmsca-33637)

on High Street. Construction began on July 16 and the hospital opened just six days later. It contained about four hundred tents aligned in six double rows, ten feet apart, with each tent capable of holding up to twelve patients. Each army corps had its own section. Named Camp Letterman after the medical director, the facility covered eighty acres and contained a cookhouse, deadhouse, embalming tent, cemetery, officers' quarters, and provisions for both the US Sanitary Commission and the US Christian Commission. The cemetery was especially needed, as the men who were left behind were those who had been the most badly wounded, and the graveyard would soon become the temporary final resting place for more than four hundred dead, including a number of Confederates. Those Confederate remains were relocated in the 1870s to cemeteries in the South. Unclaimed Union remains were eventually transferred to the new Soldiers' National Cemetery.

A staff of some four hundred doctors and attendants served the needs of as many as 1,700 wounded each week. The number changed daily when patients deemed well enough to travel were transferred by rail to permanent hospitals.

Doctors here included Acting Assistant Surgeon George W. Boughman and Assistant Surgeon William F. Breakey (both of the Sixteenth Michigan), Assistant Surgeon David M. Brubaker (109th Pennsylvania Volunteers), Acting Assistant Surgeon Benjamin F. Butcher (unknown regiment), Surgeon Louis M.

Emanuel (Eighty-Second Pennsylvania Volunteers), Acting Assistant Surgeon James B. Carpenter (US Volunteers), Acting Assistant Surgeon Charles S. Gaunt (US Volunteers), Acting Assistant Surgeon A. F. Gibbs (US Volunteers), Acting Assistant Surgeon Daniel R. Good (US Volunteers), Acting Assistant Surgeon E. F. Guth (US Volunteers), Charles A. Hamilton (Seventy-Sixth New York), Acting Assistant Surgeon William L. Hays (US Volunteers), Surgeon William B. Ward (Thirteenth Pennsylvania Reserves), Acting Assistant Surgeon Egon A. Koerper (Seventy-Fifth Pennsylvania Volunteers), Acting Assistant Surgeon J. T. Lanning (regiment unknown), Surgeon Henry Leaman (civilian contractor), Surgeon P. S. Leisenring, Assistant Surgeon Henry A. May (Forty-Fifth New York), Acting Assistant Surgeon Alex McWilliams (US Volunteers), Assistant Surgeon James Newcombe (regiment unknown), Surgeon William F. Norris (regiment unknown), Surgeon L. W. Oakley (Second New Jersey), Surgeon J. D. Osborne (Fourth New Jersey), Acting Assistant Surgeon J. R. Rowland (US Volunteers), Acting Assistant Surgeon A. B. Shekell (US Volunteers), Acting Assistant Surgeon James K. Shivers (US Volunteers), Acting Assistant Surgeon Thomas L. Smiley (US Volunteers), Acting Assistant Surgeon F. H. Smith (US Volunteers), Acting Assistant Surgeon A. B. Stonelake (US Volunteers), Assistant Surgeon Samuel B. Sturdevant (139th Pennsylvania Volunteers), Acting Assistant Surgeon H. H. Sutton (US Volunteers), Surgeon Joseph Thomas (118th Pennsylvania Volunteers), Acting Assistant Surgeon E. P. Townsend (US Volunteers), Acting Assistant Surgeon T. H. Walker (regiment unknown), Acting Assistant Surgeon R. S. L. Walsh (US Volunteers), Acting Assistant Surgeon George W. Ward (US Volunteers), Assistant Surgeon James D. Watson (Third Maine), Surgeon Daniel Baker (Twelfth Virginia), Surgeon Thomas A. Means (Eleventh Georgia), Surgeon Henry A. Minor (Eighth Alabama), Surgeon W. F. Nance (Second Florida), Surgeon D. H. Parker (regiment unknown), W. F. Richardson (Ninth Alabama), R. B. Sethall (regiment unknown), and F. J. Vance (regiment unknown).

Among the dozens of nurses who volunteered here were Cornelia Hancock, Euphemia Goldsborough, Georgeanna Woolsey, and Sophronia Bucklin.

The camp remained in operation until late November.

4. Alexander D. Buehler Farm, York Pike, 39°50.969′ N, 77°10.485′ W

Very little has been recorded about this farm, although it is known to have served as an aid station for Confederate general Edward Johnson's Division of the Second Army Corps.

Also referred to as the Eichelberger farm, the property was occupied by tenant John Z. Hartzell at the time of the battle. In his damage claim, Hartzell noted that he left the farm on July 2 in an attempt to get his horses to safety. He was overtaken by the rebels, who took the horses and allowed him to leave. Hartzell and his family did not return to the farm until after the battle. On their return, they saw that their crops had been trampled and the house used as a hospital. Hartzell was awarded $740.00 against his damage claim of $785.00.[3] The current tenant says that the modern siding on the house covers the original log structure.

Some 1,300 were treated at the various hospitals used by Johnson's Division, including the Buehler

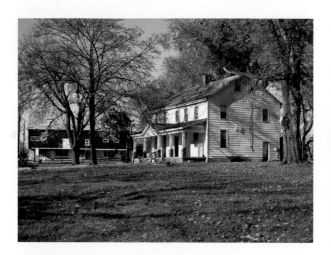

Tenant farmer John Hartzell tried to hide his horses but was overtaken by Confederate troops. They took his horses but allowed him to leave.

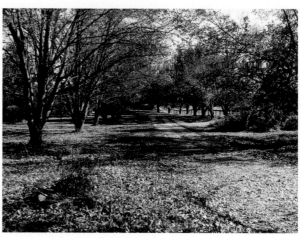

The entrance lane to the Joseph Leas farm.

farm. How many were treated here is unknown, but there were four recorded burials on the property. One of those was Seabron Solley of the Forty-Seventh Alabama. He died on July 4 and was buried in the northwest corner of the field near the county road. He was reinterred in Hollywood Cemetery in Richmond on May 17, 1873.[4] The names of the other three have been lost to history.

5. Joseph Leas Farm, 120 Hoffman Road, 39°50.892' N, 77°10.020' W

Situated near East Cavalry Field, the Joseph Leas farm treated wounded from both sides, and though not an official hospital for either, it was used primarily by General J. E. B. Stuart's Cavalry Corps. Little is known about the family or the farm, other than that there

were eleven burials on the property, six Confederate and five Union.

The names of the Union dead are unknown, but Dr. John W. C. O'Neal meticulously recorded the names of the Confederate dead wherever he found them, hoping that his records would enable Southern families to retrieve the remains of their loved ones at some point in the future. All the Confederate dead were buried in the northwest corner of Leas's field, west of the house. Presumably, the Federal dead were buried there as well.

Southern men buried on the Leas property included John R. Barrett (Green's Louisiana Battery); John H. Hoover (unknown regiment), who was killed on July 3; William Hentis (Ninth Virginia Cavalry), who may have been misidentified; an unknown man from a Virginia Cavalry troop identified only by the initials E, JE, or I; and a man named Hoye, whose troop or regiment is unknown.[5]

The medical director for the US Cavalry Corps was Surgeon George L. Pancoast, US Volunteers. Surgeon William Rulison of the Ninth New York Cavalry served as medical officer in charge of cavalry hospitals.

The Leas family filed two claims for damages. Joseph Leas claimed $633.50 for horses, bridles, halters, grain, a carriage, and whips. He was awarded $433.50. John B. Leas, believed to be Joseph's son, received full payment of $393.75 for his claim.[6]

6. Isaac Miller Farm, 240 Cavalry Field Road, 39°50.489' N, 77°10.188' W

Using a small road locally known as Stallsmith Lane, Confederate cavalry under General J. E. B. Stuart approached the East Cavalry battlefield on July 3 after

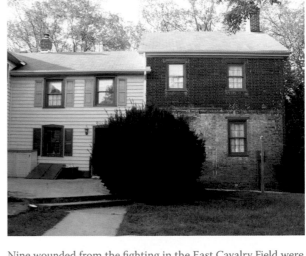

Nine wounded from the fighting in the East Cavalry Field were treated at the Isaac Miller farm.

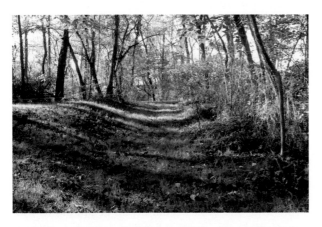

General J. E. B. Stuart used this small lane on the Miller farm to reach the East Cavalry Field.

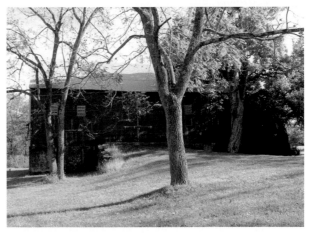

The Isaac Miller barn.

turning off the York Pike. Stuart's goal was the Low Dutch Road, at the eastern terminus of Stallsmith Lane. His route took him directly across the Isaac Miller farm, with the lane passing between the house and the barn.

Miller operated a small tannery on the farm, and the family treated wounded from the cavalry action on the nearby East Cavalry Field. Sara King and her mother, Rebecca Rinehart, came to the farm to help as nurses. They arrived with a wounded Michigan soldier named Smith. He was later moved to Elizabeth Culp's home on York Street in town.

The current owners indicated that they have learned there were nine wounded treated here, with one of them, a Confederate, dying. The wounded included men from both sides. The treating physician was Talcot Eliason, surgeon for Stuart's Division.

The original log portion of the home was built in 1771, with the brick section added in 1832.

Isaac Miller would file a claim of $415.00 for losses of horses, a buggy, and harnesses. He received full compensation.[7]

7. Jacob Rinehart Farm, 835 Hoffman Road, 39°49.981' N, 77°10.744' W

The farm of Jacob and Rebecca Rinehart and their four adult daughters is believed to have served as a headquarters for General J. E. B. Stuart during the East Cavalry Field fighting on July 3.

Before the fighting, Jacob had taken the family's stock across the Susquehanna River for safekeeping. Rebecca, a woman of feisty deportment, remained behind. On the evening of July 2, a Louisiana Tiger came to the house, saying he would like a good dinner.

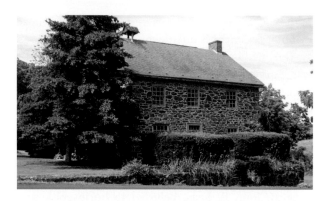

Rebecca Rinehart became an unofficial cook for men from both sides.

When Rebecca asked him what he considered a good dinner, he said he would like some chicken. She defiantly said he and his men had chased all her chickens away (actually, she had hidden them all), but if he could shoot one, he could have it. He settled for a slice of ham.

The next morning a Virginia officer named Sweet came to the house and asked which direction some of his men had gone. Rebecca pointed toward the Rummel farm and the officer thanked her and left. A short time later, Rebecca was saddened to see his men returning with his body and placing it on her porch.

Later in the morning a Confederate battery was set up in front of the house. Rebecca confronted the rebel officer, who apologized and said he thought the house was unoccupied. As he moved the battery, a Union shell dropped in their midst, prompting more protests from Rebecca. Leaving, the rebel officer apologized again and warned Rebecca that she should leave the area.

Instead, she took her family to cellar, along with some neighbors. As the fighting subsided, she left the safety of the cellar and went outside, where she saw many wounded horses, riderless and in agony. Wounded and dead littered the area. As she took in the sight, a group of Confederate soldiers brought a wounded Union soldier from Michigan and placed him on the porch. Rebecca and her daughter, Sara King, treated the man, whose name was Smith, as best they could. After giving him some bread, they took him to the nearby Isaac Miller farm, where they found several more wounded. Smith was given further treatment and moved to Elizabeth Culp's home in town.

It soon became known that the pipe-smoking Rebecca was willing to cook for men from both sides who stopped and asked for something to eat. By July 4, however, her patience was wearing thin. When a rebel soldier came by that morning and asked if she would cook up some bacon for his officer, who was asleep in the Rinehart barn, she had had enough. Drawing herself up to her full height, barely five feet, she looked the man in the eye and said, "There's the stove, you can cook it yourself. I don't know where you found the bacon but I know you got the onions out of my garden."[8]

After the war, Isaac Rinehart filed a claim of $328.40 for losses of thirty-one bushels of various grains, ten tons of hay, one hundred rails broken and burned, twelve acres of wheat, and fifteen acres of grass partially destroyed. He was awarded $218.40.[9]

8. John Rummel Farm, East Cavalry Field, 39°50.892' N, 77°10.020' W

Fifty-six-year-old John Rummel and his wife, Sarah (age fifty), purchased the farm in 1845 at a sheriff's auction, paying about $700. They lived here with their two children.

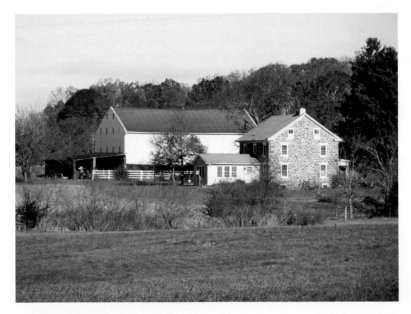

Fighting on the Rummel farm was intense, with hand-to-hand combat.

The most recognizable farm on the East Cavalry Field, Rummel's farm changed hands several times during the battle. Included on the 135-acre property were a log home, a blacksmith shop, a wagon shed, a springhouse, and a large barn that still exists. The original house is gone, replaced by the current one, which was built in 1870. John was taken prisoner on July 3 and held in the woods behind his barn. His wife, Sarah, was allowed to go to a neighbor's house.

Before using the barn for a hospital, the Confederates knocked out slats to provide openings for shooting. Fighting on the property was fierce, featuring one of the bloodiest hand-to-hand cavalry battles in all of the Civil War. Both the house and barn suffered extensive damage, not to mention the damage to the crops and fields created by the beats of thousands of hooves. The Rummels eventually filed a claim for $219.95, which was disallowed because the damage had been done by the Confederates.

After the fighting concluded, John assisted with the removal of the dead from across his farm, including thirty dead horses he personally dragged out of his lane. Nearly every building on his property was put to use in treating the wounded, with the barn carrying the brunt of the medical operation. Casualties totaled nearly five hundred, with the Union suffering about 60 percent of those. Although a Confederate hospital, like most of the others it also treated men from the opposing side. The surgeon at the Rummel home was Joseph Yates of the First South Carolina Cavalry.

9. Jacob Lott Farm, East Cavalry Field, 39°49.370' N, 77°9.749' W

The Jacob Lott farm, occupied by Jacob; his wife, Anne; and their ten children, served as an aid station for Confederate general J. E. B. Stuart's cavalry during the fighting for the East Cavalry Field. There were five

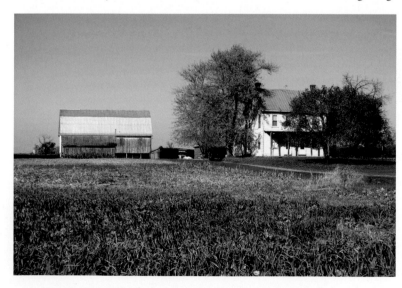

The Lott farm became an aid station for General J. E. B. Stuart's Confederates.

Confederate burials, all Stuart's cavalry men, on the farm. These were combined with six sets of remains from the southwest corner of Seminary Woods in May 1873 and sent southward.

It was in Lott's Woods that Captain William Miller of Company H, Third Pennsylvania Cavalry, etched his name in the annals of history. Miller's company sat on the Union's right flank, and they watched as the First New Jersey Cavalry, the dismounted Fifth Michigan Cavalry, and the Seventh Michigan Cavalry were all forced back by Stuart's onslaught.

After a lull in the fighting, Stuart ordered a mounted charge by the brigades of General Wade Hampton and General Fitzhugh Lee. Union general George Armstrong Custer responded by leading the First Michigan Cavalry in a countercharge. The two opposing sides met in a violent collision that Miller described as being "so sudden and violent that many of the horses were turned end over end and crushed their riders beneath them."[10]

Custer's daring countercharge temporarily slowed the Confederate advance, and with the two sides at a relative standstill, Union general David Gregg ordered parts of the Third Pennsylvania Cavalry, First New Jersey Cavalry, and Fifth, Sixth, and Seventh Michigan Cavalries into the melee in an effort to tip the advantage.

Under orders to remain on the right flank in the Lott Woods, Miller decided that he and his men could no longer stay on the sideline. His notes described what happened next, as he turned to his adjutant, Lieutenant William Brooke-Rawle and said, "If you will back me up in case I am court-martialed for disobedience, I will order a charge."[11] The adjutant immediately agreed, and Miller mounted his men and charged.

Miller's unexpected move split the lead of the Confederate column from the rear, confusing the Confederate attackers. Although Miller was shot through the right arm in the attack, overall, Company H suffered relatively few casualties.

Slowly, the Confederate charge stalled, then retreated. Miller's action would be credited by Gregg with playing a pivotal role in repelling the threat. Despite his heroism, however, Miller's name would not even be included in the Official War Department record of the battle. That oversight would eventually be corrected when, in 1897, he was awarded the Medal of Honor.

His official citation reads, "Without orders, led a charge of his squadron upon the flank of the enemy, checked his attack, and cut off and dispersed the rear of his column."[12]

Miller is one of only two Medal of Honor recipients buried in the Gettysburg National Cemetery, and the only one who received his medal for actions at Gettysburg. The other, Colonel Charles Henry Tucker Collis, received his medal for his actions at Fredericksburg.

10. Abraham Tawney Farm Site, Low Dutch Road, 39°48.694' N, 77°10.202' W

Although all traces of the Abraham Tawney farm are now gone, the 103-acre property played an important role in the East Cavalry Field fighting in 1863. When the cavalry forces of Union brigadier general David Gregg and General J. E. B. Stuart's Confederates clashed here on July 3, the farm was turned into an aid station that treated both sides. There was at least one Confederate burial, John P. Bowlin of the First Virginia Cavalry's Company C, who died on July 5

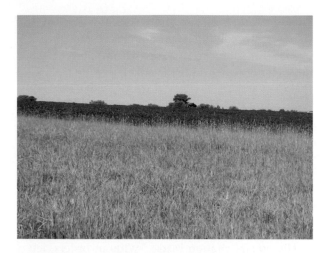

These fields once housed the Abraham Tawney farm, which was an aid station and headquarters for Union general David Gregg.

Tawney was the grandfather of James Tawney, who would eventually serve nine terms as a congressman from Minnesota.

11. Joseph Spangler Farm, 2079 Hanover Road, 39°49.065' N, 77°10.159' W

Also known as the Groft Farmhouse, the house was built in 1840 as a two-story, three-bay Georgian-style home on a stone foundation, connected to a summer kitchen by a covered walkway. It was used for hospital purposes after the battle. The present barn was constructed in 1870. The farm's buildings provided cover and concealment for the Union cavalry on July 2 and 3.[15]

Joseph Spangler, age twenty-eight, lived on the farm with his wife, Ellen, age twenty, at the time of the battle. The couple had two children at the time, including infant daughter Rosetta. The family would eventually grow to include two more children.

and was buried in an already existing cemetery on the farm, probably the Tawney family cemetery.[13]

Tawney, a fifty-two-year-old mason at the time of the battle, lived on the farm with his wife, Catherine, forty-three years old. The couple had four children, three of whom were still living in 1863: Susannah Ella (twenty), Newton Amos (nineteen), and Celina Matilda (fifteen). Their son Joseph Clinton had died in 1859 at age thirteen.[14]

The farm served as Gregg's headquarters for a time and was used as an aid station/field hospital by the Cavalry Corps, whose medical director was Surgeon George L. Pancoast, US Volunteers. The medical officer in charge of all US Cavalry hospitals was Surgeon W. H. Rulison of the Ninth New York Cavalry. The Cavalry Corps hospitals in the general area, including Tawney's, treated some three hundred wounded.

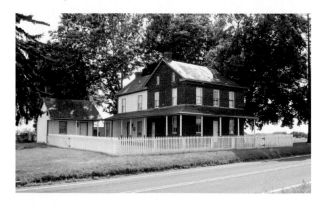

General George Custer's men took their position around Spangler's house before charging into action on the East Cavalry Field.

On the morning of July 3, General George Custer's Cavalry Brigade took a position in the fields in front of and behind the house. From there, the brigade made dramatic charges across the fields of Joseph Spangler, Jacob Lott, and Anthony Howard during the afternoon hours.

Wounded from both sides were treated here during and after the East Cavalry Field fighting, and the farm became a mental hospital for soldiers after the war.[16]

12. Jacob Brinkerhoff Farm, 1375 Hanover Road, 39°49.421' N, 77°11.657' W

Occupied by Jacob (age forty-three); his wife, Margaret (age thirty-seven); and their three-year-old son William, the Brinkerhoff farm treated wounded from both sides during the cavalry battles at the East and South Cavalry Fields. A black domestic worker, Louisa McMillan (age twenty-seven), also lived with

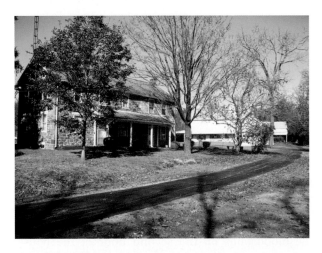

The Brinkerhoff farm was another hospital for Stuart's Cavalry.

the family.[17] Another son, Frank (age twenty at the time of the battle), does not appear to have been living with his parents in 1863. A daughter, Ida, would be born shortly after the battle.

There were at least two Confederate burials on the property, which served as a division hospital for Stuart's Confederate Cavalry. Although records are uncertain, it appears that one of those burials was Charles Harrington, of Cobb's Georgia Cavalry Legion, who may have been mortally wounded at Hunterstown. The other was believed to be Lieutenant Robert James Larew Glendy, who was severely wounded in the right thigh, leading to the amputation of his leg. He survived until July 23, probably succumbing to infection.[18]

The day before the main cavalry battle on East Cavalry Field, a smaller but no less important skirmish took place at the intersection of Hanover and Hoffman Roads, just a few hundred yards eastward. In that skirmish, the Union cavalry under Brigadier General David Gregg engaged the Confederate infantry's Stonewall Brigade in a struggle that lasted until after dusk. This effectively kept the highly respected Stonewall Brigade out of the attack on Culp's Hill, and the argument can be made that it may have had an impact on the outcome in that area of the battlefield.

13. Daniel Lady Farm, 1008 Hanover Street, 39°49.665' N, 77°12.457' W

The farm was originally part of a three-hundred-acre property owned by John Anderson from 1765 to 1767, when Samuel Hays purchased it. Hays lived on the farm for thirty years, building a log home and barn

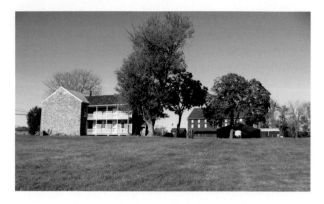

More than two thousand wounded were treated on the Lady farm. Amputated limbs were buried in the orchard.

on it. When he died in 1805, his heirs split the property in two. The northern half contained 153 acres and was owned by Hays's son James and James's wife, Sarah. This portion of the original farm became the Lady farm.

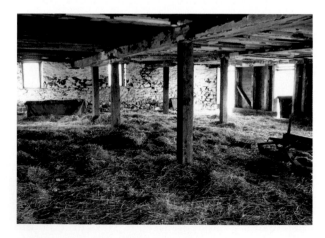

The interior of the Daniel Lady barn.

The southern portion (141 acres) was sold to Ralph Lashells, who sold it to Christian Benner in 1813. That area is now known as Benner's Hill.

The current house on the Lady farm was built in stages, beginning in the late 1820s by Moses Jenkins, at which time the original log house became a tenant house. The current barn was built in 1842, replacing an older log structure. Jacob Lady purchased the farm and some adjoining property in 1841, and son Daniel Lady became the owner of what, by then, was a 201-acre farm in 1853.

Daniel and his wife, Rebecca, lived on the farm with their seven children but were forced to leave during the fighting. This proved to be a wise move on their part when both the house and barn were struck by artillery fire. When the family returned on July 4, their farm was in shambles. The family had to bury several bodies left behind when the Army of Northern Virginia retreated. On July 4 most of Ewell's wounded were moved to the Lower Marsh Creek Presbyterian Church, where they staged for the retreat, leaving the family to find a way to cope with the wounded who could not travel.

Several hundred wounded were treated here, with officers treated in the house and enlisted men treated in the barn. Many of those wounded in the Culp's Hill fighting were first taken to Christian Benner's, then to the Lady farm. Those in the barn passed their time by carving their names or initials in the beams and window sills. They are well preserved and can still be seen. Amputated limbs were buried in the orchard and are presumed to still be there.

In 2006 the Niagara Falls Police Department asked for permission to analyze what appeared to be bloodstains on the second floor of the house. Using chemiluminescent blood reagents and special

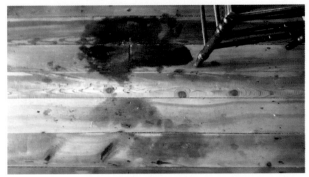

Bloodstains on the second floor of the Lady farmhouse.

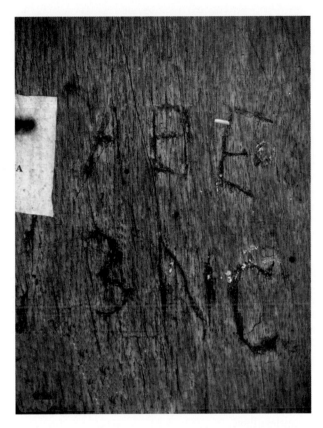

Many of the wounded carved their initials in the barn. These belonged to Private Aaron B. Eubanks of the Third North Carolina Infantry, Company G.

investigative techniques developed for historical testing, the forensic team painstakingly performed their unique task. Despite the fact that 143 years had passed, with exposure to countless outside influences, such as footsteps, cleaning agents, and other conditions that could have contaminated the "evidence," the technique was able to prove that the

stains were, indeed, blood. Similar results had been found when the team tested stains at the George Shriver house on Baltimore Street.[19]

Most of those who died on the farm were buried in temporary graves in a field across the road. A small memorial park near the barn is said to still contain the remains of twenty-six Confederate soldiers.

Doctors here included Edwin Latimer (Fourth Virginia Cavalry) and Robert T. Coleman (chief surgeon, Johnson's Division). When a badly wounded Major Joseph W. Latimer (Andrew's Artillery Battalion of Johnson's Division) was brought in, Dr. Latimer was forced into the unpleasant task of amputating his own brother's arm.

Only nineteen years old, Joseph Latimer was often referred to as the "Boy Major." He had attended Virginia Military Institute, where he had studied artillery tactics under Stonewall Jackson. Major Latimer, commanding five guns on Benner Hill, was mortally wounded when an artillery shell exploded near him, killing his horse. His men had to remove him from beneath the horse. After his brother amputated his arm in an effort to save his life, he was moved to the Warren-Sipe House in Harrisonburg, Virginia, where he died of gangrene on August 1, less than a month before his twentieth birthday.

After the war, Daniel Lady filed a claim for damages of $1,461.97 to cover losses of beds and bedding, harness, fencing, grains and crops, livestock, carpet, household goods, a county map, bags, wagon cover, books, lard, watch, tinware, crockery, yarn, foodstuffs, tallow, soap, bees, leather, rifle, clothing, boots, stoneware, pewter ware, beeswax, balances, earthenware, and a wagon, as well as damage to a carriage, the barn, and fruit trees. He was eventually awarded a reduced sum of $1,251.97.[20]

The Lady family sold the farm and moved in 1867. The farm would sustain some minor damage in 1884 from a small earthquake. The property was purchased by the Gettysburg Battlefield Preservation Association in 1999.

14. Christian Benner Farm, Hanover Road, 39°49.369' N, 77°12.678' W

Fifty-eight-year-old Christian Benner; his wife, Susannah (age fifty-six); and their sons Simon (twenty-two) and Oliver (nineteen) lived on this 208-acre farm on Benner Hill. A third son, Henry, was serving in the 101st Pennsylvania Volunteers. Also on the farm were Julia A. S. Walter (twenty-six) and her son Henry B. Walter (four). Julia may have been a domestic worker.[21]

The farm became the center of a major artillery duel and, ultimately, a Confederate field hospital. The family stayed in the house for much of the fighting, not leaving until July 3. They found nothing of value

remaining when they returned a day later, their house blood-spattered and completely plundered.

Their son Oliver claimed that bullets hit the house with such rapidity that it sounded like "taking a handful of gravel and throwing it on the roof."[22] Oliver later discovered a rebel sharpshooter who had buckled himself into one of Benner's trees with his belt. The belt had kept the man's body from falling out of the tree when he was killed.

As the number of wounded grew, they were placed in the kitchen, barn, and yard. Most of the wounded were from Early's Division, Ewell's Corps. Johnson's Division had an ambulance depot here, and many of the wounded taken to Benner's were later moved to the field hospital at the nearby Daniel Lady farm, where it was thought they may receive more advanced treatment.

At one point in the fighting, the shelling became so fierce that, to protect the wounded and those providing succor, a major asked Susannah for a red cloth to be used as a hospital flag. After some searching, she found a piece, which the major ordered a soldier to nail onto the roof. Such actions took place on farms across the area and undoubtedly saved countless lives.

After the battle, Benner collected items left around the farm by both armies, as did most of the farmers. A few weeks later, the Quartermaster Department issued orders that anyone holding such items must return them immediately. Most, including Benner, ignored the order. Benner, along with many of his neighbors, was specifically mentioned in a Quartermaster Department report that said, "Found at Christian Benner's guns, blankets, sabers, shelter-tents &c."[23]

Doctors serving here included Thomas Fanning Wood (Third North Carolina), Augustus B. Scholars

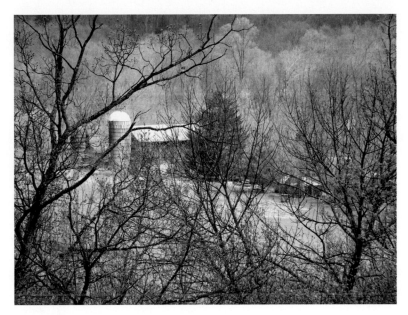

The Christian Benner farm as seen from the Culp's Hill observation tower.

(Second Louisiana), Dabney Herndon (Fifteenth Louisiana), Bushrod Taylor (brigade surgeon, Jones Brigade), Dr. Taylor (affiliation unknown), and Matthew Butler (Thirty-Seventh Virginia). Butler also served at the Henry Monfort farm on the Hunterstown Road.

There were six Confederate burials at Benner's, all from the Fourth Chesapeake Battery and all buried either in the orchard or on the back side of Rock Creek under a large walnut tree. Three were unidentified; the remaining three were interred under the names of A. J. Bryance, T. Parker, and Lieutenant PWH.[24]

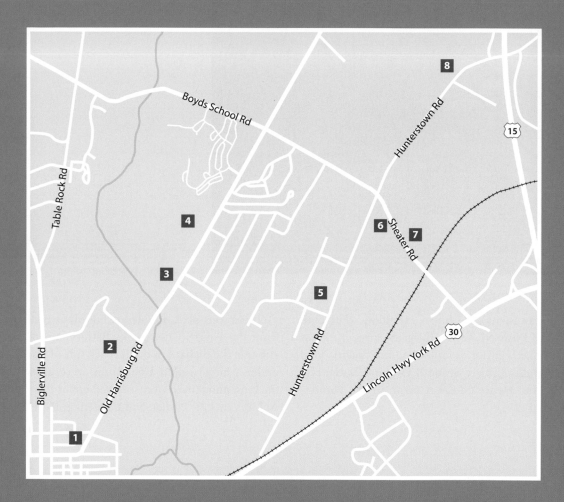

Chapter 11 sites: Old Harrisburg Road/Hunterstown Road area. (Map by Bill Nelson)

Old Harrisburg Road/Hunterstown Road Area

Most of the hospitals in this area served either *Early's Division or Johnson's Division. Doctors often helped at one or more hospitals and are often not listed specifically for any one location. Those who served Early's Division included Samuel B. Morrison (chief surgeon, Early's Division), Judson Butts (Thirty-First Georgia), and Louis E. Gott (Forty-Ninth Virginia).*

Hospitals of Johnson's Division were spread along Hunterstown Road, Fairfield Road, and possibly into Fairfield itself. Doctors here included Benjamin Cromwell (First North Carolina), Lucious C. Coke (First North Carolina), DeWilton Snowden (First Maryland Battalion), Caspar C. Henkel (Tenth Virginia), Charles W. MacGill (Second Virginia), Robert A. D. Munson (Second Virginia), John A. Hunter (Twenty-Seventh Virginia), Edwin Latimer (Andrews's Battalion), and Bushrod Taylor (Jones's Brigade).

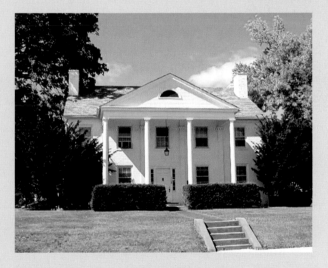

The Crawford house was used as a hospital by General Jubal Early's Division.

1. John S. Crawford House, 444 Harrisburg Street, 39°50.275' N, 77°13.671' W

The former home of Henry Baugher, president of Pennsylvania College, was being rented by John S. Crawford at the time of the battle. It would become one of the main hospitals for Major General Jubal Early's Division of the Army of Northern Virginia. Crawford also owned a farm along Plank Road.

Crawford, a sixty-six-year-old attorney, lived here with his wife, Elizabeth S. (fifty), and their children Anna D. (twenty-eight), Sarah B. (twenty-four), William (seventeen), Mary J. (fifteen), Robert S. (thirteen), and

George D. (ten), along with domestic worker Mary Johns (sixty-one).[1] Elizabeth's mother, Mrs. William Smith, and sister Jane were also here during the battle and helped with the wounded, as did a cousin, Annie Young.

Young would write a letter to another cousin, Mina, in which she described how the house opened for wounded on the first afternoon, and how both the house and yard were full of dead and wounded. She noted that General Richard Ewell, whose request for two rooms to be used as his headquarters had been refused by the Crawfords, returned the next morning with Generals Early and Rodes, this time asking for breakfast. Young accommodated their request.[2]

On July 2 General Francis Barlow was brought from the Josiah Benner farm. Barlow had been wounded on July 1 and his injury was thought to be mortal. Soon, Barlow's wife, Arabella, arrived to help her husband in his fight for his life. She also helped treat the other wounded. Barlow would survive his wounds.

There were two Confederate burials here, one behind the house and the other near the Harrisburg Road. Neither was identified.

2. Adams County Almshouse Site, Harrisburg Road, 39°50.556' N, 77°13.483' W

Built in 1820 to house nearly one hundred of Adams County's indigent and mentally ill population, the Almshouse took on a decidedly different role in the early days of July 1863, when it served as a temporary field hospital for the Union's Eleventh Corps.

On the first day of fighting, the Eleventh Corps was routed and crossed the property in a chaotic retreat into town, making a final stand around the Almshouse buildings. When Ewell's Second Corps overran the

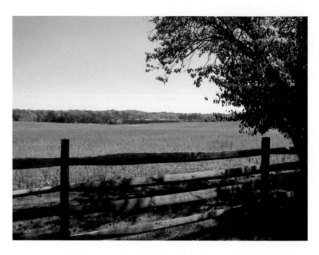

So many wounded were brought to the Almshouse that one of them noted that the only way to get a bed was to wait until someone died. The Almshouse sat in this field.

Federals, rebel wounded joined those of their enemy at this location, where their numbers would soon overwhelm the ability of the Almshouse to accommodate all of them. Some wounded waited days before their wounds were dressed, and one complained that the only way to get a bed was to wait until someone died.

The Washington bureau chief of the *New York Times*, whose wounded son had died at the Almshouse, penned the kind of scathing article only a grieving parent could write. In the piece, written July 4 and published July 6, Samuel Wilkeson chronicled the poor military decisions and poorer medical treatment that had led to his son's death, saying, in part, that his son had been "crushed by a shell in a position where a battery should never have been sent, and abandoned to death in a building where surgeons dared not to stay."[3]

Late in the morning of July 3, a Confederate signal corpsman climbed to the roof, from where he began to send messages. Union artillery responded, placing those in the Almshouse in grave danger. The Union wounded complained to their captors that signals should not be sent from a hospital, and the Southerners agreed. An officer proceeded to the roof and had the man removed at gunpoint before any further damage could be done.

Civilian doctor John W. C. O'Neal served here during and after the battle, and Union surgeon Henry K. Neff of the Eighth Pennsylvania Reserves assisted, even after he was taken prisoner. Jacob Culp and his family lived at the Almshouse as caretakers and assisted in treating the wounded. Culp lost a wagon when it was confiscated by a Confederate officer who said he needed it to take his wounded father to Virginia. He was not reimbursed.

There were several Confederate burials on the property. Sergeant G. H. Gamble (Thirty-First Georgia), Bradford Harrison (Fourth Georgia), and J. J. Bond (Twelfth Georgia) were all killed on July 1 and buried under a walnut tree near the Almshouse graveyard. Sergeant William P. White (Thirteenth Georgia) was killed on July 1 and was buried on a hill behind the graveyard. Joseph H. White (Forty-Ninth Virginia) was killed on July 3 and buried in the "poorhouse orchard." Lieutenant R. W. Meacham and J. Pinkney Lynch (both from the Thirteenth Georgia) were killed on July 1 and 2, respectively. Both were buried in the Almshouse cemetery.[4]

Remains identified as those of a Lieutenant Blume, from an unnamed Georgia regiment, were buried in the woods in the same area as William White. Blume actually may have been confused with Lieutenant F. J. Theodore Blume (Second New York Light Battery), who also was killed on July 1. This speculation arises because no Southerner named Blume was found to have been killed at Gettysburg. To add to the confusion, the New York Blume was also shown to have been buried south of the brickyard.[5]

In July 1911 a relic hunter discovered what proved to be the graves of three Union soldiers near the Almshouse. Unidentifiable, they were transferred to the national cemetery. Burial records indicate that there was a fourth Federal soldier also interred on the property.

The Almshouse cemetery remains at its original location on Barlow Knoll and contains the graves of civilians from the Almshouse complex. No Civil War soldiers' remains are believed to be in the cemetery today.

A fire in the 1950s destroyed several of the buildings on the complex. Others were razed over the next several years, with the last one removed circa 1974. Today nothing exists except the cemetery to provide mute testimony to what sat here during the battle.

3. Josiah Benner Farm, 980 Old Harrisburg Road, 39°50.785' N, 77°13.302' W

This 123-acre farm dates to 1776, when it was owned by John Reid, who named it Spring Garden. In July 1863 it became one of the main hospitals for Major General Jubal Early's Division of the Army of Northern Virginia's Second Corps.

Period buildings on the farm include the two-story house, whose second-story porch was added postwar, a frame Pennsylvania bank barn, and a springhouse. The south side of the barn has initials carved into the stonework. Those initials are often said to be those of the men treated there, but a more likely explanation is

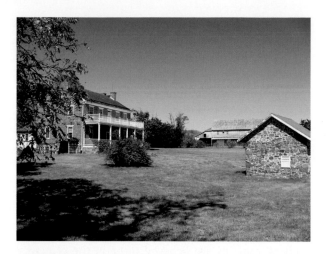

The Benner farmhouse was struck eight times by artillery fire during the battle.

that they are simply the initials of the Benner children. In the 1930s a fire caused significant interior damage to the structure.

The springhouse provided not only cool drinking water for the wounded but also cover for skirmishers on both sides. Confederate general Richard Ewell, who had lost a leg at Brawner's Farm a year earlier, was said to have bathed his pain-wracked stump in the cooling waters of the springhouse as he passed by.

The Benner family fled the property during the fighting and, considering the farm's location, probably were not surprised to see the house and barn filled with wounded when they returned. On the afternoon of July 1, the farm sat in the line of advance for Early's Division. The Seventeenth Connecticut formed a skirmish line near the house and barn, and as the fight ebbed and flowed, skirmishers from both sides used the buildings as cover. The house was struck eight times by artillery shells, one causing a fire that was extinguished by the building's occupants. Another shell remains embedded in a rear wall of the house. A damage claim for $551.50 was honored but at the reduced rate of $471.50.[6]

Although it was a Confederate hospital, arguably the best-known patient at the Benner farm was Union general Francis Channing Barlow. The twenty-nine-year-old was badly wounded on the nearby knoll that today bears his name. He was carried to Benner's on a blanket used as a stretcher. The stretcher bearers were his own men who had been captured. Confederate surgeons probed Barlow's wound and told him it was unlikely he would survive. Barlow was later move closer to town, to the home of John Crawford.

Barlow's wife, Arabella, came to Gettysburg to nurse her husband back to health, much as she had done when he had been badly wounded at Antietam. Unfortunately, she would succumb to typhus in 1864. Whether it was due to Arabella's nursing is open to conjecture, but Barlow not only survived but also went on to a highly successful legal career, prosecuting Boss Tweed in the Tammany Hall scandal and becoming a founder of the American Bar Association. Barlow eventually remarried, this time to Ellis Shaw, sister of Robert Gould Shaw of the famed Fifty-Fourth Massachusetts.

There were twenty-five Confederate burials on the farm, as well as fourteen Union ones.

4. Jacob Kime Farm Site, Table Rock Road, 39°50.999' N, 77°13.176' W

Thirty-six-year-old Jacob Kime and his wife, Elizabeth (age thirty-three), lived on this farm as tenants of Josiah Bringman. The couple had been married sixteen years and had four children. The afternoon of July 1, General John B. Gordon launched an attack from the Kime fields toward Union troops on Blocher's Knoll (now Barlow Knoll). The farm soon became a hospital for wounded Georgians.

The farm consisted of 168 acres and included a four-room log house, barn, and several outbuildings. The barn that was on the property during the battle was replaced in 1876. The replacement barn suffered minor damage in 1929 when it was struck by lightning. All the buildings are now gone, but the original farm lane looks much as it did in 1863. Three to four feet deep, it provided cover for Gordon's brigade. Much of the property today is occupied by the campus of Gettysburg Area High School.

Early in the afternoon of July 1, Confederate officers warned Jacob that he should move his family for safety. He returned that evening to find his crops trampled, clothing scattered, linens and blankets ripped for bandages, the house and other buildings damaged, and his animals butchered. Kime retired to the cellar, where he remained throughout the fighting. He could only listen helplessly as the wounded cried out for morphine that was not available. After the fighting ended, the family discovered piles of amputated arms and legs scattered around the house, presumably many of them from the men Jacob had heard begging for relief.

Three identified burials were found on the farm, all of them under a peach tree in the orchard. Major Peter Brennan and William Young (both of the Sixty-First Georgia) were buried with Lieutenant Colonel William McLeod of the Thirty-Eighth Georgia.[7] Eleven additional burials were unidentified.[8] It was McLeod's story that was most compelling.

The twenty-one-year-old McLeod had been shot in the temple during an attack on Blocher's Knoll. His servant, Moses, wrapped McLeod's body in a blanket

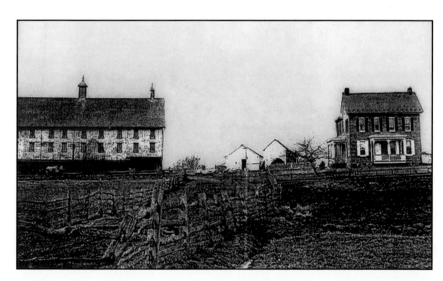

The Kime farm as it appeared in 1863. (Courtesy of Gettysburg Area High School waymark)

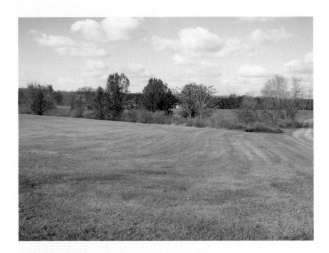

Site of the Jacob Kime farm. Jacob Kime took refuge in his cellar during the battle.

and personally buried him with the two casualties from the Sixty-First Georgia just mentioned. In 1865 Moses and McLeod's brother-in-law, John Prescott, returned to Gettysburg to retrieve the body. When they got back to Georgia with the body, McLeod's grieving mother said he had been alone in the ground for two years and she vowed he would never be alone again. She refused to have him buried until another family member died, so they could be buried together. McLeod's casket was kept in the house until then. Ironically, it was McLeod's brother-in-law, Prescott, who had brought him home from Gettysburg, who would be the next family member to die. In 1872 they were buried side by side.[9]

The Kimes filed a damage claim in the amount of $821.25 for losses of crops, livestock, poultry, salt, horse gear, saddles, windmill and horse rake, lard, and other items. They would be awarded full compensation.[10]

5. Henry Monfort (Montford) Farm, 248 Hunterstown Road, 39°50.764' N, 77°12.598' W

This 125-acre farm was occupied by fifty-three-year-old W. H. (Henry) Monfort; his wife, Catherine (age fifty-two); and at least one child. Built in 1848 by Henry and his brother Jacob, the farm served as a hospital for Confederate general Edward Johnson's Division.

The wounded were placed in the house, barn, and several outbuildings. The house received extensive damage, and the second floor of the barn still contains residual bloodstains.

Doctors treating the wounded here included William R. Whitehead (Johnson's Division), Robert T. Coleman (chief surgeon, Johnson's Division), Bushrod Taylor (chief surgeon, Jones's Brigade), and several others. Taylor is credited with saving the life of General John Marshall Jones, commander of Jones's

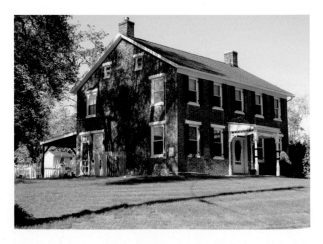

The Monfort home became a hospital for Confederate general Edward Johnson's Division.

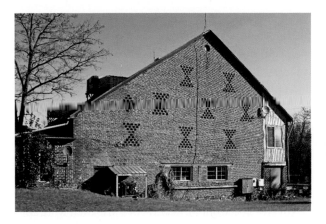

Bloodstains remain on the second floor of the Monfort barn.

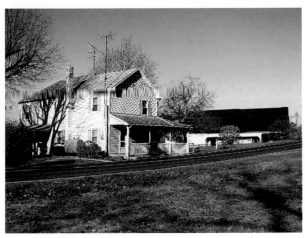

Martin Shealer's barn featured a thatched roof until it was torn down in the 1930s.

Brigade, when Jones suffered a severe wound to the thigh while fighting on Culp's Hill. Several months later, Jones would be wounded again in the Mine Run Campaign. He would be killed at the Wilderness in 1864.

There were fifty-two recorded Confederate burials on the property.

6. Martin Shealer Farm, Shealer Road, 39°50.984' N, 77°12.358' W

Built in 1792, the barn on the Martin Shealer farm uniquely featured a thatched roof. It kept that feature until its demolition in the early 1930s. The mows, stalls, and barn floor were filled with the wounded of Johnson's Division for several weeks after the battle, and forty-four Confederates died in the barn and were buried just outside in the adjoining field. A few years after the battle, the remains were disinterred and taken to Hollywood Cemetery in Richmond.

Owned by forty-two-year-old Martin Shealer and his wife, thirty-six-year-old Amanda, it was Amanda who was running the farm in 1863 while raising their five children. Martin had been serving in the 165th Pennsylvania Volunteers and did not muster out until July 28, 1863, nearly four weeks after the fighting ended at Gettysburg. Not knowing what to expect, Martin returned home to find his house and barn filled with wounded, most of them Confederates. Ignoring their philosophical differences, Martin immediately began treating his former enemies alongside his wife.

The farm served as a Confederate hospital for about four weeks. The Shealers received a full award of $585.00 for their claim of damages and losses to the farm and crops of corn, hay, grass, oats, and rye; a mare; livestock (cows, sheep, hogs); grain; fences; and lumber.[11]

7. Elizabeth Weible Farm, Shealer Road, 39°50.931' N, 77°12.313' W

Previously owned by the Walters family, the farm was owned by fifty-five-year-old widow Elizabeth Weible in July 1863 when it served as another hospital of Early's Division, most likely for the brigades of General Harry T. Hays and Colonel Isaac Avery. It would fill that capacity until the middle of August. The barn no longer exists but the house remains.

Records indicate that there were 311 wounded treated between Weible's and Monfort's, but the breakdown between the two is not known. It is also likely that some of those 311 would have been treated at Shealer's.

There were thirteen Confederate burials around Elizabeth Weible's barn: Corporal Marshall H. Walker (Sixth North Carolina, killed while carrying

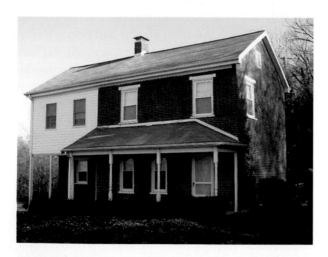

Widow Elizabeth Weible's farm contained thirteen Confederate graves.

his company's colors), Andrew Jackson Hutchins (Sixth North Carolina), Hinton Coslett Glenn (regiment unknown), Thomas J. Delozier (First Maryland Infantry Battalion), Lieutenant R. A. Oursler (Seventeenth Mississippi), Captain L. A. Comier (Sixth Louisiana), J. L. Simmons (Eighth Louisiana), L. A. Thebedau (regiment unknown, killed July 1), Corporal M. H. Walker (Sixth North Carolina), Sergeant J. Maynard (Sixth North Carolina), Sergeant M. McKinney (Sixth North Carolina), Lieutenant V. W. Southall (Twenty-Third Virginia), and Captain James H. Burns (Sixth North Carolina). Several of these men were able to be returned to their families after requests were made to Dr. John W. C. O'Neal, who had documented grave locations and body descriptions of hundreds of Confederate dead.[12]

8. Henry A. Picking Farm and Schoolhouse, Hunterstown Road, 39°51.436' N, 77°12.107' W

Henry (age forty-six) and Charlotte (age thirty-eight) Picking and their four children lived on this farm, which became a Confederate field hospital for Johnson's Division. The house is original (with some alterations), but the barn is postwar. The schoolhouse is also believed to be a replacement for the one used in 1863.

Major Henry Kyd Douglas, formerly of Stonewall Jackson's staff, was wounded in the shoulder and was brought here for treatment. Wounded six times during the war, Douglas was placed on the floor of the parlor, where he said at least six doctors examined him, including Hunter McGuire (medical director of Ewell's Corps), an old friend. Douglas would go on after the war to gain a measure of fame with his memoirs, *I Rode*

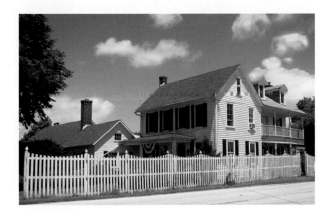

Recovering Confederates helped the Pickings harvest their crops later in the summer.

with Stonewall. Before then, however, he wrote glowingly about his treatment at the hands of the Pickings.

There were sixteen burials on the property, nearly all of them from the Stonewall Brigade. They were located along a fence near the Hunterstown Road, opposite the schoolhouse.

Many of the Confederates who were unable to be moved when the retreat began signed their paroles and assisted the Pickings in their harvest several weeks later.

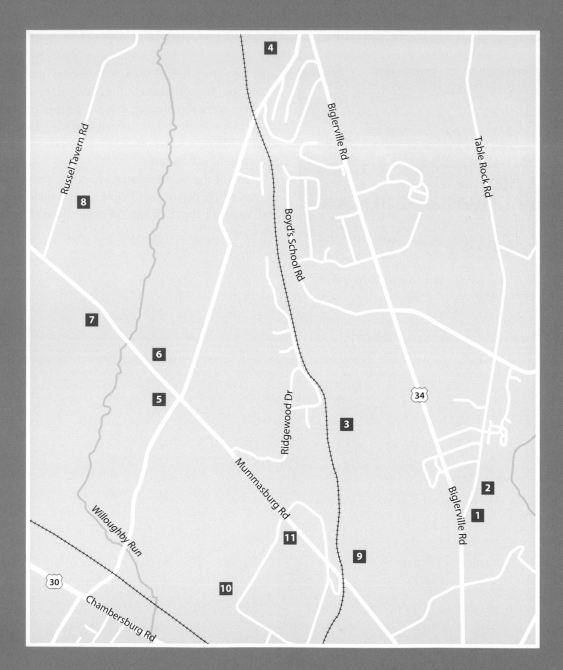

Chapter 12 sites: Biglerville Road/Mummasburg Road area. (Map by Bill Nelson)

Biglerville Road/Mummasburg Road Area

1. John and David Blocher Farm, 15 Table Rock Road, 39°50.862' N, 77°13.809' W

This property is actually two properties in one, with the main farm being the home of David Blocher and the small structure to the right of the driveway entrance serving as the home of his father, John Blocher (39°50.845' N, 77°13.859' W). John's house is the only prewar structure on the property.

The entire farm covered slightly more than twenty-three acres. John Blocher's small house, which became Ewell's headquarters, was built in the 1820s when Blocher purchased the farm from John Patterson. A weaver by trade, seventy-year-old John Blocher lived alone in the one-and-a-half-story structure, which was later raised to two stories. His wife, Catherine, had died just three years earlier. Early in the battle, the house was used by the Seventeenth Pennsylvania Cavalry as it performed picket duty on Carlisle Road. On July 1 the cavalrymen were driven off the farm by soldiers of Brigadier General George P. Doles's Brigade. Later in the day, the Georgians were part of the rebel forces that pushed the Union Eleventh Corps back through town. After the Pennsylvanians were driven off, the house became a Confederate aid

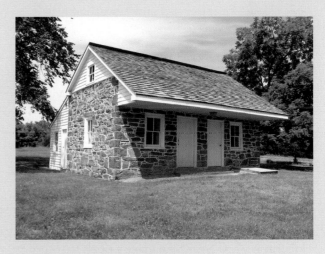

John Blocher's house served as headquarters for Confederate general Richard Ewell and was the site for the meeting of General Robert E. Lee and several of his corps commanders.

station and was purported to be the site of a meeting the night of July 1 between Robert E. Lee and his corps commanders Ewell, Early, and Rodes to plan the next day's offensive.[1]

The nearby house and barn are the site of Rev. David Blocher's farm. David, the thirty-five-year-old son of John, lived on the farm with his wife, Maria, also

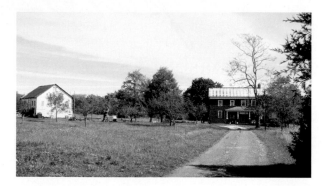

David Blocher's home became a small hospital during the first day of fighting.

thirty-five. David served as a minister in the German Brethren church. The house and barn are both replacements for structures sitting on the farm in 1863. On July 1 the battle line of Doles's Brigade moved across the farm to attack Blocher's Knoll, named for the Blocher family. The name has since been changed to Barlow Knoll, after General Francis Channing Barlow, who was severely wounded there during the battle.

The map drawn by S. G. Elliot shows as many as twenty-eight Confederate burials on the farm, but that number is not supported by any other source.[2] Dr. John W. C. O'Neal, who made a point to record as many Confederate burials as he could, identified two on the property. Both were from the Fourth Georgia Infantry and were buried under a tree near the house. The two were Lieutenant Colonel David R. E. Winn and Josiah H. Law, whose rank is unknown. Winn was killed leading a charge on Blocher's Knoll.[3]

After the war, the Winn family attempted to retrieve Winn's body, but David Blocher refused unless they paid a fee for the exhumation. Eventually Dr. Rufus Weaver, in charge of retrieving Southern dead, got involved and was able to negotiate a fee of five dollars so Winn's lower jaw, which included a gold plate that held a set of dentures, could be included when the body was sent home. Blocher had originally insisted on ten dollars to cover his cost of maintaining the grave and had refused to relinquish the jaw until he was paid.

David Blocher filed a claim for losses of grain, blacksmith tools, a heifer, and fifteen feet of fencing. He requested $351.00 and received the full amount.[4]

2. William Ross Farm, Biglerville Road, 39°51.091' N, 77°13.994' W

This 114-acre farm, including 15 acres of crops, was occupied by William and Sarah Ross and served as a field hospital for General Robert Rodes's Division, and possibly others, during the battle. The house, barn, and outbuildings were used to house Confederate wounded, although it is unlikely that all or any of the present buildings existed in 1863. The exception would be a small shed that is thought to be the one used during the seventy-fifth anniversary celebration.

There is only one Confederate burial shown on the Ross farm. He was an unnamed soldier from the Twelfth Alabama. A review of Confederate casualty records indicates two possibilities as to the man's identification. William M. Johnston was wounded on July 1, was captured, and died on July 8. No other pertinent information is available for Johnston. The second possibility is that the unfortunate man was Robert Rogers, who suffered a severe injury of the right shoulder on July 1. The twenty-year-old was captured and subsequently died on August 21 at a location listed only as "a field hospital."

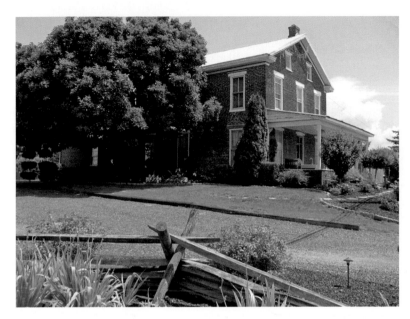

The Ross farm became a hospital for Confederate general Robert Rodes's Division.

The Rosses, following the advice of a Union officer, left the farm on July 1. They returned to find fifteen acres of crops destroyed, as well as losses of a horse, a colt, four steers, four sheep, bedding, clothing, lard, foodstuffs, furniture, hay, wheat, and 350 rails. William Ross's damage claim for $742.00 was reduced to $676.00. In support of the claim, his neighbor Isaac Deardorff testified that he observed Confederates on Ross's property throughout the entire three days of fighting, and wounded were brought into the house.[5]

3. Samuel Cobean Farm, Biglerville Road, 39°51.229' N, 77°14.391' W

Widower Samuel Cobean lived on this 136-acre farm with his niece after his wife, Eliza, died in 1860. He had two sons serving in the Union army in Virginia. On the morning of the first day of fighting, Cobean was advised by the Union to leave while he still had the chance. He refused, choosing to spend the next three days in his cellar.

The house was built in 1805 by David Dunwoody, who sold the property to Cobean's father, Samuel Alexander Cobean. Ultimately the elder Cobean transferred ownership to his son Samuel, who owned it during the battle. The house sat immediately behind Reese's Alabama Battery, whose position near the house drew Union artillery fire from Barlow Knoll. The house suffered extensive damage inside and out as a result, but the damage was repaired quickly after the battle. The rapid repairs were made somewhat easier by Cobean's financial standing as one of the wealthiest men in Adams County. Sitting on an

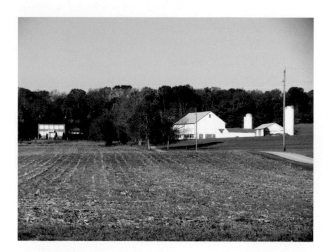

The Cobean farm. Today the farm is used by the National Park Service for administrative offices.

old Native American trail, the farm has two natural springs that continue to provide water. The barn has since been replaced but the house remains, although a frame addition on the west side of it is postwar. The farm served as a hospital for Ewell's Corps and, as it was situated behind the Confederate line, wounded from both sides were treated here.[6] When the house and barn filled with wounded, two large wall tents, a large hospital tent, and several small shelter halves were used to shelter the wounded.

Doctors here included William R. Whitehead (Johnson's Division), Harvey Black (Fourth Virginia, who commanded the hospital at Cobean's), J. William Walls (Fifth Virginia), Frank L. Taney (Tenth Louisiana), John A. Straight (affiliation unknown), Hunter McGuire (Ewell's Corps), John M. Hayes (Twenty-Sixth Alabama), and Samuel B. Morrison (chief surgeon for Early's Division).

General Isaac Trimble was brought here after his July 3 wounding, his leg being amputated in the parlor by McGuire, Black, and Hayes. Trimble was moved to Robert McCurdy's home in town, then to Schmucker Hall on the Lutheran Seminary campus, where he recuperated until healthy enough to be sent to a military prison in Baltimore.

Before Pickett's Charge on July 3, 1863, Confederate artillery prepared to fire from Seminary Ridge or Oak Ridge in the area of the Cobean farm toward Cemetery Hill. The Union artillery returned fire, and a significant amount of their overshots landed on the Cobean farm. A few of the shells struck the house and barn, killing some of the wounded.

Despite the large number of wounded here, there was only one known burial west of the house, along the Almshouse fence. According to Dr. John W. C. O'Neal, this was Captain James T. Davis of the Twelfth Alabama.[7]

Cobean filed a damage claim for losses of farm equipment, grain, meat, and flour; rails and fences burned and broken; and damage to his house and crops, and said all his cattle had been slaughtered to feed the rebels. Like so many others, he received only a partial payment.[8]

Today the farm is owned by the National Park Service and is used for administrative offices.

4. John Hamilton Farm Site, Biglerville Road, 39°52.732' N, 77°14.827' W

This farm of 150 acres, owned by John and Sarah Hamilton, was occupied by the Confederate army in the days immediately preceding the battle, with their wounded remaining until mid-July. The barn and

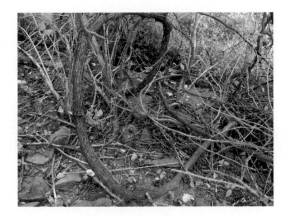

The Hamilton barn's foundation is being overtaken by nature and is barely discernible as it extends from the upper left to the center right.

grounds were used as a hospital by Rodes's Division of Ewell's Second Corps. Sarah was listed as the owner.

The farm had a large barn and blacksmith shop, with the shop operated by the Hamiltons' son John Eline Hamilton. The younger John, twenty-two years old, had become a blacksmith at the age of eighteen, working as an apprentice under a Mr. Thomas.

On June 26, 1863, officers of Early's Division stopped at the shop while on their way to Gettysburg, asking young John to shoe their horses. He was kept under guard for two days to ensure that he did not leave. When he overheard one of the Confederates say to another that he would be taken with them to do their smithing, he waited for his chance. Noticing a guard dozing off, John fled to the hills about a mile away, telling only his mother where he was going so she could bring him food. He returned after the battle and resumed his trade until he enlisted in the 195th Pennsylvania Volunteers. His brother, Marcus Jerome

Hamilton, also served in the army, with the 138th Pennsylvania Volunteers.[9]

The large barn on the property housed most of the wounded, although there were some in the house and in tents around the barn. None of the 1863 buildings remain and, although parts of the barn's foundation can still be seen, the entire barn area is being reclaimed by the surrounding woods and cannot be seen without assistance from someone who knows the location. The current owner of the property was gracious enough to conduct a tour of the land and allow the author to spend a considerable amount of time exploring the area. The accompanying photo shows the extent to which the trees and undergrowth have overtaken the area.

John Hamilton claimed $494.00 in damages, receiving an award of $444.00 for flour, shelled corn, hay, eight acres of wheat, blacksmith tools, and three horses, including one taken by the rebels as early as June 26.[10]

5. Samuel Hartzell Farm, Mummasburg and Herrs Ridge Roads, 39°51.262′ N, 77°15.248′ W

Readers may recognize the name of Samuel Hartzell but from a different context. Hartzell owned the orchard that sat across Chambersburg Pike from the Mary Thompson house, which served as headquarters for Robert E. Lee. Some place Lee's headquarters in the orchard itself, although this has not been proved.

The Hartzell farm sat at the intersection of Mummasburg and Herrs Ridge Roads amid a complex of farms that all served as aid stations or field hospitals in some manner. Samuel, forty-seven years old, had lost his first wife, Rebecca, in 1849 when she was thirty years old. He would later remarry twice, to Eliza and

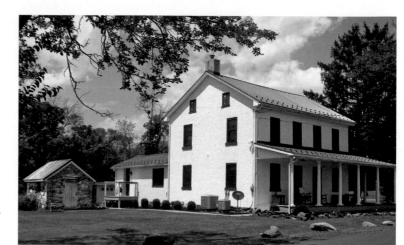

The Hartzell farm was one of many in this immediate area that served as hospitals during the battle.

Elizabeth. It is not certain which of these was his wife at the time of the battle, if either was. Hartzell's son, Elias, would be killed at the Battle of Sailor's Creek in April 1865 as the war neared its end.

The farms in this area treated as many as one thousand wounded. Some of those were wounded in the first day's fighting, while others were among those left behind when the retreat began.

Hartzell claimed that his farm was used by the rebels and that he had suffered losses of $630.10 for bees, livestock, farm implements, grains, horse gear, rails, and thirty-five acres of fields and meadows. The $25.00 damage he claimed for his fields and meadows was disallowed, leaving him with an award of $605.10. His neighbor David Schriver was a witness for Hartzell's claim, stating that he had personally witnessed rebels burning Hartzell's rails and that he had put out the fire himself.[11]

There were no known burials on the property.

6. David Schriver (Shriver) Farm, Mummasburg Road, 39°51.365' N, 77°15.341' W

David and Susan Schriver, both fifty-one years old, lived here with their three adult children, Jacob, John, and Hannah. Their son David was not home, as he had enlisted in the Twenty-First Pennsylvania Cavalry just two weeks before fighting broke out in Gettysburg.

The 150-acre farm became a Confederate hospital for O'Neal's Brigade during the battle, overflowing with more than 750 wounded. Initially, only three surgeons were available to treat the throng, using only a couple of makeshift operating tables. Eventually, several more physicians arrived, including S. W. Mitchell (chief surgeon, Rodes's Division, who floated between Schriver's and the Hankey farm), Hunter McGuire (medical director of Ewell's Corps), George W. Briggs (Thirtieth North Carolina), John M. Hayes

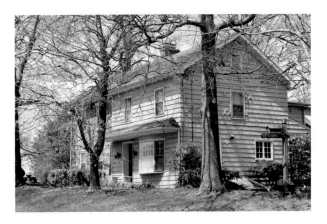

Only three physicians were on hand to treat more than 750 wounded when Schriver's farm opened as a hospital.

(Twenty-Sixth Alabama and chief surgeon of O'Neal's Brigade), William H. Philpot (chief surgeon, Doles's Brigade), William T. Brewer (Forty-Third North Carolina), J. W. C. O'Neal (local civilian doctor), and Abner Embry McGarity (Forty-Fourth Georgia). Hayes was the medical officer in charge.

While treating the wounded here, McGarity learned of the death of his wife's brother, Lieutenant Barnett Hardeman Cody (Fifteenth Alabama).

Colonel Samuel H. Lumpkin of the Forty-Fourth Georgia was one of the highest-ranking officers treated here. His shattered leg was amputated. Ironically, he had been a doctor before leaving civilian life to serve in the Confederate army.

The stone portion of the house is original. The barn, which sat on the opposite side of Mummasburg Road, no longer stands. The farm was used as a hospital for more than a month, with sixteen Confederate burials in the orchard.

Schriver claimed damages of $1,291.50 for two hundred pounds of ham and shoulders, lard, apple butter, tinware, bedding, clothing, furniture, poultry, horse gear, farm tools and implements, livestock, fencing and rails, and grains and grass fields, as well as damage to the barn, house, and outbuildings. He was awarded $891.50.[12]

7. Jacob Hankey Farm, Mummasburg Road, 39°51.598' N, 77°15.618' W

Although referred to as the Jacob Hankey farm, Jacob had died at age sixty-two just three years before the battle. It is believed that the farm was being operated by Jacob's son David during the battle. Living on the farm at the time were Jacob's widow and David's mother, Elizabeth (age fifty-seven), and two adult daughters, Susan and Elizabeth. Sons Frederick and Jacob C. were both serving in the Union army and were not present.

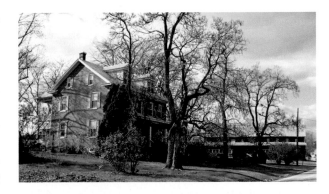

Wounded survivors from Iverson's Brigade, cut down in large numbers on Oak Ridge on July 1, were treated here at Hankey's farm.

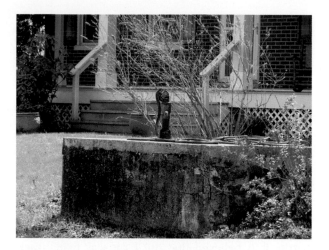

This pump sits at the location of Hankey's original front porch.

The 230-acre farm had buildings on both sides of the road and served as a major Confederate hospital for Rodes's Division, with at least 145 burials on the property. Although the barn was used to treat and shelter the wounded, the house is a replacement. The location of the original house is easily determined by the presence of a hand pump that sits in front of the current home. This pump sat on the porch of the original house. During the battle, thirsty soldiers drained the well and an armed guard had to be placed at the pump to allow time for the well to refill.

When Dr. Charles Krauth and his family fled their home on the campus of the Lutheran Theological Seminary, they walked to the Hankey farm. The Krauths were not alone. In addition to nearly one thousand wounded, the Hankeys took in about thirty neighbors who had also been forced out of their homes.

One of those caught here before she could leave was Samuel Hartzell's domestic worker, an African American known only as Mrs. Isaac Smith. When the Confederates arrived, Mrs. Smith went to the cellar and crawled to the darkest corner she could find, piling up crates and furniture in front of her. "I was the only colored person there, and I didn't know what might happen to me," she recalled later. A wounded Confederate officer asked Hankey to have the women all come up from the cellar and help cook and care for him and his men. Hankey told the man that one of the women was an African American and asked how she would be treated. The officer promised she would not be bothered, and issued a written order to his men to that effect. He ordered that the door to the kitchen be boarded up halfway, so food could be cooked and handed out without the need for any Confederates to enter.[13]

Another civilian at Hankey's was a Mr. Boyde, who had come to search for the body of a friend, H. B. Slade of an unnamed North Carolina regiment. Despite information that Slade had been buried under a peach tree at Hankey's, Boyde was unsuccessful in locating the remains. After several weeks he was forced to return home, not having achieved his goal.

Many of the wounded here were members of General Alfred Iverson's and General Junius Daniel's Brigades, who had been mauled in the first day's fighting on Oak Ridge. With so many wounded, it became necessary to erect tents throughout the farmyard.

Doctors here included Simon Branch (Twenty-Third North Carolina and chief surgeon of Iverson's Brigade), Frank Patterson (Second North Carolina Battalion and chief surgeon of Daniel's Brigade), David Russell (Twenty-Third North Carolina), J. H. Purefoy (Twenty-Third North Carolina), Isaac F. Pearson (Fifth North Carolina), John Henry Hicks (Twentieth North Carolina), J. Robinson Godwin (Second North Carolina Battalion), William Brewer (Forty-Third North Carolina), W. S. Mitchell (chief surgeon, Rodes's Division, who was also at the David Schriver farm), Leonidas Kirby (Second North Carolina), Robert G. Southall (Sixth Alabama), George Whitfield (Twelfth Alabama), William Proby Young (Fourth Georgia), James Etheridge (Twelfth Georgia), Abner Embry McGarrity (Forty-Fourth Georgia), John M. Hayes (Rodes's Division), and John F. Shaffner (Fourth North Carolina).

Among the wounded of Iverson's Brigade brought here for treatment were three high-ranking officers from the Twenty-Third North Carolina Infantry, Colonel Daniel Harvey Christie, Lieutenant Colonel Robert Daniel Johnston, and Major Charles C. Blacknall. All three would die here.

8. The Grove, Russell Tavern Road, 39°52.026' N, 77°15.793' W

Neighbors around the Hankey farm said that as many as one thousand Confederate wounded were at Hankey's and adjoining properties. One of those properties was said to be a large grove of trees on a slight elevation just north of the Hankey property. A review of the US Sanitary Commission map showing hospital locations corroborates this.[14] There appear to be no additional references, so the location of this grove of trees is not certain, although, coincidentally, this grove of trees appears at about the same location shown on

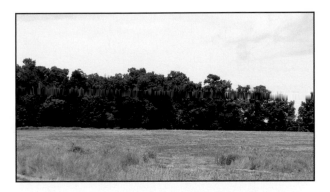

An outdoor Confederate hospital was established at this approximate location.

the Sanitary Commission map. While tree growth and development have changed the appearance of the area, this is a likely location for the field hospital. A visit to the area indicates that it has all the elements that both sides sought when establishing field hospitals in open areas: a protected location, shade from the sun, and a reliable source of water nearby in the form of Willoughby Run.

While there is little doubt that there was a Confederate field hospital in this general area, the exact location will remain a mystery until additional information becomes available.

There were no recorded burials on the site.

9. Moses McClean Farm, Mummasburg Road, 39°50.751' N, 77°14.431' W

Period documents spell the name as either McClean or McLean. Most National Park Service documents use the spelling McClean, so that is the one used in this work also.

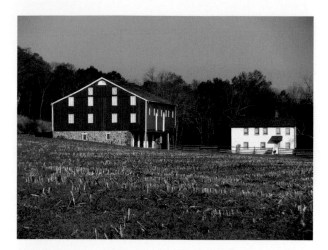

The McClean barn became an aid station for Confederate wounded, as well as wounded Union prisoners.

The farm was owned by fifty-nine-year-old attorney Moses McClean, who also owned a house on Baltimore Street in town. McClean was active in local politics, serving at various times as county commissioner, state assemblyman, and US congressman. Also in the family home were his wife, Hannah (fifty-two); their three daughters, Maggie (twenty-six), Sallie (twenty-one), and Elizabeth (fifteen); two of their sons, Robert (eighteen) and Colin (thirteen); and their domestic worker, Lucy Butler.[15]

The farm was being rented by David H. Beams at the time of the battle. Beams was serving with the 165th Pennsylvania Volunteers, and his wife, Harriett, was forced to flee with their three-year-old child. All the family belongings were either stolen or destroyed.

The farmhouse was a two-story L-shaped structure built between 1820 and 1830. A two-story red Pennsylvania bank barn, wagon shed, and corncrib, all built between 1850 and 1854, also sat on the property. Generals Ewell and Early had their headquarters in the barn, a well-known landmark for modern-day visitors on Oak Ridge.[16]

Located on the lower eastern slope of Oak Hill, the house and barn were occupied by Union skirmishers from the Eleventh Corps on the first day of fighting but were overrun and captured by soldiers of Rodes's Division. The Confederates held the position until they retreated from the battlefield on July 3. Although it was long thought that the farm was not used as a hospital, it is now believed that the house and barn were used as a temporary aid station for wounded Union prisoners and Confederates throughout the battle.

Companies A and B of the Forty-Fifth New York held the McClean barn early in the battle, where they had captured a number of rebels, one of whom was twenty-one-year-old Bernhard Schwarz. One of his captors was his younger brother Rudolph, a member of Company B. The two had not seen each other for some time, and they embraced and got reacquainted in the brief time they had together. When the Union line collapsed, Bernhard Schwarz was freed with the other Confederate prisoners. In the New Yorkers' chaotic retreat through town, several of them fell captive themselves. Not seeing his brother among the prisoners, Bernhard asked some members of Company B about his brother, only to learn that he had been killed in the battle earlier that afternoon.

The McClean family stayed in their home on Baltimore Street throughout the battle. On the evening of July 2, a shell struck the house, entering the garret through a side wall. Failing to explode, the shell

tumbled down the stairs and through an open doorway to the first landing, stopping where five-year-old
Hannah, granddaughter of Moses McClean, had been
sitting just moments before.

The farm suffered damage even before the battle began, when the Southern army camped in the
McClean fields on June 26, followed by Union cavalry just four days later. McClean would file a damage
claim of $1,138.35, claiming damage to the house and
barn, eight acres of oats, ninety bushels of wheat, one
ton of hay, twenty-seven acres of grass, fifty bundles of
long straw, a stone fence, 4,546 rails, thirty-five posts,
ten fence boards, ten and a half acres of corn, forty
pounds of ham, and ten pounds of beef, as well as
damages caused by driving over the farm. He received
full reimbursement.[17]

As many as thirty-five Confederates were buried
on the farm, most of them from North Carolina and
Alabama.

10. James Wills Farm, Buford Avenue, 39°50.615' N, 77°15.181' W

This farm dates to 1798, when it was owned by William
McPherson. James Wills acquired the property in
1859, building a barn in 1860 that survived the war
but burned down not long after. During the battle,
the farm was owned by Wills but occupied by a black
tenant named William Job. The house occupies the
approximate site of the original eighteenth-century
settlement homestead of William McPherson that
stood on the site during the battle. In 1867 Theodore
Bender purchased the farm from Wills, who could not
maintain the farm because of financial losses from

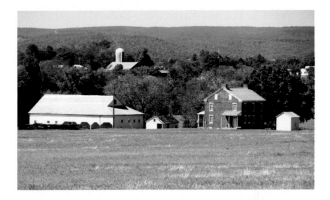

The Wills farm was one of many that had to be sold after the
battle because owners could not afford to repair the battle
damage.

battle damages, leading to the farm's later names: the
Theodore Bender farm and the Leroy Winebrenner
farm, after a later owner. Bender's farm had a house
that he built in 1868, a barn, a wagon shed, a carriage
house, and what Bender described as a "never failing
well at the door."[18]

On the first day of the battle, the Army of Northern
Virginia marched across the farm to attack the Union
troops in the fields and woods to the west and south.
The Confederates set up artillery near the buildings
and used the farm as a field hospital for several days
after the battle. The buildings provided badly needed
cover for Confederate infantry and artillery, but at
the same time they also became obstacles to troop
movements.

A postwar map drawn by S. G. Elliott shows about
250 Confederate burials, although that is believed to
be a high estimate.[19]

11. John S. Forney Farm Site, Buford Avenue, 39°50.837' N, 77°14.728' W

Although all portions of the John S. Forney farm are long gone, the site is very easy to locate. Just a few yards south of the Mummasburg Road–Buford Avenue intersection sits the monument to the Seventeenth Pennsylvania Cavalry. This monument is in what was the front yard of the Forney farmhouse in 1863. Having deteriorated badly, the house was torn down in 1938 to clean up the area in time for the dedication of the Eternal Light Peace Memorial.

Forney, born in 1830, was married to Mary Schriver. The youngest of eleven children, Forney had spent ten years in California mining gold before returning to Gettysburg, his hometown, in 1859. He had married Mary and also purchased the farm in 1862. Forney, his wife, and their infant daughter left the farm when the battle was imminent, traveling farther out Mummasburg Road to stay with Mary's father, David Schriver. The Forney farm was nearly destroyed in the battle, with only the badly damaged house and barn still standing when the Forneys returned. The buildings were all used as field hospitals for General Robert E. Rodes's Division.

The 150-acre farm was the site of the slaughter of General Alfred Iverson's North Carolina Brigade when Iverson ordered a poorly planned assault, not knowing what was in front of him. As his brigade approached a stone wall that runs roughly along the line of Doubleday Avenue, Union troops rose up from behind the wall and delivered a withering volley, killing as many as nine hundred of Iverson's men. The dead fell in a perfect row, just as they had been marching across the field, now known as Iverson's Pits. Another four hun-

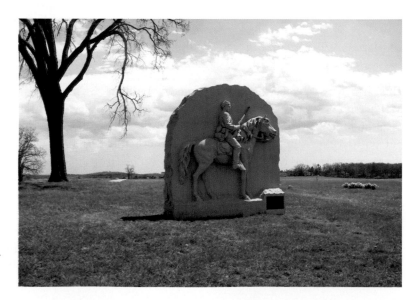

The Seventeenth Pennsylvania Cavalry monument sits in what was formerly the Forney front yard.

dred were taken prisoner. Iverson was relieved of his command shortly after, and only intervention by Confederate president Jefferson Davis prevented Iverson from being court-martialed.

Forney said he lost his entire stock to the rebel army, although he claimed they had treated him with civility. His damage claim of $1,162.00 asked for payment to cover his losses of 3,891 rails burned, shell and bullet damage to the house, window curtains, sixty-two acres of grains, trampled fields, fences used for fuel, and much household property carried away or destroyed. He was eventually awarded $1,031.46.[20]

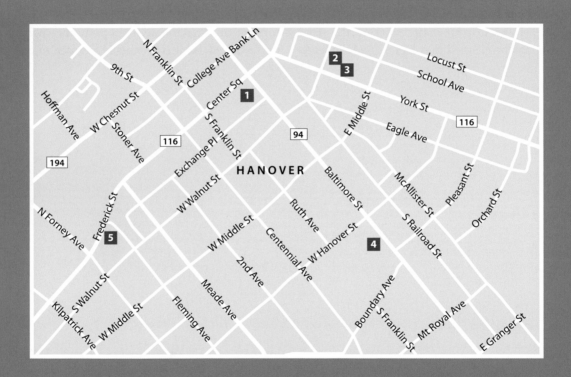

Chapter 13 sites: Hanover. (Map by Bill Nelson)

ON THE MORNING OF JUNE 25, 1863, *Confederate major general J. E. B. Stuart took six thousand troops and left the main body of Robert E. Lee's Army of Northern Virginia. Headed north under vague orders from Lee that empowered him to select his own route, Stuart and his column planned to move eastward and ride between the Union Army of the Potomac and Washington, destroying telegraph lines and railroad routes along the way. Ultimately, he intended to meet with General Richard Ewell at York, Pennsylvania.*

That plan was thwarted, however, when Union troop movements forced him to move farther eastward than he had planned. This path took him through Rockville, Maryland, where detachments from Brigadier General Wade Hampton's and Colonel J. R. Chambliss's brigades captured a large Union wagon train. The wagon train, eight miles long, added 125 wagons, nine hundred mules, and four hundred prisoners to Stuart's responsibilities. The wagons were loaded with oats, whiskey, bacon, hams, and sugar, and while the capture deprived the Yankees of needed supplies, it ultimately proved to be a detriment, slowing Stuart's advance and delaying his eventual arrival in Gettysburg.

Delaying him even further, Stuart's scouts reported Union cavalry in his path just outside Littlestown, Pennsylvania, forcing him to again alter his route. His revised travel plan would take him to Hanover, where he hoped to find Ewell's troops.

Meanwhile, Union cavalry under General Judson Kilpatrick was also searching for Ewell, following a path from Frederick, Maryland, toward York, where Ewell had been on June 28. Kilpatrick and his men spent the night of June 29 at Littlestown, moving out at daybreak on June 30. Still not sure of Ewell's position, Kilpatrick reached Hanover at about eight o'clock that morning, where enthusiastic citizens, still reeling from a raid three days earlier by Confederate cavalry under Lieutenant Colonel Elijah V. White, provided the Union troops with food.

The head of Kilpatrick's column, comprising the brigades of General Elon Farnsworth and the flamboyant George Armstrong Custer, had already passed through Hanover when Stuart observed the Yankees. When the Thirteenth Virginia Cavalry encountered the Union rear guard, comprising two companies of the Eighteenth Pennsylvania Cavalry, they ordered the Union troopers to surrender. The Pennsylvanians, however, made a dash to rejoin the main body of their regiment. The Virginians were joined by elements of the Ninth Virginia Cavalry, who pursued the fleeing Federals into town, with the Second North Carolina Cavalry joining the fight.

Quickly, the Fifth New York Cavalry attacked the North Carolinians while the Eighteenth Pennsylvania Cavalry regrouped. Terrified townspeople found themselves in the midst of the fighting, and citizens and soldiers alike rushed for cover wherever they could find it. In the chaos, ambulance guard Bradley Alexander of the Fifth New York Cavalry was run over by one of his ambulances, suffering injuries that eventually led to his death at his home near Black Creek, New York. Soon, the Confederates had control of Hanover.

Bolstered by reinforcements from the First West Virginia Cavalry and First Vermont, a Union counterattack drove the Confederates back, regaining control of the town for the Union. In this counterattack several Confederate prisoners were taken. Among them was Lieutenant Colonel William Payne, whose dying horse had thrown him into a tanning vat at the Winebrenner Tannery, where the sheepish officer was pulled out by his captors. The fierce fighting in this segment of the battle also saw the Fifth New York Cavalry's Private Thomas Burke capture a Confederate battle flag, earning him the Medal of Honor.

The Ninth and Tenth Virginia troopers threw up fierce resistance, and Stuart himself evaded capture in the hand-to-hand fighting near the Karl Forney farm only by spurring his horse to jump a wide water-filled ditch as he was pursued by several Yankee soldiers.

Stuart placed artillery south of the town and began moving his wagon train. Union artillery batteries from the First and Fourth US Artillery moved into position on the opposite side of town, precipitating a two-hour-long artillery duel, with shells striking a number of buildings in town. As darkness closed in, Stuart withdrew his men, ending the battle.

Stuart's Hanover encounter, coupled with the delay caused by the slow-moving captured wagon train and another brief skirmish at Carlisle, proved costly to General Robert E. Lee at Gettysburg. Stuart's cavalry would not arrive there until late in the day on July 2, with the battle already having been fought for two days. His absence deprived Lee of important intelligence regarding the location of Union forces.

Union casualties in the Hanover fighting totaled 215, with 86 suffered by the Eighteenth Pennsylvania Cavalry in its first taste of combat. The Fifth New York Cavalry saw 42 casualties. On the Southern side, Stuart lost at least 117 men, with 55 of those noted by the Second North Carolina Cavalry. Of the 332 casualties suffered by the two sides, 28 were killed, 123 wounded, and 181 missing. Those wounded required treatment, and the town of Hanover responded.

"I saw a man lying on the street issuing profusely from his head. He was a Confederate soldier, but as he was a fellowman supposed to be dying, I went to his assistance," Rev. Dr. William K. Zieber, pastor of Emmanuel Reformed Church, later recalled.[1] Local physicians William Bange (surgeon dentist), George Hinkle, John Culbertson, Henry Eckert, Jacob Smith, and Horace Alleman immediately offered assistance, as did Dr. Perin Gardner (assistant surgeon, First West Virginia). Gardner assumed command. The local Ladies' Aid Society also helped treat the wounded, as did many area residents.

One of those killed at Hanover was Corporal John Hoffacker of the Eighteenth Pennsylvania Cavalry. He was killed instantly in the first Confederate attack, almost within sight of his home in nearby West Manheim Township. He had enlisted just two months earlier. His brother William would be killed at Spotsylvania Courthouse a year later.

1. Concert Hall Site, Southwest Corner of Town Square, Hanover, 39°48.015' N, 76°58.998' W

Situated on the southwest corner of the town square, the Concert Hall became one of the first public buildings to be pressed into service as a hospital.

Built by V. C. S. Eckhart, the hall served as a social, musical, and entertainment center. More than sixty wounded were treated here.

The building was razed in the early 1900s.

2. Marion Hall Site, Southwest Corner of E. Walnut Street and School Avenue, Hanover, 39°48.071' N, 76°58.821' W

Built in 1840 by the congregation of the Emmanuel Reformed Church, Marion Hall was originally used as a Sunday school and lecture room. In 1854 local citizen William Barnitz conducted a private school in the two rooms.

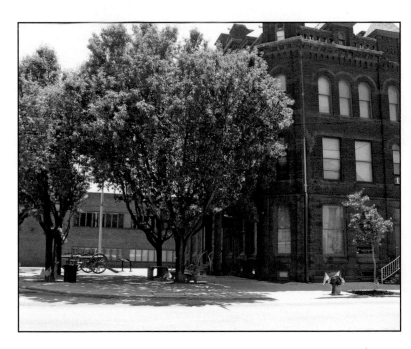

Site of the Concert Hall. The Concert Hall's central location made it an ideal site for a hospital after the Hanover fighting.

In 1860 the Marion Rifles, a volunteer militia, bought the property, named it Marion Hall, and used it as an armory and drill room. The Marion Rifles were named for Francis Marion, a Revolutionary War militia leader known as the Swamp Fox.

During the battle it became a short-term hospital. About twenty Union soldiers were brought here after being wounded in hand-to-hand fighting. Those who died were taken to the Flickinger Foundry across the street, then buried in the nearby Reformed Church graveyard.

After the Civil War the building was bought by railroad magnate Cyrus Diller, who used it as a boarding house for the men who worked for him on the railroad. In 1913 the building was converted into a stable, and it was razed in 1996 for parking for the nearby Trinity Reformed Church.[2]

3. Flickinger Foundry Site, 116 York Street, Hanover, 39°48.031' N, 76°58.814' W

Now the Trinity Reformed Church, the Flickinger Foundry played a somewhat unique role in the Battle of Hanover, serving as both a hospital and a morgue. Beginning on the evening of the battle, the dead were brought here and prepared for burial, while one room in the building was also set aside as a hospital to treat the wounded.

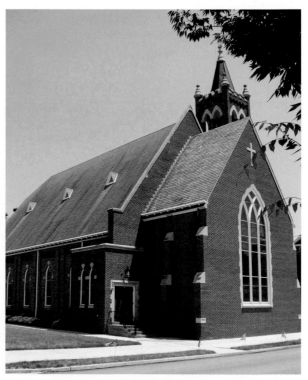

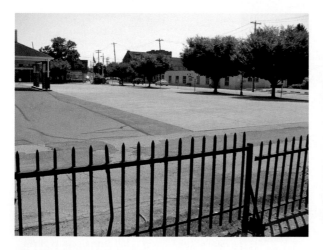

The home of the Marion Rifles is now a parking lot for the Trinity Reformed Church.

The foundry sat on space now occupied by the Trinity Reformed Church.

Henry Wirt, a leading citizen of Hanover, ordered caskets made, with most of the Union remains placed in the nearby graveyard of the Trinity Reformed Church. A few were buried in the cemetery of St. Matthew's Church. Rev. Dr. William K. Zieber performed the burial ceremonies. The bodies were later removed and transferred to the national cemetery in Gettysburg. Confederate dead were buried by civilians on various properties around town. Those remains were later removed and sent south.

The Flickinger Foundry was razed and the present Trinity Reformed Church was constructed on the site in 1884, with renovations in 1910, 1932, 1954, and 1995. A tornado in 1915 damaged the church's spire so badly that it had to be removed and replaced by the present spire.

4. Pleasant Hill Hotel Site, 319 Baltimore Street, Hanover, 39°47.767' N, 76°58.723' W

Before the fighting in Hanover, the Pleasant Hill Hotel was being used as a private academy. Sitting on what is now the side lawn of the Warehime-Myer Mansion, the hotel was rented by the government after the battle and set up as the official hospital for the wounded. All the wounded being treated in the various smaller hospitals in town were brought here for treatment. Eventually, the hospital also treated about 150 wounded from the fighting in Gettysburg. Dr. Perin Gardner, an army surgeon, was placed in charge. The facility remained in use as a hospital from July 10 through August 15.

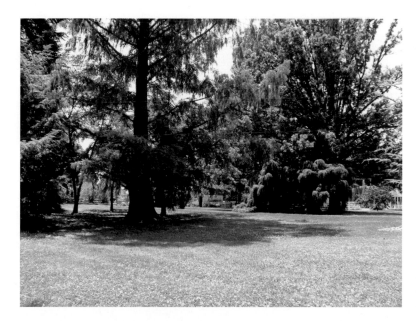

All the temporary hospitals in Hanover were consolidated into one larger hospital at the Pleasant Hill Hotel, which sat on this site.

The structure was built in 1810 by Adam Forney, who operated it as the Forney Tavern. At the time of the battle, the facility was owned by Adam Fisher.

The four-story property contained thirty-six rooms, with the first floor used as a bar and smoking room, the second floor as a parlor and sitting room, and the third and fourth floors as sleeping rooms. While the building was in use as a hospital, the second-floor parlor served as the operating room.[3]

After the battle, every room in the building was filled with the wounded. Several of those being treated there ultimately died and were transferred to the Flickinger Foundry for preparation for burial.

After the tavern closed, the building was used as a school and private dwelling. It was torn down in 1915.

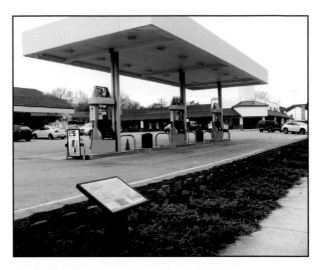

The beginning of the battle at Hanover took place at what is now a convenience store.

5. Karl Forney Farm Site, Frederick Street at Forney Avenue, 39°47.744' N, 76°59.318' W

Now a convenience store, the Karl Forney farm fields saw the Second North Carolina Cavalry and the Thirteenth Virginia Cavalry mount a charge that culminated in the two smashing into the Eighteenth Pennsylvania Cavalry's column, pushing the Pennsylvanians back into town. A Union counterattack pushed the Southern forces back across the same fields.

The fighting raged back and forth around the Forney farmhouse, which sat here at the time of the battle. When the fighting ended, the wounded were strewn over a wide area, with three Confederates and one Union soldier lying in the road immediately in front of the house. The four were brought inside, where they were treated by the Forney family.

One of the Confederate wounded was Sergeant Sam Reddick of the Second North Carolina Cavalry. He had been wounded in the road in front of the house, shot through the breast. Gathering his strength, Reddick dragged himself into Forney's yard, then onto the porch, where he lay for several hours before the family noticed him and brought him inside. Along with the other three found in the road, Reddick was treated in the Forney living room.

Reddick's condition worsened despite the care given him, and just before he died, he asked Mrs. Forney to return his New Testament to his sister, who had given it to him when he left home two years earlier. When his family received it in North Carolina, Reddick's father, a clergyman, asked Forney to mark the grave, which was recorded as having been about "100 yard southwest of Hanover near a red barn covered with slate, along a fence under a locust tree by the roadside." The red barn presumably was Forney's. Family members came to Hanover and retrieved the body about a year later and took it home.[4]

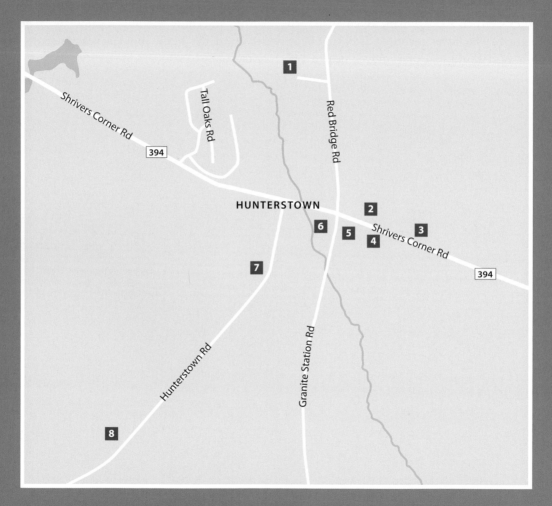

Chapter 14 sites: Hunterstown. (Map by Bill Nelson)

Hunterstown

BEFORE 1863 THE LITTLE HAMLET of Hunterstown was known primarily for two things. First, in 1794 General George Washington had stopped at John Tate's blacksmith shop to reshoe his horse while returning to Philadelphia after quelling the Whiskey Rebellion. Second, it had once been in contention to be selected as the county seat for Adams County, losing out on the honor to Gettysburg. Then, in the summer of 1863, fate intervened.

At dawn on July 2, while the main body of the Union Army of the Potomac was preparing for another day of fighting at Gettysburg, portions of the Sixth Corps and the Union cavalry, under Brigadier General George Armstrong Custer, were deployed elsewhere to protect the flanks from Confederate attack. These detachments were particularly concerned about J. E. B. Stuart's cavalry, which had attacked Union troops in nearby Hanover just two days earlier.

Early in the afternoon, Stuart approached Gettysburg with three brigades of his cavalry, capping the end of an arduous eight-day ride during which he had had no communication with Confederate general Robert E. Lee. As Stuart passed through Hunterstown, a contingent of his rear guard, under the command of Brigadier General Wade Hampton, encountered an advance cadre of Union cavalry.

A running battle through the streets of Hunterstown developed between the two, the Union mounting a charge and pushing the Confederates toward the town square. There, the Southerners, part of Cobb's Georgia Legion, reformed their ranks. Once that was done, Colonel Pierce Young ordered his legionnaires to mount a countercharge. With both sides slashing with their sabers, the Union troops weathered the attack. After passing through the square, the Georgians turned southward along a road that no longer exists, attempting to get to the main body of Hampton's brigade, consisting of men from Phillips's Georgia Legion, the Second South Carolina Cavalry, and the First North Carolina Cavalry.

Meanwhile, Kilpatrick met briefly with Custer at the Grass Hotel on the town square. There, Kilpatrick gave Custer orders to attack the Confederates as soon as he came upon them. Custer and his men found that opportunity south of the town near the farm of John Felty.

Observing the Confederates ahead, troopers from the Seventh Michigan Cavalry and most of the Sixth Michigan Cavalry set up their positions on either side of the road, using Felty's wheat fields for cover. Others moved into the Felty barn to get into elevated positions, while the Second US Artillery's Battery M, under Lieutenant A. C. M. Pennington, set up behind the barn.

Recognizing that fences on both sides of the road would prevent Hampton's cavalrymen from spreading out into adjoining fields, Custer decided to lure the Southerners into an ambush. He ordered the Sixth Michigan Cavalry's Company A to attack, choosing to lead the charge himself into what now was the bulk of Hampton's brigade.

At the farm of John "J. G." Gilbert, Custer's men and those from Hampton's brigade clashed in hand-to-hand combat. In the brutal fighting, Custer's horse was shot, falling onto Custer and trapping him under the dead weight. As Custer struggled to free himself, Lieutenant Colonel William Delony, the Cobb's Legion commander, led his men into the fight at full gallop. Nearly surrounded, Custer continued to struggle. Ironically, Delony's horse also was killed, trapping its rider much as Custer had been trapped. Delony soon broke free, however, and reentered the fray.

As Custer pulled himself to his feet, his orderly, Private Norvell Churchill, raced in and swept Custer onto his own horse and turned back toward the Felty farm. The rest of the Sixth Michigan followed, pursued closely by the Confederate cavalry in a mad dash along the road to Hunterstown.

As the Federal troops approached the starting point of their charge, the Sixth Michigan's men who had remained in position at the Felty farm, along with the Seventh Michigan, arose from their hidden positions and began providing covering fire. Pennington's guns joined the fight, forcing the Confederates back. As the daylight began to fade, the Louisiana Guard Artillery arrived in support of the Georgians and challenged the Union's guns.

Continuing well after dark, the artillery duel took its deadly toll until Hampton withdrew his men. The Confederates had nine men killed, most of them officers who had been leading the pursuit. Another five were wounded and seven were missing. Kilpatrick had thirty-three men killed, wounded, or missing, with most of those from the Sixth Michigan Cavalry's Company A.

The wounded were moved to several locations in the Hunterstown area while the survivors moved toward Gettysburg. The two sides were destined to meet again in less than twenty-four hours.

The fight at Hunterstown, which would become known as the North Cavalry Field, was only a very small part of the Gettysburg Campaign, but it had a significant impact on the main battle. It prevented Wade Hampton's cavalry from reaching Lee's left flank via the Hunterstown Road, where they had been expected to protect General Richard Ewell during the assault on Culp's Hill. This delayed the Confederate attack, forcing Ewell to move some three thousand infantry to the Hanover Road, weakening his forces in the main assault.

In the game of "What if . . . ," the battle at Hunterstown may also have revised history. Slightly more than two hours before the encounter at Hunterstown, the Union Signal Corps on Little Round

Top had seen Longstreet's countermarch. Incorrectly believing the column of ten thousand Confederates was moving toward the Union right flank, they alerted Union headquarters, which responded by ordering David Gregg to take some of his cavalry north from Hanover Road toward Hunterstown. Gregg's orders were to determine whether that Confederate column intended to use what today is Route 394 to launch an attack on Culp's Hill and the Union supply lines near Baltimore Pike. It was these cavalry troopers who met the Confederate cavalry at Hunterstown.

Had they not been dispatched toward Hunterstown, Gregg's cavalry would most likely have been placed on General Daniel Sickles's lightly protected left flank. Under such a scenario, instead of fighting in Hunterstown, the Union cavalry would almost certainly have challenged Longstreet's column and delayed it long enough to allow Meade time to adjust Sickles's line of advance into the Peach Orchard. What became the infamous Meade-Sickles controversy would have, in that case, never occurred, thus depriving historians of one of the great story lines of the second day of battle.

Doctors who are known to have performed their services in the Hunterstown area included Benjamin Cromwell (First North Carolina Cavalry), Lucious C. Coke (First North Carolina Cavalry), DeWilton Snowden (First Maryland Battalion), Caspar C. Henkel (Tenth Virginia Cavalry), Charles W. MacGill (Second Virginia Cavalry), Robert A. D. Munson (Second Virginia Cavalry), John A. Hunter (Twenty-Seventh Virginia Cavalry), Edwin Latimer (Andrews's Battalion), and Bushrod Taylor (Jones's Brigade).

1. Great Conewago Presbyterian Church, 174 Red Bridge Road, 39°53.256' N, 77°9.746' W

The origins of this church extend back to 1747, when the congregation worshiped in a log cabin near the cemetery gate. The present church was built during the pastorate of Rev. Joseph M. Henderson, using stones taken from the church property. In honor of the original pastor, it was given the name of Henderson Meeting House. In 1849 the present entrance was constructed, allowing three other entrances to be closed. At the same time, a foyer and choir loft were added and the pulpit and pews were replaced.

During the battle, the church served as a Confederate field hospital and binding station. The minister at the time was Rev. John R. Warner, who also served Lower Marsh Creek Presbyterian Church. Warner

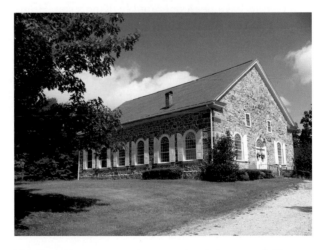

The Great Conewago Presbyterian church became a field hospital during the battle.

would go on to become a lecturer and battlefield guide.

Two of the six original oil chandeliers are still in use, although they are now electric. The other four are replicas. In 2002 a major renovation was undertaken, including a complete rebuild of the balcony. Timbers salvaged from the old balcony were used to construct a Celtic cross, which now hangs behind the pulpit.[1]

The cemetery holds the remains of thirty Revolutionary War veterans and also serves as a monument to the Civil War dead buried there.

2. Abraham (Hugh) King House and Store Site, 10 Hunterstown-Hampton Road, 39°52.938' N, 77°9.610' W

Owned by eighty-year-old Abraham King, the store is believed to have been operated by King's son, Hugh. The wounded from the early part of the battle were

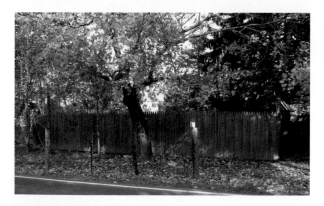

The King family operated a store in their home, which became a small field hospital in the early stages of the Hunterstown fighting.

brought here. Little else has been recorded about those treated here or the occupants of the property.

3. Methodist Episcopal Church, Hunterstown-Hampton Road, 39°52.883' N, 77°9.422' W

The Methodist Episcopal Society dates to 1739 in Hunterstown, when itinerant ministers Henry Furlong and John M. Jones arrived and began conducting services for the few Methodists living there. It would be another one hundred years before steps were taken to organize a church in Hunterstown, when services were held in various houses in the village. Eventually, services were held in an old schoolhouse.

In 1858 a brick church was built by the Methodist Society. Dedicated a year later, it suffered significant damage in 1879 during a major storm.

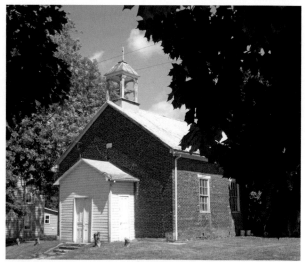

Those wounded in the early Hunterstown fighting sought shelter in the Methodist Episcopal church.

In 1863 the church was used as a small aid station. Most of those brought to it were wounded in the opening phase of the battle, which occurred not far from the church on Schrivers Corner Road.[2]

4. Deatrick's Store Site, Hunterstown-Hampton Road, 39°52.935' N, 77°9.619' W

Conveniently located next to the town square, Deatrick's Store was operated by Boreas Deatrick, a cabinetmaker by trade who also served as the town undertaker. His store sat adjacent to the J. G. Gilbert Store, which was used as the morgue during the battle. The Deatrick store is no longer standing. Bodies from the various hospitals in Hunterstown were brought to Deatrick's for burial preparation.

Deatrick would go on to enlist in Company K of the 184th Pennsylvania Infantry in 1864. He died in 1917 following a stroke at the age of eighty-eight and is buried in the graveyard of the Great Conewago Presbyterian Church.[3]

5. J. G. Gilbert Store, 39°52.938' N, 77°9.632' W

Situated immediately beside Dietrick's Store, the J. G. Gilbert Store quickly became the town morgue for those bodies prepared by Dietrick for burial. The dead were laid out on the porch beneath the overhang as they awaited transport to nearby railheads.

Some period maps show the property as being that of Jacob King.

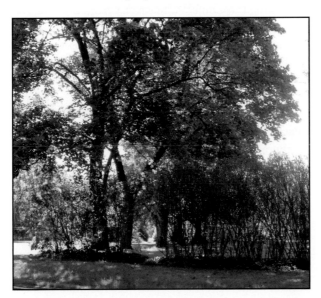

Boreas Deatrick served as the town's undertaker. His store sat on this site.

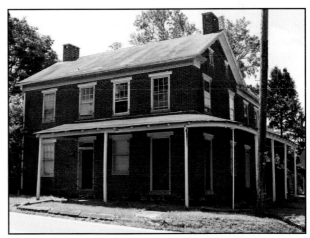

The dead were placed under the porch overhang at Gilbert's store.

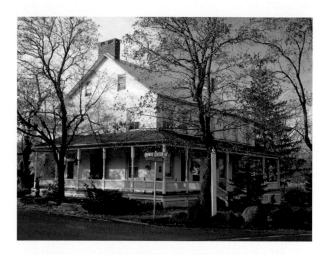

The Grass hotel became the largest hospital in town during and after the battle. It served as General Judson Kilpatrick's headquarters and still has a bullet hole in the front door.

6. Jacob L. Grass Hotel, Shrivers Corner Road, 39°52.940′ N, 77°9.656′ W

At this hotel, owned by Jacob and Harriett Grass, wounded from both sides were treated. The hotel served as General Judson Kilpatrick's headquarters, and it was here that Custer received orders to charge the Confederate line located just over the ridge on the Hunterstown Road.

A bullet hole remains in the front door, and the hotel is listed on the National Register of Historic Places.

7. John Felty Farm, Hunterstown Road, 39°52.691′ N, 77°9.960′ W

Central to the battle, the Felty farm was the scene of Custer's ambush of the Confederates. Felty's fences played a major role in the success of Custer's attack by

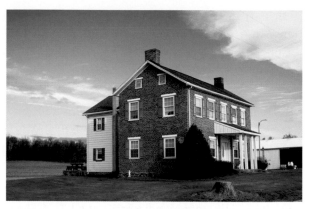

John Felty's farmhouse served as a hospital, with eight Confederate burials.

preventing the Confederate cavalry from utilizing the fields on either side of the road.

The barn, which housed Union troops from the Sixth and Seventh Michigan Cavalries, as well as the Second US Artillery's Battery M, no longer exists, having been torn down in 2007.

The wounded were carried into the farmhouse for treatment. Several would succumb to their injuries.

There were eight Confederate dead buried under a cherry tree in the corner of the Felty field, as well as at the Presbyterian Church cemetery. There are no records of which of the eight were buried in either location. All were from Cobb's Georgia Legion of Cavalry, and the names of two were unrecorded. The others were Thomas Riley Barrett, Second Lieutenant Cicero C. Brooks, Brevet Second Lieutenant John Weaver Cheeseboro, Second Lieutenant Thomas Howze, Junior Second Lieutenant Nathan S. Pugh, and Ebenezer F. Smith.[4]

Please note that the Felty farm is private property and visitors are asked to respect the owner's wishes that nobody wander on it.

8. John Gilbert Farm, 1736 Hunterstown Road, 39°52.459' N, 77°10.226' W

The John Gilbert farm was the scene of some of the most vicious fighting of the Hunterstown battle. There, General George Armstrong Custer's horse was shot from under him, the mortally wounded animal falling onto the general and pinning him. Only quick thinking by aide Norvell Churchill and a dose of good fortune saved Custer, as young Churchill rushed into the melee and pulled Custer onto his horse. Rushing back toward the Felty farm with Custer holding on to Churchill, the Sixth Michigan troopers raced toward the trap that had been set. The Confederates gave chase, as Custer had hoped they would, and soon the brutal fighting had moved back to the Felty farm. The Gilbert farm became a hospital, rather than a battleground.

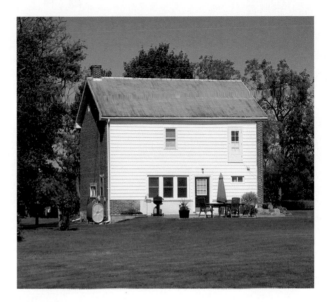

The Gilbert farm saw fierce hand-to-hand fighting virtually in the front yard.

Men from both sides were treated in the Gilbert farmhouse. Considering the ferocity of the hand-to-hand fighting, casualties were relatively light. No burials were recorded on the Gilbert property.

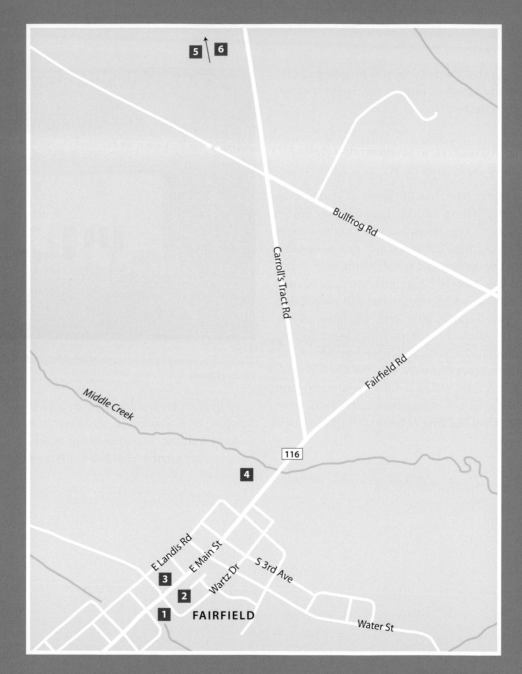

Chapter 15 sites: Fairfield area. (Map by Bill Nelson)

ON THE MORNING OF JULY 3, 1863, *the Sixth US Cavalry, under the command of Major Samuel Starr, was dispatched to Fairfield by Union brigadier General Wesley Merritt. Starr's orders were to locate and cut off a Confederate supply train reported to be in the area. Unknown to the Union cavalry, the train was being escorted by a portion of the Laurel Brigade, consisting of the Sixth, Seventh, and Eleventh Virginia Cavalry and Preston Chew's Battery of horse artillery, commanded by Brigadier General William E. "Grumble" Jones.*

At about the same time that the Confederate artillery was opening the artillery barrage that preceded Pickett's Charge, the two sides met on Carrolls Tract Road in the vicinity of the Benjamin Marshall and Hugh Culbertson farms. A charge by the Seventh Virginia Cavalry was pushed back at about the same time as Chew's artillery unlimbered and fired on the Federals. The Seventh Virginia charged again, this time with support from the Sixth Virginia Cavalry. The fighting devolved into a vicious hand-to-hand struggle, with Starr's men being driven off.

In the fighting, the flag bearer for Company H of the Sixth US Cavalry was killed. Private George C. Platt, an Irish immigrant, picked up the colors, stuffed them inside his coat, and carried them the rest of the battle, despite suffering a saber wound to his head. On July 12, 1895, Platt was awarded the Medal of Honor for his actions. His citation reads, "Seized the regimental flag upon the death of the standard bearer in a hand-to-hand fight and prevented it from falling into the hands of the enemy."[1]

A second Medal of Honor was awarded to Sergeant Martin Schwenk of the Sixth US Cavalry's Company B. Born in Germany, Schwenk tried to fight his way through Confederate fire to deliver a dispatch. He later successfully rescued one of his officers while under severe fire. His citation, awarded in 1889, reads, "Bravery in an attempt to carry a communication through the enemy's lines; also rescued an officer from the hands of the enemy."[2]

Union losses were six killed, twenty-eight wounded, and 208 missing, with most of the missing actually having been taken prisoner. Confederate losses were eight killed, twenty-one wounded, and five missing.

Temporary field hospitals were set up in the immediate vicinity of the fighting. Many of the wounded were later moved into the town of Fairfield for treatment.

The people of the town, with a population of only 218, had to wonder why their village was attracting so many wounded. Less than two weeks earlier, a skirmish outside town between the Fourteenth Virginia Cavalry and the Union's First Troop, Philadelphia City Cavalry, had brought wounded into Fairfield for the first time, and over the three days of the larger battle in Gettysburg a steady stream of Confederate wounded had been brought to Fairfield, further taxing the already meager resources of the town. When the Union army passed through Fairfield on July 6, they found 871 Confederate wounded in the buildings and fields of Fairfield, about four wounded for every man, woman, and child living in Fairfield.

The Confederate victory at Fairfield, albeit a relatively minor skirmish, had far-reaching consequences. Had the Union forces been victorious, they would have held Fairfield Gap, a major line of retreat for Lee's army. Lee's badly bloodied and demoralized army would have had to fight its way through well-defended positions, possibly delaying him sufficiently that Union pursuers could have boxed him in from the rear. Had that happened, Lee could possibly have been defeated, ending the war.

Surgeon Benjamin Franklin Ward of the Eleventh Mississippi Infantry was the surgeon in charge at Fairfield. Other doctors who are known to have served in Cashtown, in Fairfield, or along the Chambersburg Pike were LeGrand J. Wilson (Forty-Second Mississippi), James H. Southall (Fifty-Fifth Virginia), A. G. Emory (Fourteenth Tennessee), W. S. Parker (Fifty-Fifth North Carolina), James Parks McCombs (Eleventh North Carolina), William G. McCreight (Forty-Second Mississippi), Franklin J. White (Forty-Seventh North Carolina), E. N. Hunt (Second Mississippi), John H. G. Turkett (Seventh Tennessee), William B. Shields (Eleventh Mississippi), Joseph Holt (Second Mississippi), P. Gervais Robinson (Twenty-Second North Carolina), Robert Gibbon (Twenty-Eighth North Carolina), John Tyler McLean (Thirty-Third North Carolina), R. S. Baldwin (Sixteenth North Carolina), George Trescott (First South Carolina Rifles), Francis LeJau Frost (First South Carolina), William H. Scarborough (Fourteenth South Carolina), and W. P. Hill (Thirty-Fifth Georgia).

1. Rufus C. Swope House, 10 W. Main Street, 39°47.222' N, 77°22.153' W

Rufus C. Swope, a forty-one-year-old tanner, lived here with his wife, Evelyn, and several children. In the fall of 1862, Governor Andrew Curtin appointed

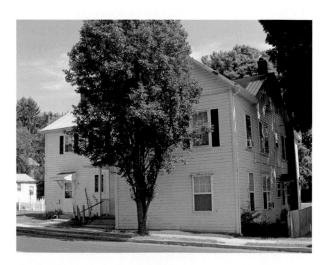

The Swope house became a hospital for at least two Union wounded. One died, and the other survived and rose to the rank of major general.

Swope as the draft commissioner for the Fairfield District, overseeing the selection of young men in the area for military service. As such, he was very unpopular, and in the matter of a few weeks after the first draft, his stable was burned down by two men, one of whom had been drafted into what had become known as the Drafted Militia.[3] A month later Swope was appointed assistant quartermaster for the US Volunteers. He later served as quartermaster of the Fifth Corps, Second Division.

As the fighting wound down along Carrolls Tract Road, Lieutenant Christian Balder of the Sixth US Cavalry attempted to escape the pursuing rebels by riding through the village. Witnesses said Balder rode madly up the street with a Confederate in close pursuit. The Union cavalryman suddenly wheeled his horse into what today is South Miller Street and turned to meet his enemy. A rifle shot knocked Balder from his horse. The critically wounded Balder dragged himself to Swope's porch, where the family took him inside. Knowing that death was near, Balder asked Swope to send his personal belongings to his family in Connecticut.

Friends said Balder had refused to surrender because of an incident earlier in the war, when he had been accused by his superior officer of cowardice. He declared then that never again would any man make such an accusation.[4]

Lieutenant Adna R. Chaffee, also of the Sixth US Cavalry, was another of the wounded to be treated by the Swope family. Chaffee recovered and rose to the rank of major general, commanding the US forces in the Boxer Rebellion.

In August 1903, a tablet was placed on the Swope house to commemorate its use as a hospital.

2. McKesson House (a.k.a. Blythe House), 18 E. Main Street, 39°47.254' N, 77°22.107' W

Originally a log and fieldstone house, the home has been modernized with the addition of siding. The house was built in 1801 by William McKesson and was a popular tavern. There were brick additions to the structure circa 1830 and 1860. During the war, the house was owned by Sarah Amanda McKesson Blythe, widow of Ezra Blythe, who died in 1844. An 1872 map identifies the home as that of Mrs. Bly.[5]

Among others, Major Samuel Starr of the Sixth US Cavalry was treated at the McKesson House. Starr had been shot in the arm and had suffered a saber wound to his head. He was originally taken to the Marshall House but was later moved to the McKesson House in town, where his arm was amputated. Locals tell the unconfirmed story that, when Starr was brought to the house, Blythe inquired of those who had brought him, "Does he have lice?" before allowing him into the house.

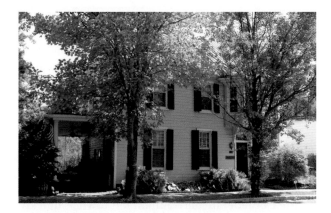

Major Samuel Starr's arm was amputated in this house.

As is often the case when stories are passed down, the final disposition of Starr's arm has a number of versions. One version claims that the arm was buried in the garden but the major complained of so much pain afterward that it was dug up and placed in a more comfortable box. Another version has the major taking the disinterred arm with him when he left Fairfield.

A variation of that story tells that Starr recovered and left Fairfield (without the arm) but had a great deal of pain from the amputation. He supposedly returned some time later with friends, who dug up the arm. Finding it in a cramped position, they repositioned it and reburied it. Starr is said to have never had pain from the arm again. The three versions are quite similar, so the story may have some level of validity.[6]

3. St. John Lutheran Church, 13 E. Main Street, 39°47.246' N, 77°22.131' W

Known as Zion Evangelical Lutheran Church at the time of battle, the church shared a pastor with a church in Emmitsburg. On Sunday, June 28, 1863, Rev. Washington Van Buren Gotwald, a student of the Lutheran Theological Seminary in Gettysburg, was conducting the service. As it concluded, a Confederate detachment under the command of Lieutenant John H. Chamberlayne rode up. Looking for horses, Chamberlayne's men unhitched those in the yard while Chamberlayne entered the church with his pistol drawn. He gave a receipt to each person whose horse was taken, telling them that they would be paid for their animals on the conclusion of a treaty of peace between the Confederate States and the federal government.

The Confederate detachment left town as quickly as it had entered, but encountered a squad of Union troops near Fountaindale. After a short skirmish, the horses were recaptured and returned to the citizens.[7]

The church was used as a hospital for the Sixth US Cavalry and the Sixth Virginia Cavalry following the cavalry action east of town, with both Confederate and Federal soldiers cared for. Boards were placed across the backs of the pews and covered with blankets. A Dr. Price of the Confederate army and Dr. William Henry Forwood, assistant surgeon of the Sixth US Cavalry, treated the wounded.

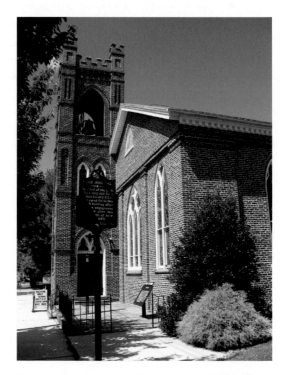

The church treated wounded from both sides, with a Confederate doctor and a Union doctor working side by side.

4. Daniel Musselman Farm, 203 E. Main Street, 39°47.399' N, 77°21.945' W

On the northeast end of town, outside historic town boundaries but within the historic district, is the Daniel Musselman farm, occupied by thirty-seven-year-old Daniel Musselman; his wife, Sarah; and their three children. The Musselmans had purchased the one-hundred-acre farm in 1854, although, because of a fire in 1848, it is not known whether any of the original house remains.

The 1863 US Sanitary Commission map of the Gettysburg area shows a Confederate field hospital, marked "Johnson's Division," located on the fields of the farm. The hospital must have been of significant size, because the bulk of the 871 wounded Confederates captured when the Union army passed through Fairfield on July 6 are believed to have been found here.

Musselman had been one of the townspeople who had lost horses to J. E. B Stuart when he came through in October 1862. Musselman also served as a witness for Daniel Mickley in his loss of a horse at the same time.[8]

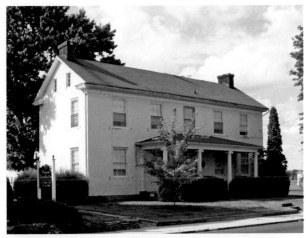

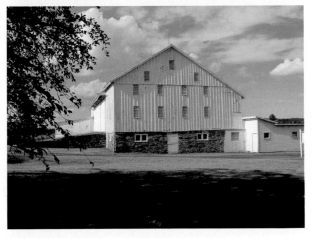

The Musselman farm is still an operating farm today.

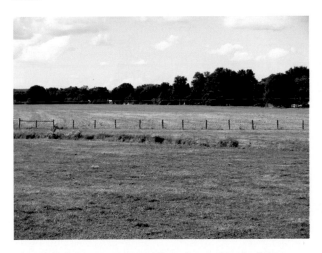

The Confederate army set up a large hospital in the field behind Musselman's barn.

Musselman filed an extensive damage claim for $1,770.52, saying he lost fence posts and rails, grains and crops (both stored and in the field), three mares, four fat cows, eight head of young cattle, harnesses, farm equipment, a straw cutter, a carriage, bacon, sausage, lard, butter, shad, clothing, and dishes and tableware, and he claimed that his real estate suffered damage from troops' encamping on and driving over it. His claim was denied by the federal government because the claims were inflicted by the rebels. Eventually, the State of Pennsylvania did honor most of his claim, awarding him $1,570.69, although he may never have actually received payment.[9]

5. J. A. (Benjamin) Marshall Farm, 1054 Carrolls Tract Road, 39°49.796' N, 77°22.129' W

The area along Carrols Tract Road near the Marshall farm saw significant fighting on July 3. A large plaque in front of the Marshall house, placed by surviving members of the Sixth US Cavalry, points out the hand-to-hand nature of the fighting, and that the regiment suffered 242 casualties out of the 400 engaged, a casualty rate of 60.5 percent. The plaque was placed here in 1909, and the Sixth US Cavalry held a reunion here on July 3, 1911, the forty-eighth anniversary of the battle.

Wounded in this area, Major Starr and others were first taken to the Marshall house before being taken to town for further treatment.

There were at least six Confederate burials on the Marshall farm: three in the corner of the orchard and another three under a locust tree near the house.[10]

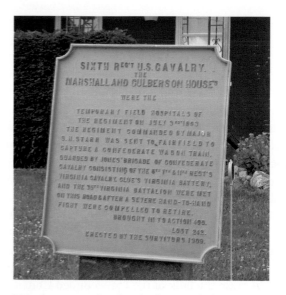

This plaque was placed in the front yard of the Marshall farm by surviving members of the Sixth US Cavalry.

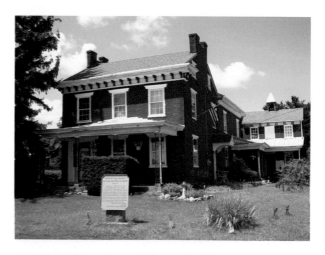

The Marshall farm became a hospital while the two armies were still fighting in front of the farm.

6. Hugh Culbertson Farm, 1240 Carrolls Tract Road, 39°48.846' N, 77°22.042' W

Hugh and Sally Culbertson lived on this farm in 1863. Much like the Marshall farm, the Culbertson farm served as a hospital for the wounded of both sides for a time on July 3. Later in the day, most of the wounded were moved into town.

It was in the general vicinity of the Culbertson farm that Private George Platt of the Sixth US Cavalry saved the regimental colors when the flag bearer was killed. When the flag bearer fell, Platt quickly scooped up the colors and stuffed them inside his coat to prevent them from falling into rebel hands. He was awarded the Medal of Honor for his actions.

The Culbertson farm also served as a collecting point for some 150 Union prisoners. Hugh and Sally Culbertson are both buried in the graveyard of the Lower Marsh Creek Presbyterian Church.

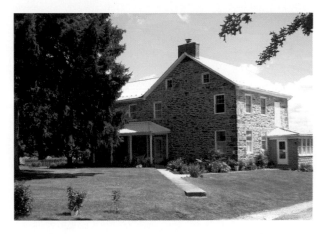

The Culbertson farm sat just a short distance from the Marshall farm and saw similar fighting.

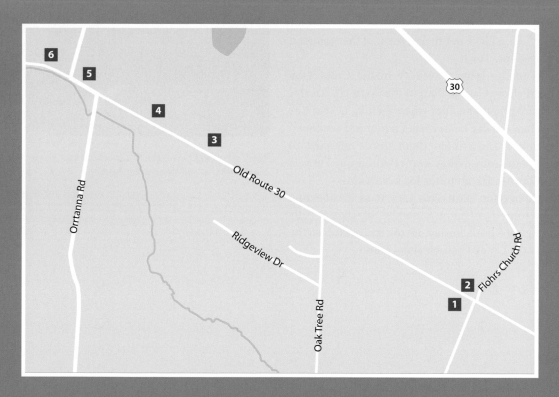

Chapter 16 sites: Cashtown. (Map by Bill Nelson)

Cashtown

ALTHOUGH THE TINY VILLAGE OF CASHTOWN had been laid out in the late 1700s as part of the newly formed Franklin Township, it had no official name of its own early in its history. Travelers began referring to it as Cashtown when the innkeeper at what is now the Cashtown Inn insisted on nothing but cash for the services he provided at his tavern and inn. He also was the toll collector for the highway passing his establishment, and cash was the only acceptable means of payment for passage along that route.

While the tiny village of Cashtown saw little fighting, local lore contends that the area was the site of the first bloodshed in Adams County before the fighting at Gettysburg. On June 26, 1863, at ten o'clock in the morning, four local residents, Henry Hahn, Henry Shultz, David Powell, and Uriah Powell, decided to ambush the advancing column of approaching rebel soldiers just west of Cashtown near what is now Old Route 30. As the troops passed, Hahn fired a heavy load of buckshot at the column of Confederates, knocking one of them from his horse. The soldier died later that evening, and Hahn and the other men fled into an area known as Gallagher's Knob, where they hid for the next ten days.[1]

Despite the lack of fighting in the area, Cashtown did play a pivotal role in the Battle of Gettysburg. The village's first brush with the Confederate army had come in October 1862 when General J. E. B. Stuart launched a raid into the area. Eight months later the bulk of the Army of Northern Virginia came to town, first with the arrival of Early's Division of the Second Corps on June 26, followed by General A. P. Hill's Third Corps on June 29.

While in Cashtown on June 30, Hill ordered General Henry Heth's Division to go to Gettysburg on a foraging and reconnaissance probe. Along the way, a brigade from Heth's Division, commanded by Brigadier General Johnston Pettigrew, was spotted by the Eighth Illinois Cavalry, which reported its observations to Union brigadier general John Buford. Buford knew of the presence of other Confederates in the area and set up pockets of his troops along the roads to the north and west of town, suspecting that any rebel advance would come from one of those directions.

The next day, July 1, Buford's suspicions were confirmed when Heth's entire division moved from Cashtown toward Gettysburg. As history now knows, Heth's men encountered Buford's cavalry along the ridges west of town. The next three days would become known as the Battle of Gettysburg. Throughout the battle the Southern supply and ammunition wagons were parked around Cashtown, and after the battle the town become a hospital for Confederate casualties.

When Lee's army began its retreat, Lee split it into two columns. One column of mostly infantry would go southwest through Fairfield. The second column, which grew to be seventeen miles long, would go northwest through Cashtown with the supply wagons and the wounded. When the ambulance train reached Cashtown, many of the wounded could go no farther. Dr. Willliam P. Powell (Fifth Texas) volunteered to stay behind with them. About 171 Confederate wounded were treated at various places in town, most of them from Pender's Division of the First Corps, with a few from McLaws's Division. The surgeon of McLaws's Division, Dr. Wilson, was in charge.

Two other doctors known to have assisted at Cashtown were William Montgomery (assistant surgeon of Archer's Brigade) and William A. Spence (Forty-Seventh Virginia). Others who are believed to have served in Cashtown, in Fairfield, or along the Chambersburg Pike were James H. Southall (Fifty-Fifth Virginia), A. G. Emory (Fourteenth Tennessee), W. S. Parker (Fifty-Fifth North Carolina), James Parks McCombs (Eleventh North Carolina), William G. McCreight (Forty-Second Mississippi), Franklin J. White (Forty-Seventh North Carolina), E. N. Hunt (Second Mississippi), John H. G. Turkett (Seventh Tennessee), William B. Shields (Eleventh Mississippi), Joseph Holt (Second Mississippi), P. Gervais Robinson (Twenty-Second North Carolina), Robert Gibbon (Twenty-Eighth North Carolina), John Tyler McLean (Thirty-Third North Carolina), R. S. Baldwin

(Sixteenth North Carolina), George Trescott (First South Carolina Rifles), Francis LeJau Frost (First South Carolina), William H. Scarborough (Fourteenth South Carolina), and W. P. Hill (Thirty-Fifth Georgia).

1. Flohrs Church, 595 Flohrs Church Road, 39°52.563' N, 77°20.398' W

Dating to 1822, when it was known as the Reformed and Lutheran Union Church, Flohrs Evangelical Lutheran Church served as a temporary hospital in the days following the battle, as the Confederate army moved back toward Virginia.

There were three known Confederate burials in the church's cemetery: William Nuckle (Sixth Virginia Cavalry) and First Lieutenant Jacob G. Shoup (Seventh Virginia Cavalry), who were both casualties of the July 3 battle along Carrolls Tract Road in Fairfield, and an

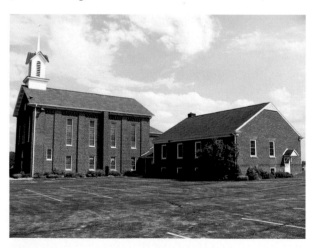

Flohrs Church served as a temporary hospital for wounded Confederates.

unidentified set of remains, likely those of E. Dinkle (Seventh Virginia Cavalry). Dinkle would also have been mortally wounded at Fairfield.[2]

An unmarked grave in the cemetery contains the remains of Henry Hahn, mentioned earlier as the shooter of the first known casualty of the Gettysburg Campaign in Adams County, a Confederate soldier. Hahn died in 1879 at age fifty-five.

2. Henry Mickley House, 616 Flohr's Church Road, 39°52.571' N, 77°20.398' W

The owner of the Cashtown Inn at the time of the battle, Henry Mickley lived in this home. Mickley's son Jacob ran the inn, which Henry Mickley sold in 1864 to Daniel and Mary Heintzelman. Confederate general George Steuart, father of General George Hume Steuart, stayed at Mickley's home after Mickley volunteered to house the seventy-three-year-old general as a possible deterrent to any damage to his property. If that indeed

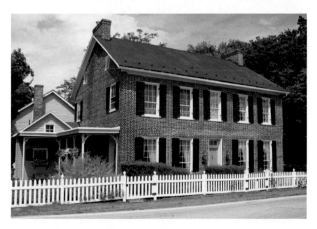

Henry Mickley offered to house the elderly general George Hume Steuart in hopes of minimizing damages to his home.

was Mickley's motive, it apparently did not work, as he claimed damages of $2,331.00. He was awarded $1,705.90 for his claim of losses of vinegar, butter, buckets, cow chain, chickens, corn, bags, salt and sundries, crops, fencing, wagon and horse, and cherries.[3]

With ambulances and wagons lining the roads and fields throughout the area, it was inevitable that Mickley's house would be used to treat the wounded. His 1817 house was one of the larger homes in the Cashtown area and provided ample room to house numerous wounded. The exact number is unknown, although it is known that there were no burials on the property.

3. Isaac Rife Farm, 1013 Old Route 30, 39°52.916' N, 77°21.216' W

Sixty-six-year-old Isaac Rife had three adult children, one of whom, David, had died nine years earlier at age nineteen. Rife's daughter Mary had married Jacob Shank, son of Christian Shank, whose farm had also served as a hospital. Rife's youngest daughter, Elizabeth, had married Israel Mickley and lived on the farm adjacent to Isaac's.[4]

There were two known Confederate burials on the Isaac Rife farm. Eli Joyner (Forty-Seventh North Carolina) had been wounded in the side on July 3, probably in Pickett's Charge. He died on July 6, indicating that he had been left behind when the ambulance train left Cashtown under General John Imboden's command. First Lieutenant Albert Thomas Traylor (Seventh South Carolina) had been wounded in the chest on July 2 and died on July 8, having also been left behind when the ambulances moved southward. Traylor was buried under a chestnut tree on the Rife property.[5]

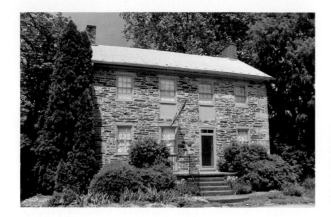

Two of those left behind when the Confederates retreated eventually died and were buried on the Rife property.

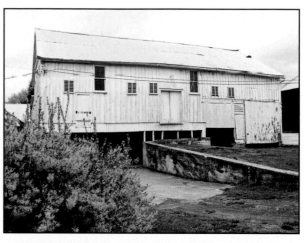

The Mickley barn was filled with wounded. It is still used today as part of a fifth-generation fruit farm.

Isaac Rife filed a claim for $661.00 for losses of three horses, grains, fencing, rails, fields and pastures, livestock, provisions, harnesses, wagon wheels, flour, tongue and lock, and chains.[6]

4. Israel and Elizabeth Mickley Farm, 1047 Old Route 30, 39°52.943' N, 77°21.281' W

Elizabeth and Israel Mickley operated a fruit farm until Israel's death a year before the battle, at age thirty-three. As a widow and single mother, Elizabeth was raising five children, ranging in age from two to eight years, when the Confederates came to her farm to use her barn and property as a hospital. Elizabeth would later remarry, this time to Henry Young, husband of her sister, who, when she was dying, asked Elizabeth to marry Henry and take care of him.[7]

The Confederates used the Mickley farm for two weeks as a hospital, filling the barn with wounded and placing the others around the barn and house.

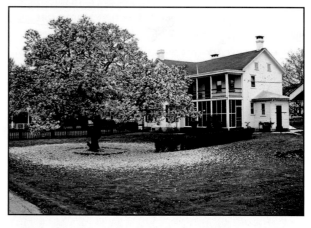

The Mickley farm housed and treated wounded Confederates for two weeks after the battle.

The barn still stands today and is part of the Kuhn Orchards.

Elizabeth filed a damage claim for $74.00 for losses of wheat, fencing, wood, hay, and corn fodder, as well as damage to the barn. She complained that the rebels had done "at least $10 damage to her barn." Her claim was honored in full.[8]

5. Dr. William C. Stem House, Cashtown-Ortanna Road Junction, 39°53.026' N, 77°21.484' W

Cashtown physician William Stem, thirty-nine years old, lived here with his wife, Eliza, and their two children. The house was built in 1826 and sat on a one-acre lot. When Henry Heth and his staff took possession of the property on June 29, 1863, and made it their division hospital, every square foot of Stem's land was placed into service treating Confederate wounded. Tents covered the front and rear yards, and Stem's office was opened to treat the sick and wounded.

At least two general officers were believed to have been treated here: Alfred M. Scales and William

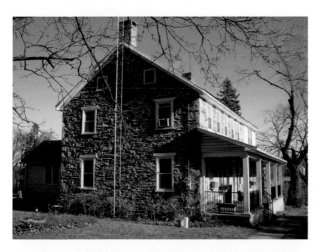

The house and office of Dr. Stem became the official hospital for General Henry Heth's Division.

Dorsey Pender. Pender rested here until ambulances were ready to resume the journey back to Virginia. Pender was evacuated to Staunton, Virginia, where an artery in his leg ruptured on July 18. Surgeons amputated his leg in an attempt to save him, but he died a few hours later. Scales survived and went on to become a congressman and governor of North Carolina.

Stem claimed losses of medicines (chloroform, ether, morphine, alcohol, and sulfur), hay, grass, sleigh bells, a scythe, seven cords of oak wood, bees, shelled corn, oats, a new halter, a harness set, buggy curtains, one fat hog, a clothes basket, a door, and lost and damaged farm equipment. His claim of $212.95 was accepted.[9]

6. Cashtown Inn, 1325 Old Route 30, 39°53.074' N, 77°21.619' W

The inn was believed to have been built circa 1804 by Peter Mark, who opened a tavern here in 1815 that served as a rest stop for travelers for the next thirty years. The facility was owned by Henry Mickley during the battle and was known as the Mickley Hotel, operated by his son Jacob. Mickley sold the property in 1864 to Daniel and Mary Heintzelman.

General A. P. Hill's Third Corps passed the inn on its way to the battle on June 29. Watching them, innkeeper Jacob Mickley noted that it looked as if "the entire force under Lee . . . passed within twenty feet of [his] bar room dore [*sic*]."[10] The previous October, the cavalry under J. E. B. Stuart had taken a similar route.

With two brick ovens used to feed the troops, as well as a basement with a natural spring, the inn became the headquarters for Generals A. P. Hill,

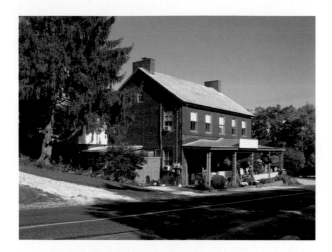

A hospital and headquarters for three generals, the inn's stable was used to house the wounded.

Henry Heth, and John Imboden. An adjoining stable, no longer standing, housed the wounded. Amputated limbs were tossed out windows and were said to be stacked so high that they blocked the incoming light.

At about four o'clock in the afternoon on July 4, the ambulance train finally left Cashtown. Stretching seventeen miles, the train completed its departure more than twenty-four hours later when the last wagon passed the inn.

Mickley filed a damage claim for $2,331.00, claiming losses of a wagon, a horse, a steer, fifty chickens, one hundred apple trees, and 480 gallons of whiskey and brandy. He was awarded $1,705.90.[11]

Glossary of Civil War–Era Medical Terms

Anyone researching records of sick or wounded soldiers on either side will often encounter unfamiliar medical terms. Some of the terms that were quite common during the Civil War have since fallen into disuse. Others are still commonly used today but may not be familiar to the layman. The following list of medical terms used during the Civil War may be helpful to those studying the treatment of the wounded.

Ablepsy—Blindness.

Abscess—Swollen, inflamed area of body tissue with a localized collection of pus.

Ague—Fever, often caused by malaria. Marked by sudden onset of fever, chills, shivering, and perspiration.

Amputation—Removal of a limb or portion of a limb.

Anasarca—Abnormal accumulation of fluid in tissues and cavities of the body, resulting in swelling. Also known as dropsy.

Anodyne—Drug used to lessen pain through reducing the sensitivity of the brain or nervous system. The term was common in Civil War-era medicine, but such drugs are now more often known as analgesics or painkillers.

Apoplexy—Stroke. Sometimes used to refer to an internal discharge or leakage of blood.

Ascetics—Accumulation of fluid in the abdominal cavity.

Asphyxia—Loss of consciousness due to suffocation, inadequate oxygen, and too much carbon dioxide.

Black fever—Acute infection with high temperature and dark red skin lesions and high mortality rate. This was common among wounded soldiers, particularly those who did not receive immediate treatment.

Blood poisoning—Bacterial infection; septicemia.

Blue mass—A mercury compound usually administered to facilitate a bowel movement. See *Calomel*.

Boil—Pus filled skin nodule caused by staphylococci bacteria. Usually painful and susceptible to often fatal infection in unsanitary conditions.

Cacospysy—Irregular pulse.

Calomel—Mercurous chloride given to facilitate a bowel movement or to treat a variety of diseases. If given in large doses, or over an extended period of time, it caused severe side effects, including death from mercury poisoning. Two months before the Battle of Gettysburg, Union surgeon general William A. Hammond had ordered the removal of all calomel from the US Army formulary, believing that it caused more deaths than lives saved. He was court-martialed for his efforts.

Camp fever—Serious illness commonly found in populations with less than sanitary conditions, such as camp, prisons, and field hospitals. Many cases were reported in the field hospitals around Gettysburg. More commonly known today as typhus, the disease was often fatal.

Catarrh—Inflammation of mucus membranes of nose and throat, causing increased flow of mucus (common cold).

Chloroform—Drug used as an anesthesia. Chemically known as trichloromethane. The vapor depresses the central nervous system and allowed surgeons to perform otherwise painful procedures. Some of the wounded survived the surgical procedure but succumbed to fatal side effects of the chloroform, such as cardiac arrhythmia. It was also eventually found to be carcinogenic in large doses.

Cholera—Bacterial disorder characterized by severe cramps and watery diarrhea. Often fatal to weakened prisoners.

Chronic—Continuing for a long period of time.

Comminuted fracture—Break or splinter of the bone into more than two fragments caused by high-impact trauma. In the Civil War that trauma was usually caused by a bullet or shrapnel.

Compound fracture—Fracture in which the bone protrudes from the skin. This was quite common with Civil War battle wounds.

Consumption—A form of tuberculosis.

Debilitation (debilitas)—A weakened condition usually related to chronic exhaustion and poor diet.

Debridement—Removal of dead, damaged, or infected tissue to improve the healing potential of the remaining healthy tissue.

Diarrhea—Watery stools, often resulting in dehydration. May also be symptomatic of more serious medical conditions.

Diphtheria—Acute, highly contagious disease. Characterized by abdominal pain and intense diarrhea.

DOW—Abbreviation for "died of wounds," often seen on medical records.

Dresser—Surgeon's assistant in a hospital.

Dropsy—See *Anasarca*.

Dysentery—Various intestinal inflammations characterized by abdominal pain and intense diarrhea.

Dyspepsia—Condition accompanied by feeling of bloating, regurgitation of food, and upper abdominal discomfort. Usually occurs following a meal. More commonly referred to as indigestion today.

Embalming surgeon—Individual who embalmed bodies in preparation for burial. Usually only done for those remains being sent to the family for burial at home.

Enteritis—Inflammation of intestines.

Erysipelas—Acute infectious disease of skin or mucus membranes. Characterized by local inflammation, fever, and swelling at the wound. Modern term is *cellulitis*.

Excision—Removal by cutting. Often done in lieu of full amputation. See *Resection*.

Exsanguination—Severe blood loss.

Febris—Fever.

Flux—Discharge of fluid from the body (for example, hemorrhage or diarrhea).

Gangrene—Localized death and decomposition of body tissue, resulting from either obstructed circulation or bacterial infection. Treated by amputation.

Gastritis—Inflammation of the stomach.

Gathering—Collection of pus.

Heat stroke—Condition in which the body temperature elevates because of the surrounding environmental temperature. Brought on when the body does not perspire to reduce temperature. Coma and death result if not reversed. High heat and humidity contributed to the deaths of some soldiers at Gettysburg either during the battle itself or on the long marches many had to take to reach the battlefield.

Hematemesis—Vomiting blood.

Hemophthis—Spitting of blood.

Hemorrhia—Heavy bleeding.

Icterus—Characterized by yellowish skin, eyes, and urine. Also known as jaundice.

Ictus solis—Major disturbance of the body's ability to regulate its cooling mechanism. Usually caused by prolonged exposure to excessive heat from the sun. It is made worse when air circulation is limited. This condition was responsible for many of the deaths at Gettysburg.

Intermittent fever—Term often used to describe malaria.

Laryngitis—Inflammation of the larynx.

Laudable pus—Pus that formed in wounds, often after surgery or amputation. In the mid-nineteenth century this was thought to be a sign of healing and was looked on favorably by attending surgeons. In reality, it was a sign of infection and was often fatal.

Laudanum—Mixture of opium and alcohol. Although used most often as a pain reliever, some physicians prescribed it for fever reduction or as a treatment for diarrhea. Many of the wounded became addicted as a result of their treatments.

Miasma—Poisonous vapors thought to infect the air.

Morsal (mormal)—Gangrene.

Mortification—Tissue death. Usually due to obstruction, loss, or diminution of blood supply; it may be localized to a small area or involve an entire extremity or organ.

Necrosis—Mortification of bones or tissue, usually skin.

Nephritis—Acute or chronic disease of the kidneys, characterized by inflammation and degeneration.

Noxious effluvis—Hospital or camp odors thought to make wounded soldiers sicker.

Osteomyelitis—An infection of the bone. In the Civil War it was most commonly caused by bullet wounds that resulted in fractures. Osteomyelitis often resulted in death despite the original wound's relatively minor damage by today's standards. The fear of this infection was an underlying reason for many amputations.

Paronychia—Painful, pus-producing inflammation at the end of a toe or finger.

Pellagra—Disease characterized by changes in mental stability, diarrhea, and darkening of those parts of the skin exposed to sun. Caused by lack of niacin. Widespread among the wounded who had supplemented their rations while on the march by foraging, resulting in a diet consisting substantially of corn products, which contain no niacin.

Peritonitis—Inflammation of the internal membrane lining the abdomen or pelvic wall. Common with abdominal wounds and often fatal if the patient somehow survived the wound.

Phthiriasis—An infestation of lice. Not uncommon in camps and field hospitals.

Pleurisy—Inflammation of membranes covering the lungs and the lining of the chest cavity. Characterized by difficult and painful breathing. Also known as pleuritis.

Primary amputation—Surgery done following the period of shock but before inflammation sets in.

Prostration—Extreme exhaustion. Common after long marches in periods of high heat and humidity, such as that experienced at Gettysburg.

Pyemia—Condition that often followed a serious wound, characterized by rapid pulse, fever, sweating, and chills. Often the next stage following erysipelas and nearly always fatal. Later known as blood poisoning. The modern term is *septicemia*.

Quinine—Drug derived from cinchona tree bark. Used to treat malaria but often accompanied by undesirable side effects after prolonged use, such as hearing or vision impairment and gastrointestinal symptoms.

Resection—The surgical removal of part or all of a damaged organ, tissue, or bone. Most often, battlefield wounds requiring surgery involved either resection or amputation. With resection, a limb could be saved but would either be limited in its ability to function or even useless. Also referred to as excision.

Rheumatism—Inflammation of joints, muscles, or connective tissue. More commonly referred to as musculoskeletal diseases today.

Rubeola—Measles. Not unheard of at Gettysburg, but more common in the early stages of the war when soldiers were exposed to illnesses for the first time.

Scorbutus—Disease resulting from deficiency of ascorbic acid (vitamin C), which is found in fresh fruits and vegetables. Characterized by weakness, spongy gums, and bleeding from mucus membranes. Also known as scurvy. This was a very common health issue in Civil War hospitals and prison camps.

Scrofula—Swelling of the lymph nodes due to tuberculosis.

Scurvy—See *Scorbutus*.

Seat of injury—Physicians' designation in notes or reports to designate the location of a wound (for example, "seat of injury, thigh," or "seat of injury, head").

Siriasis—Brain inflammation due to sun exposure.

Smallpox—Acute, highly contagious, and often fatal disease. Characterized by chills, prolonged high fever, vomiting, and pustular skin eruptions.

Soldier's disease (a.k.a. **soldier's sickness**)—Addiction to opium or other painkillers. Also referred to symptoms that appeared during withdrawal. Addiction was not uncommon among those whose wounds produced severe pain.

Sulphate of morphia—Painkiller made from mixing morphia (derived from opium) and diluted sulfuric acid. Civil War surgeons liked to prescribe it because it was water soluble and therefore easily administered in weaker doses by cutting it with water.

Sunstroke—Form of heat stroke resulting from prolonged exposure to the sun. Can be fatal in extreme cases. Common to soldiers on the march, or to the wounded who lay in the sun until treatment could be obtained.

Supperation—Formation of pus. Often referred to as laudable pus, a desirable condition during the Civil War era

that was thought to be a sign of healing but was actually a symptom of infection.

Tartar emetic—Antimony potassium tartrate, administered to induce vomiting.

Tetanus—Clinical condition associated with wounds, caused by the release of bacterial toxins that grow in the wound. Resulted in stiffness of skeletal muscles, particularly those in the jaw. This gave rise to its alternate name, lockjaw. This condition was nearly always fatal during the Civil War.

Tonsillitis—Inflammation of tonsils.

Typhoid—Acute infectious disease characterized by fever and diarrhea. A cause of many deaths among the wounded. Caused by fecal contamination of food or water.

Ulcus—Ulcer.

Venesection—Bleeding, or bloodletting, as a form of treatment for disease.

Vulnus incisum—Relating to a wound caused by a cut.

Vulnus punctum—Relating to a wound caused by a puncture.

Vulnus sclopeticum—Gunshot wound. Often appeared on hospital records as "vuls. sclo."

Sources: US Army Medical Department (Office of Medical History), Mayo Clinic, National Museum of Civil War Medicine.

The question can reasonably be asked, What is a table of money value comparisons doing in a book about field hospitals? The rationale for such a table becomes more apparent when one considers that the Bureau of Labor Statistics Consumer Price Index, on which this table is based, calculates that the dollar has experienced an average inflation rate of 1.94 percent a year from 1863 until 2020, the most recent year available. That translates to a cumulative price change of 1,948.53 percent.

Throughout this book, the damage claims for those whose properties served as aid stations or field hospitals are mentioned, and it may elicit a chuckle when we read that Elizabeth Mickley was angry because the rebels did at least $10 of damage to her barn, but her anger is easier to understand when we recognize that her loss was actually $204.85 at today's rate. Similarly, Francis Bream's $7,000 loss escalates to a loss of more than $143,000 at today's values. Numbers like these make it apparent why many farms had to be sold after the war.

The following table will aid the reader in better understanding the financial burden imposed by the treatment of the wounded.

1863 dollars	Equivalent 2020 dollars
1	20.49
100	2,048.53
200	4,097.06
300	6,145.60
400	8,194.13
500	10,242.06
600	12,291.19
700	14,339.72
800	16,388.25

1863 dollars	Equivalent 2020 dollars
900	18,436.79
1,000	20,485.32
1,500	30,727.98
2,000	40,970.63
2,500	51,213.29
3,000	61,455.95
3,500	71,698.61
4,000	81,941.27
4,500	92,183.93
5,000	102,426.59
5,500	112,669.25
6,000	122,911.90
6,500	133,154.56
7,000	143,397.22
7,500	153,639.88
8,000	163,882.54
8,500	174,125.20
9,000	184,367.86
9,500	194,610.52
10,000	204,853.17

Source: "CPI Inflation Calculator: 1863 Dollars in 2020," Bureau of Labor Statistics, accessed April 21, 2020, https://www.officialdata.org/1863-dollars-in-2020.

Acknowledgments

Nobody writes a book alone. Nobody. And I am no exception. Without the help of many people, this book never would have seen the light of day.

The entire idea for the book originated with my beautiful wife, Suzanne. She planned to write it herself, and she shared the idea with me one day while we were hiking on the Gettysburg battlefield. I thought it was a great project. We worked on it together until it became apparent that writing it was going to interfere with some of her other personal projects, so we agreed that I would take on the writing. We had done most of the research together, including the "detective work" of locating farms that no longer existed. Without her input, support, and hard work, this book would never have been written.

My son, Mike, assisted in locating some of the more obscure sites that were needed to flesh out the stories. On at least three occasions, Mike and I bushwacked our way through some pretty rugged terrain, only to find out that there was a hiking trail or lane that would have brought us to the same place, minus the scrapes and scratches, but without the fun and memories.

My daughter, Cheryl, provided moral support and inspiration despite a serious health scare. I am happy to note that she is now well on the way to recovery, and that is more important to me than any book could ever be.

Aside from immediate family, countless people had a hand in bringing this project to fruition. Not the least of these was the late Greg Coco. I met Greg several years ago at a book signing and enjoyed our conversations at subsequent ones. Our common ground, aside from a love of Civil War history, was the fact that he had written reviews of some of my earlier books. Greg was a pioneer in researching the field hospitals of Gettysburg, and I wish I had known him better so we could have shared information. Greg, I hope this work measures up to your challenge.

I asked five very busy people if they would review the manuscript and offer their critical comments. John Heiser (Gettysburg historian); licensed battlefield guides Dr. Richard Schroeder, Fran Feyock, and Susan Strumello; and licensed town guide Lisa Shower all agreed with no hesitation to take on the task, and their patience and expertise made this book much better than it would have otherwise been. Thanks for your hard work and, more importantly, your friendship. I would be remiss, too, if I did not acknowledge John Heiser's invaluable assistance in locating research materials, and he went beyond the call of duty in patiently answering questions and providing documents that Suzanne and I would never have found on our own.

Dr. Schroeder, in addition to being a licensed battlefield guide and reviewer of the manuscript, is a descendent of the Kime family, whose farm on the Old Harrisburg Road was one of the hospitals discussed in this book. He provided some excellent background information and source material about the family farm that made the Kime story much more interesting. Thank you, Rick.

Thanks to the National Museum of Civil War Medicine in Frederick, Maryland; the Pry House Field Hospital Museum in Sharpsburg, Maryland; the Clara Barton Missing Soldiers Office Museum in Washington; the Seminary Ridge Museum in Gettysburg; and the National Library of Medicine in Bethesda, Maryland, all of which provided valuable information on Civil War medicine in general, as well as specific information on Gettysburg field hospitals.

Maps and photos are an integral part of any book of this type, and I am indebted to Bill Nelson for his excellent maps, and to the National Archives and the Library of Congress for the period photos.

The people of Gettysburg showed amazing hospitality and a willingness to share the history of their properties. More times than I can count, what was intended to be a brief visit to take a photograph of a farm turned into an impromptu tour of their home, sometimes accompanied by an invitation to stay for a meal. These invitations came from complete strangers whom I had never met before. Where else does that happen?

Property owners, caretakers, and others who proved to be invaluable information sources and gracious hosts included Butch Poe (John Crawford farm), Chris O'Hare (John Cunningham farm), Jim Crane (John Crist farm), Mr. and Mrs. Lloyd Smith (Daniel Lady farm), Julie Aha (Isaac Rife farm), Dean Schultz and the Adams County Land Conservancy (John Cunningham, Jonathan Young, and Jacob Schwartz farms), John Repasky (Jonathan Young farm), Stephani Maitland (William Douglass farm), Sheri Beitzel and Ken Dayhoff (Jonathan Young farm), Rich Winkelmann (David Stewart farm), Peggy and Dennis Bair (Isaac Miller farm), Karl Orndorff (Jonathan Young and John Cunningham farms), John Pannick (Daniel Sheaffer farm), Mary Barnes and her son Chris (Peter Conover farm), Sally Thomas (Fairfield hospitals), Marvin Muhlhausen (Hanover hospitals), and Katherine Jeschke of the Gettysburg Foundation (railroad station and surrounding warehouse hospitals). I can never thank all of you enough.

Licensed battlefield guide Tim Smith and the Adams County Historical Society helped in a number of areas, and Main Street Gettysburg provided valuable information on hospitals in town. National Park Service ranger Dennis Flake provided important information on troop movements and activity on what is now the Eisenhower National Historic Site in a very enjoyable telephone conversation. I must also thank Carolyn Fouts for taking time out of her busy day to escort Suzanne and me on a personal tour of the Memorial Church of the Prince of Peace and explaining the historical significance of the memorial wall, and Rev. Dr. Herbert Sprouse, rector, for providing the photo of the David McCreary House, which stood on the church site at the time of the battle.

My publishers have been a pleasure to work with and deserve their own accolades. Lynn York and Robin Miura and the staff at Blair Publishing, and my contacts at Westchester Publishing Services, copyeditor Ashley Moore and production editor Kimberly Giambattisto, have all patiently made corrections, endured my questions, and offered suggestions that undoubtedly made the final product much better than it would have been otherwise. Callie Riek must also be recognized for the job she did in designing the book's cover.

Finally, as always, I must thank my agent, Rita Rosenkranz, for her diligence and expertise in guiding the project from manuscript to published book. I could not have done it without you, Rita.

If I missed anyone, please know that it was inadvertent, and your assistance is no less appreciated.

Notes

Prologue

1. Display, National Museum of Civil War Medicine, Frederick, Maryland.
2. Gregory Coco papers, Box B-69, File 8-a, Gettysburg National Military Park Archives.
3. Sarah Broadhead, *Diary of a Lady of Gettysburg, Pennsylvania: From June 15 to July 15, 1863* (Ithaca, NY: Cornell University Library, 1864), 23.
4. William A. Rupp, diary entry, July 10, 1863, Special Collections and College Archives, Gettysburg College.
5. Diary of Wilfred McDonald, Sergeant, Co H, 118th PVI, Gregory Coco Papers, Box B-69, File 43, Gettysburg National Military Park Archives.

Chapter 1

1. J. J. Woodward and George A. Otis, eds., *The Medical and Surgical History of the War of the Rebellion* (Washington, DC: US Government Printing Office, 1870), Part II, Vol. 1, p. 643.
2. Display, National Museum of Civil War Medicine, Frederick, Maryland.
3. "Townshend in the Civil War," William L. Clements Library, University of Michigan, accessed March 27, 2020, http://dev.clements.umich.edu/exhibits/online/townshend/civilwar.html.
4. Carol Adrienne, "John Meck Cuyler, M.D., A Confederate Surgeon's Sacrifice," Civil War Rx blog, n.d., accessed May 18, 2020, http://civilwarrx.blogspot.com/2013/05/john-meck-cuyler-md.html.
5. Walter F. Beyer and Oscar F. Keydel, *Deeds of Valour*, vol. 1 (Detroit: Perrien-Keydel, 1901).
6. Jonathan Letterman, *Report on the Operations of the Medical Department during the Battle of Gettysburg*, October 3, 1863.
7. Letterman.
8. Justin Dwinell, unpublished, undated medical report of the Battle of Gettysburg, n.p., MSC 129, National Library of Medicine, Bethesda, MD.
9. Cyrus Bacon Jr., *A Michigan Surgeon at Gettysburg 100 Years Ago—the Daily Register of Dr. Cyrus Bacon, Jr.*, Cyrus Bacon manuscript collection, University of Michigan, July 2–August 3, 1863.
10. Obituary of L. P. Warren, *Confederate Veteran* 22 (1914): 472.
11. Display, National Museum of Civil War Medicine.
12. Ethel Grace Alison, "The Work of the Sisters of Charity in the Battle of Gettysburg," Adams County Historical Society, Gettysburg.
13. Sarah Broadhead, entry for July 9, 1863, *Diary of a Lady of Gettysburg, Pennsylvania: From June 15 to July 15, 1863* (Ithaca, NY: Cornell University Library, 1864).

14. Eileen F. Conklin, *Women at Gettysburg, 1863* (Gettysburg: Thomas, 1993), 412–413.
15. Cornelia Hancock, *Letters of a Civil War Nurse*, ed. Henrietta Stratton Jaquette (Lincoln: University of Nebraska Press, 1998), 12.
16. Conklin, *Women at Gettysburg*, 182.
17. Conklin, 121.
18. Camp Letterman wayside marker.
19. H. S. Peltz, "Two Brass Buttons," *Gettysburg Compiler*, March 15, 1887.
20. Quoted in Roland Maust, *Grappling with Death: The Union Second Corps Hospital at Gettysburg* (Dayton, OH: Morningside, 2001), excerpts at http://www.gdg.org/Research/Authored%20Items/maust.html.
21. Maust.
22. Display, National Museum of Civil War Medicine.
23. Hancock, *Letters*, 8.
24. Letterman, *Report on the Operations*.
25. Display, National Museum of Civil War Medicine.
26. Display, National Museum of Civil War Medicine.
27. Allie Ward, "Burying the Dead," Civil War Institute blog, Gettysburg Compiler, August 2, 2012, https://gettysburgcompiler.org/2012/08/02/burying-the-dead-by-allie-ward-54463/.
28. Robert P. Nevin, *Pittsburgh Chronicle*, July 18, 1863.
29. Quote on Camp Letterman wayside marker.
30. Maust, *Grappling with Death*.

Chapter 2

1. Records of the Department of the Auditor General, "Records Relating to Civil War Border Claims: Damage Claims Applications," Roll 137, Record Group 32, Pennsylvania State Archives, Harrisburg, Pennsylvania (hereafter cited as Damage Claims).
2. "Landmark for 109 Years Gone (photo)," *Gettysburg Times*, June 9, 1967.
3. Felix Blanchard to Mrs. Worthy, July 24, 1863, Gregory Coco Papers, Box B-69, File 7, Gettysburg National Military Park Archives.
4. Felix Blanchard to his mother, August 6, 1863, Gregory Coco Papers, Box B-69, File 7, Gettysburg National Military Park Archives.
5. "Gettysburg 150th: July 1, 2013 Battlefield Experience Programs," *From the Fields of Gettysburg*, blog of Gettysburg National Military Park, National Park Service, April 27, 2013, https://npsgnmp.wordpress.com/2013/04/27/gettysburg-150th-july-1-2013-battlefield-experience-programs/.
6. Georgeanna Woolsey, wayside marker at Gettysburg Railroad Depot.
7. 1860 United States Federal Census, Borough of Gettysburg, Adams County, Pennsylvania, p. 53, lines 2–3, dwelling 364, family 414.
8. Liberty Augusta Hollinger Clutz, *Some Personal Recollections of the Battle of Gettysburg* (privately printed, 1925), 12.
9. Clutz.
10. 1860 United States Federal Census, p. 52, lines 8–17, dwelling 359, family 409.
11. National Park Service, *List of Classified Structures at Gettysburg National Military Park*, structures 36–45.
12. John W. Busey and Travis W. Busey, *Confederate Casualties at Gettysburg: A Comprehensive Record* (Jefferson, NC: McFarland, 2016), 2104.
13. "I. E. Avery's Words for His Father, the 'Letter From the Dead,'" North Carolina Department of Natural and Cultural Resources, accessed April 26, 2020, https://www.ncdcr.gov/blog/2015/07/03/i-e-averys-words-for-his-father-the-letter-from-the-dead.
14. 1860 United States Federal Census, p. 51, lines 14–22, dwelling 352, family 402.
15. Clutz, *Some Personal Recollections*. The use of Jeremiah Culp's shop as a hospital is corroborated in David A. Culp's unpublished family history, "Gettysburg Culp

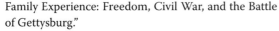

Family Experience: Freedom, Civil War, and the Battle of Gettysburg."

16. 1860 United States Federal Census, p. 45, lines 20–24, dwelling 307, family 354.

17. 1860 United States Federal Census, p. 45, lines 20–24, dwelling 307, family 354.

18. 1860 United States Federal Census, p. 44, lines 11–14, dwelling 299, family 346; *Star and Sentinel* (Gettysburg), April 26, 1887.

19. George Grenville Benedict, *Vermont in the Civil War: A History of the Part Taken by Vermont Soldiers and Sailors in the War for the Union, 1861–1865*, published in 2 vols. in 1886 and 1888 (repr., n.p.: Nabu, 2012).

20. *Proceedings of the Reunion Society of Vermont Officers, with Addresses Delivered at Its Meetings*, vol. 1 (repr., n.p.: Nabu, 2010).

21. William McSherry, *History of the Bank of Gettysburg, 1814–1864, the Gettysburg National Bank, 1864–1914* (Gettysburg: Gettysburg National Bank, 1914), 92.

22. 1860 United States Federal Census, p. 43, lines 12–15, dwelling 293, family 339.

23. Charles A. Fuller, *Personal Recollections of the War of 1861 as Private, Sergeant and Lieutenant in the Sixty-First Regiment, New York Volunteer Infantry* (Sherborne, NY, 1905), 96–97.

24. 1860 United States Federal Census, p. 50, lines 2–6, dwelling 341, family 389.

25. David Wills to Governor Andrew Curtin, July 24, 1863, Gettysburg National Military Park Archives.

26. Judge David Wills to Abraham Lincoln, November 2, 1863, manuscript letter, p. 2, Robert Todd Lincoln Papers, Manuscript Division, Library of Congress Digital ID # alo181p2, www.loc.gov/exhibits/gettysburg-address/exhibitionitems/Assets/alo181p2_725.jpg.

27. H. C. Bradsby, *1886 History of Adams County* (Chicago: Warner, Beers, 1886), 144.

28. 1860 United States Federal Census, p. 49, lines 27–39, dwelling 339, family 387.

29. Chaplain William C. Way, 24th Michigan Infantry, to *Detroit Tribune*, July 15, 1863.

30. Fannie J. Buehler, *Recollections of the Rebel Invasion and One Woman's Experience during the Battle of Gettysburg* (Gettysburg: Star and Sentinel Printing, 1896), 19–20.

31. Buehler, 26–27.

32. Buehler, 20–21.

33. Union Provost Marshals' File of Papers Relating to Individual Citizens, Roll 255, Publication Number M345B, Record Group 109, War Department Collection of Confederate Records, National Archives and Records Administration.

34. 1860 United States Federal Census, p. 38, lines 17–24, dwelling 258, family 302.

35. *Gettysburg Compiler*, January 15, 1908.

36. *Gettysburg Compiler.*

37. Sarah Broadhead, wayside marker at the Presbyterian Church on Baltimore Street.

38. Agnes Barr, "Account of the Battle of Gettysburg," Adams County Historical Society, Gettysburg.

39. Historical marker, Alumni Park.

40. William R. Kiefer, *History of the 153rd Pennsylvania Volunteer Infantry* (Easton, PA: Chemical Publishing, 1909), 216.

41. 1860 United States Federal Census, p. 41, lines 12–16, dwelling 277, family 323.

42. James Purman, Medal of Honor citation, US Army Center of Military History, Fort Leslie J. McNair, District of Columbia.

43. YWCA Gettysburg and Adams County, Survivors, Inc., Association of Licensed Battlefield Guides, Gettysburg Licensed Town Guides, and For the Cause Productions, *Women behind These Walls—Stories of the Civil War in Gettysburg, through the Eyes of Women*, walking tour information posters in windows of Samuel Witherow House.

Chapter 3

1. 1860 United States Federal Census, Borough of Gettysburg, Adams County, Pennsylvania, p. 59, lines 4–11, dwelling 410, family 461.

2. Murdock McGregor, Assistant Surgeon, 33rd Massachusetts Infantry, to George George, n.d., Gettysburg National Military Park Archives.

3. US Department of the Interior, National Park Service, Nomination Form, National Register of Historic Places—Dobbin House, Adams County, Pennsylvania; Fredrick Tilbeg and Harry Pfanz, Documentation for Historical Base Map, June 23, 1958, Gettysburg National Military Park Archives.

4. 1860 United States Federal Census, p. 58, lines 37–40, and p. 59, lines 1–3, dwelling 409, family 460.

5. 1860 United States Federal Census, p. 35, lines 9–14, dwelling 234, family 276.

6. YWCA Gettysburg and Adams County, Survivors, Inc., Association of Licensed Battlefield Guides, Gettysburg Licensed Town Guides, and For the Cause Productions, *Women behind These Walls—Stories of the Civil War in Gettysburg, through the Eyes of Women*, walking tour information posters in windows of specific women's homes.

7. YWCA Gettysburg and Adams County et al., *Women behind These Walls.*

8. Nicholas Paonessa, supervisor, *Case Report: Bloodstains of Gettysburg: The Use of Chemiluminescent Blood Reagents to Visualize Bloodstains of Historical Significance* (Niagara Falls, NY: Forensic Identification/Crime Scene Unit, Niagara Falls Police Department, 2006), accessed August 14, 2019, https://www.bluestar-forensic.com/medias/content/gettysburg_iabpanews.pdf.

9. 1860 United States Federal Census, p. 41, lines 22–29, dwelling 279, family 325.

10. Matilda (Tillie) Pierce Alleman, *At Gettysburg; or What a Girl Saw and Heard of the Battle* (New York: W. Lake Borland, 1889), 88–90.

11. Alleman, 90–91.

12. YWCA Gettysburg and Adams County et al., *Women behind These Walls.*

13. 1860 United States Federal Census, p. 22, lines 29–37, dwelling 146, family 176.

14. Peter C. Vermilyea, "The Effect of the Confederate Invasion of Pennsylvania on Gettysburg's African American Community," *Gettysburg Magazine*, July 2001, p. 120.

15. "A Mother's Story," *Gettysburg Compiler*, July 4, 1906.

16. "A Mother's Story."

17. Church history of the Memorial Church of the Prince of Peace church files.

18. Ethel Grace Alison, "The Work of the Sisters of Charity in the Battle of Gettysburg," Adams County Historical Society, Gettysburg.

19. Congressional Medal of Honor Society, Henry S. Huidekoper citation, accessed April 27, 2020, http://www.cmohs.org/recipient-detail/669/huidekoper-henry-s.php.

20. Albertus McCreary, "Gettysburg: A Boy's Experience of the Battle," *McClure's*, July 1909.

21. YWCA Gettysburg and Adams County et al., *Women behind These Walls.*

22. Elizabeth Salome "Sallie" Myers, "How a Gettysburg School Teacher Spent Her Vacation in 1863," *San Francisco Sunday Call*, August 16, 1903.

23. Myers.

24. Alleman, *At Gettysburg*, 29.

25. Alleman, 14.

26. 1860 United States Federal Census, p. 34, lines 38–40, and p. 35, lines 1–5, dwelling 232, family 274.

27. J. Howard Wert, "Little Stories of Gettysburg," *Gettysburg Compiler*, January 8, 1905.

28. "Terrible Accident," *Gettysburg Compiler*, November 20, 1863.

29. David A. Murdoch, "Catherine Mary White Foster's Eyewitness Account of the Battle of Gettysburg, with Background on the Foster Family Union Soldiers," *Adams County History* 1 (1995): article 5, p. 48.

30. YWCA Gettysburg and Adams County et al., *Women behind These Walls*, James and Catherine Foster House.

31. Murdoch, "Catherine Mary White Foster's," 51–52.

32. Murdoch, 53.

33. 1860 United States Federal Census, p. 11, lines 10–15, dwelling 70, family 87.

34. Pennsylvania House of Representatives, *Revised Report of the Select Committee Relative to the Soldiers' National Cemetery* (Harrisburg, PA: Singerly and Myers, State Printers, 1865), 149.

35. 1860 United States Federal Census, p. 11, lines 4–9, dwelling 69, family 86.

36. Quoted in US Department of the Interior, National Park Service, *Impact of War: The Slyder Family Farm*, NPS Teachers' Guide (Gettysburg: US Department of the Interior, National Park Service, n.d.), 24.

37. Quoted in US Department of the Interior, National Park Service, 25.

38. Doug Gelbert, *Look Up, Gettysburg!* (Cruden Bay Books, 2009), 8.

39. Fannie J. Buehler, *Recollections of the Rebel Invasion and One Woman's Experience during the Battle of Gettysburg* (Gettysburg: Star and Sentinel Printing, 1896), 26.

40. Buehler, 26.

41. Fahnestock store wayside marker.

42. 1860 United States Federal Census, p. 2, lines 30–34, dwelling 14, family 15.

43. "A Woman's Story of the Battle," *Gettysburg Compiler*, June 24, 1903.

44. 1860 United States Federal Census, p. 2, lines 8–12, dwelling 10, family 11.

45. YWCA Gettysburg and Adams County et al., *Women behind These Walls*.

46. 1860 United States Federal Census, p. 30, lines 34–40, and p. 31, lines 1–3, dwelling 204, family 245.

47. Charles M. McCurdy, *Gettysburg, a Memoir* (repr., Scotts Valley, CA: CreateSpace Independent Publishing Platform, 2013), 18.

48. McCurdy.

49. McCurdy.

50. 1860 United States Federal Census, p. 2, lines 2–7, dwelling 9, families 9–10.

51. Patriot Daughters of Lancaster, *Hospital Scenes after the Battle of Gettysburg* (repr., London: Forgotten Books, 2018), 22–24.

52. "Gettysburg 150th—July 1, 2013 Battlefield Experience Progams," *From the Fields of Gettysburg*, blog of Gettysburg National Military Park, National Park Service, April 27, 2013, https://npsgnmp.wordpress.com/2013/04/27/gettysburg-150th-july-1-2013-battlefield-experience-programs/.

53. William C. Way, letter, *Detroit Advertiser and Tribune*, July 24, 1863.

54. 1860 United States Federal Census, p. 18, lines 31–39, dwelling 124, family 146.

55. "Thomas James Shorb," Find a Grave, accessed March 27, 2020, https://www.findagrave.com/memorial/158811128/thomas-james-shorb.

56. "Joseph Michael Shorb," Find a Grave, accessed March 27, 2020, https://www.findagrave.com/memorial/6923229/joseph-michael-shorb.

57. Timothy H. Smith, *John Burns, the Hero of Gettysburg* (Gettysburg: Thomas, 2000), 82–84.

Chapter 4

1. *Detroit Advertiser and Tribune*, July 24, 1863.

2. Obituary of Alexander Spangler, *Adams County News*, April 30, 1910.

3. David McConaughy to Governor Andrew Curtin, July 25, 1863, Gettysburg National Military Park Archives.

4. 1860 United States Federal Census, Borough of Gettysburg, Adams County, Pennsylvania, p. 29, lines 7–15, dwelling 194, family 233.

5. YWCA Gettysburg and Adams County, Survivors, Inc., Association of Licensed Battlefield Guides, Gettysburg

Licensed Town Guides, and For the Cause Productions, *Women behind These Walls—Stories of the Civil War in Gettysburg, through the Eyes of Women,* walking tour information posters in windows of specific women's homes.

6. 1860 United States Federal Census, p. 31, lines 27–32, dwelling 209, family 250.

7. Jennie Croll, "Memoir of Mary A. Horner," *Philadelphia Weekly Press,* November 16, 1887.

8. 1860 United States Federal Census, p. 29, lines 16–18, dwelling 195, family 234.

9. YWCA Gettysburg and Adams County et al., *Women behind These Walls.*

10. 1860 United States Federal Census, p. 3, lines 24–30, dwelling 20, family 24.

11. 1860 United States Federal Census, p. 3, lines 31–32, dwelling 21, family 25.

12. 1860 United States Federal Census, p. 4, lines 17–24, dwelling 25, families 31, 32.

13. "Story of Elizabeth and Jacob Gilbert, Residents of Gettysburg during the Civil War," *Gettysburg Compiler,* September 6, 1905.

14. Civil War Vertical File Manuscripts, Special Collections and College Archives, Musselman Library, Gettysburg College.

15. "Story of Elizabeth and Jacob Gilbert."

16. "Story of Elizabeth and Jacob Gilbert."

17. 1860 United States Federal Census, p. 32, lines 28–30, dwelling 217, family 258.

18. YWCA Gettysburg and Adams County et al., *Women behind These Walls.*

19. Sarah Broadhead, *Diary of a Lady of Gettysburg, Pennsylvania: From June 15 to July 15, 1863* (Ithaca, NY: Cornell University Library, 1864), 20–21.

20. Broadhead, 23.

21. US Department of the Interior, National Park Service, "Gettysburg College and the Battle," *Sentinel,* 150th anniversary ed., 2013.

22. Charles H. Glatfelter, *A Salutary Influence: Gettysburg College, 1832–1985* (Gettysburg: Gettysburg College, 1987), 184. Some sources attribute the quote to Professor Michael Jacobs.

23. Eileen F. Conklin, *Women at Gettysburg, 1863* (Gettysburg: Thomas, 1993), 412–413.

Chapter 5

1. 1860 United States Federal Census, Borough of Gettysburg, Adams County, Pennsylvania, p. 56, lines 16–22, dwelling 390, family 441.

2. H. C. Bradsby, *1886 History of Adams County* (Chicago: Warner, Beers, 1886), 201.

3. Timothy H. Smith, *The Story of Lee's Headquarters* (Gettysburg: Thomas, 1996), 38.

4. Damage Claims, Roll 134.

5. *Adams Sentinel,* July 18, 1859.

6. Sheads Family Papers, Box 1, Accession Number 8595, Adams County Historical Society, Gettysburg.

7. Damage Claims, Roll 139.

8. Elizabeth A. Sheffer, "The Sheads House," *Gettysburg Times,* January 23–24, 1988.

9. 1860 United States Federal Census, p. 8, lines 37–40, and p. 9, lines 1–5, dwelling 52, family 68.

10. Damage Claims, Roll 133.

11. Smith, *Story of Lee's Headquarters,* 5.

12. Informational display inside the Thompson house.

13. 1860 United States Federal Census, p. 56, lines 23–27, dwelling 391, family 442.

14. "Family Left Because Wounded Filled Home," *Gettysburg Times,* August 31, 1985. Greg Coco Papers, Box B-72-1, file 162, Gettysburg National Military Park Archives.

15. *Gettysburg Times.*

16. Damage Claims, Roll 136.

17. "Surgeons at the Lutheran Seminary," Seminary Ridge Museum records.

18. "Surgeons at the Lutheran Seminary."
19. 1860 United States Federal Census, p. 33, lines 13–21, dwelling 222, family 264.
20. Lydia Catherine Ziegler Clare, "A Gettysburg Girl's Story of the Great Battle," memoirs, 1900, Gregory Coco Papers, Box B-72-1, File 187, Gettysburg National Military Park Archives.
21. Clare.
22. *Report of the Chairman of the Faculty*, August 11, 1863, Lutheran Theological Seminary Archives.
23. Gregory A. Coco, *Wasted Valor: The Confederate Dead at Gettysburg* (Gettysburg: Thomas, 1990), 61.
24. Seminary Ridge Museum burial records.
25. 1860 United States Federal Census, p. 56, line 40, and p. 57, line 1, dwelling 393, family 444.
26. *Report of the Chairman of the Faculty*.
27. Scott D. Hartwig, "I Have Never Seen the Like Before: Herbst Woods, July 1, 1863" (essay 5, presented at the National Park Service Symposia, Gettysburg Seminars), Gettysburg, March 23, 1996.
28. Damage Claims, Roll 135.
29. Mary Rose and Lillian Rose, "Jacob Herbst and His Descendants," *Adams County Sentinel*, September 7, 1904, Herbst Family File, Adams County Historical Society, Gettysburg.
30. National Park Service, *List of Classified Structures, Gettysburg National Military Park (PA)*, structure 72.
31. National Park Service, structure 72.
32. Francis Bacon Jones, "Chronicles of Captain Francis Bacon Jones," Gregory Coco Papers, Box B-69, File 34, Gettysburg National Military Park Archives.
33. Kathleen R. Georg, "Edward McPherson Farm: Historical Study," Gettysburg National Military Park, October 14, 1977.
34. Damage Claims, Roll 139.
35. Damage Claims, Roll 137.
36. Georg, "Edward McPherson Farm."
37. Obituary of Basil Biggs, *Gettysburg Compiler*, June 13, 1906.
38. LeGrand J. Wilson, *The Confederate Soldier*, ed. James W. Silver (Memphis: Memphis State University Press, 1973).
39. Damage Claims, Roll 135.
40. John W. Busey and Travis W. Busey, *Confederate Casualties at Gettysburg: A Comprehensive Record* (Jefferson, NC: McFarland, 2016), 2012.
41. Warner, Beers, and company staff, et al., *History of Cumberland and Adams Counties, Pennsylvania*, pt. 3, *Adams County* (Chicago: Warner, Beers, 1886), 208–210.
42. Busey and Busey, *Confederate Casualties at Gettysburg*, 2116, 2136, 2598.
43. Damage Claims, Roll 133.
44. Damage Claims, Roll 131.
45. Damage Claims, Roll 133.
46. Busey and Busey, *Confederate Casualties at Gettysburg*, 2098, 2113, 2136.
47. Mark H. Dunkelman, *Gettysburg's Unknown Soldier: The Life, Death, and Celebrity of Amos Humiston* (Westport, CT: Praeger, 1999), 9, 202.
48. Damage Claims, Roll 140.
49. Damage Claims, Roll 132.
50. Busey and Busey, *Confederate Casualties at Gettysburg*, 2016.
51. Busey and Busey, 2016.
52. Busey and Busey, 2136.
53. Damage Claims, Roll 136.
54. Damage Claims, Roll 135.
55. Damage Claims, Roll 139.
56. Damage Claims, Roll 139.

Chapter 6

1. *Adams Sentinel*, January 15, 1862.
2. John William Crapster O'Neal, "List of Marked Confederates Buried upon the Battlefield of Gettysburg," Gettysburg National Military Park Archives, n.d.

3. John W. Busey and Travis W. Busey, *Confederate Casualties at Gettysburg: A Comprehensive Record* (Jefferson, NC: McFarland, 2016), 266–268.

4. Busey and Busey, 266–268.

5. O'Neal, "List of Marked Confederates."

6. Damage Claims, Roll 132.

7. Michael Peffer, *Crossing the Threshold* (Grand Rapids, MI: Inner Workings, 2014), 33.

8. US Department of the Interior, National Park Service, Nomination Form, National Register of Historic Places—Black Horse Tavern, Adams County, Pennsylvania.

9. Some sources say that DeSaussure was killed instantly when he was shot on the George Rose farm.

10. Damage Claims, Roll 132.

11. Damage Claims, Roll 133.

12. Lizzie Beard, unpublished memo, Gregory Coco Papers, Box B-72-1, File 170, Gettysburg National Military Park Archives.

13. *The War of the Rebellion: A Compilation of the Official Records of the Union and Confederate Armies*, ser. 1, vol. 27, pt. 2 (Washington, DC: US Government Printing Office, 1889).

14. Busey and Busey, *Confederate Casualties at Gettysburg*, 2015–2016.

15. O'Neal, "List of Marked Confederates."

16. Busey and Busey, *Confederate Casualties at Gettysburg*, 2010.

17. Damage Claims, Roll 133.

18. Gabor Borritt, "History of the Farm by the Ford," *Gettysburg Times*, June 12, 2015.

19. O'Neal, "List of Marked Confederates."

20. Damage Claims, Roll 131.

21. Damage Claims, Roll 133.

22. O'Neal, "List of Marked Confederates."

23. Damage Claims, Roll 132.

24. Busey and Busey, *Confederate Casualties at Gettysburg*, 802.

25. Damage Claims, Roll 138.

26. Busey and Busey, *Confederate Casualties at Gettysburg*, 2128.

27. Damage Claims, Roll 140.

28. Busey and Busey, *Confederate Casualties at Gettysburg*, 2011.

29. Mrs. George F. Harper, "The Scotts and Cunninghams See the Battle," *Gettysburg Times*, April 22, 1941.

30. Damage Claims, Roll 133.

31. US Department of the Interior, National Park Service, Nomination Form, National Register of Historic Places—Lower Marsh Creek Presbyterian Church, Adams County, Pennsylvania.

32. Church history, dedication service printed program, June 26, 1988.

33. Damage Claims, Roll 134.

34. Busey and Busey, *Confederate Casualties at Gettysburg*, 2055.

35. George T. Stevens, Surgeon George T. Stephens Report, Camp Letterman Papers, Gettysburg National Military Park Archives.

36. Damage Claims, Roll 139.

37. Damage Claims, Roll 141.

38. Damage Claims, Roll 137.

Chapter 7

1. National Park Service, *List of Classified Structures, Gettysburg National Military Park (PA)*, structures 33–35.

2. John W. Busey and Travis W. Busey, *Confederate Casualties at Gettysburg: A Comprehensive Record* (Jefferson, NC: McFarland, 2016), 2005.

3. Damage Claims, Roll 138.

4. US Department of the Interior, National Park Service, *Daniel Klingel Farmhouse Historic Structure Report*, August 2016 (Philadelphia: US Department of the Interior, National Park Service).

5. US Department of the Interior, National Park Service.

6. File 214-772, Record Group 92, "Records of the Office of the Quartermaster General (OQMD)," Quartermaster General Files, National Archives and Records Administration.

7. National Park Service, *List of Classified Structures at Gettysburg National Military Park*, structures 87–96.

8. Daniel A. Skelly, *A Boy's Experience during the Battles of Gettysburg* (Gettysburg: privately printed, 1932).

9. Charles W. Reed, Medal of Honor citation, August 16, 1895, for actions of July 2, 1863, Congressional Medal of Honor Society.

10. Busey and Busey, *Confederate Casualties at Gettysburg*, 2050.

11. Damage Claims, Roll 140.

12. Busey and Busey, *Confederate Casualties at Gettysburg*, 2050–2051.

13. Damage Claims, Roll 140.

14. Internal report, National Park Service, *Record of Land Ownership for the Eisenhower National Historic Site*, vol. 1, pp. 16–18.

15. Dennis Flake, National Park Service ranger, Eisenhower National Historic Site, conversation with the author, June 15, 2018. Ranger Flake painstakingly traced the troop movements across the farm and described the damage done in great detail during our discussion. He also made me aware of his article on the subject in the *Civil War Monitor*, which provides more information.

16. Dennis Edward Flake, "The Eisenhower Farm during the Battle of Gettysburg," *Civil War Monitor*, March 9, 2018.

17. Historic American Buildings Survey, Library of Congress, Survey Number HABS PA-5373; National Park Service, *Record of Land Ownership*, 17.

18. Elliott's map of the battlefield of Gettysburg, Pennsylvania (Philadelphia: S. G. Elliott, 1864).

19. National Park Service, *Record of Land Ownership*, 27.

20. National Park Service, 20.

21. Kathleen R. Georg Harrison, "Longstreet's Headquarters Re-examined, or the Significance of a Piece of Painted Wooden Signboard!," Gettysburg National Military Park, February 19, 1981.

22. Stan Wolf, "Pitzer's School: "Schoolhouse to Residence," Cumberland Township Historical Society, October 2014.

23. John William Crapster O'Neal, "List of Marked Confederates Buried upon the Battlefield of Gettysburg," Gettysburg National Military Park Archives.

24. Damage Claims, Roll 138.

25. Busey and Busey, *Confederate Casualties at Gettysburg*, 2011.

26. O'Neal, "List of Marked Confederates."

27. Damage Claims, Roll 139.

28. Busey and Busey, *Confederate Casualties at Gettysburg*, 2116.

29. National Park Service, *List of Classified Structures at Gettysburg National Military Park*, structure 150.

30. Damage Claims, Roll 139.

31. Stephen M. Hood, *The Lost Papers of Confederate General John Bell Hood* (El Dorado Hills, CA: Savas Beatie, January 2015), e-book version, p. 48.

32. National Park Service, *List of Classified Structures at Gettysburg National Military Park*, structures 25–31.

33. Historic American Buildings Survey, Library of Congress, Survey Number HABS PA-365.

34. Damage Claims, Roll 132.

35. US Department of the Interior, National Park Service, *Impact of War: The Slyder Family Farm*, NPS Teachers' Guide (Gettysburg: US Department of the Interior, National Park Service, n.d.), 42.

36. National Park Service, *List of Classified Structures at Gettysburg National Military Park*, structures 77–85.

37. Damage Claims, Roll 139.

38. Busey and Busey, *Confederate Casualties at Gettysburg*, 2049.

39. Adams claimed to have amputated four legs and one finger among his several operations. It is unlikely that any of those were in the field, however.

40. Timothy H. Smith, *Farms at Gettysburg: The Fields of Battle* (Gettysburg: Thomas, 2007), 31.

41. National Park Service, *List of Classified Structures at Gettysburg National Military Park*, structures 158, 166–169.

42. John Blair Linn, diary, Centre County Library and Historical Museum, Bellefonte, PA.

43. Smith, *Farms at Gettysburg*, 33.

44. State and federal claims for all three men are itemized in National Park Service records at Gettysburg National Military Park.

Chapter 8

1. Ziba B. Graham, "On to Gettysburg" (paper presented to Michigan Military Order of the Loyal Legion of the United States, Detroit, March 2, 1889), Gregory Coco Papers, Box B-69, file 26, Gettysburg National Military Park Archives.

2. Mary Tepe's name appears in the Library of Congress archives as Mary Tippee. *Vivandières*, common in European armies, especially in France, were women who were part of a regiment and sold spirits, tobacco, and other comforts and attended to the sick.

3. O'Rorke's name is often spelled O'Rourke, which is the more common spelling in his native Ireland.

4. Harry Smeltzer, "Gettysburg's Jacob Weikert Farm," Bull Runnings Digital History Project blog, accessed May 5, 2020, https://bullrunnings.wordpress.com/2018/02/20/gettysburgs-jacob-weikert-farm/.

5. Damage Claims, Roll 132.

6. National Park Service, *List of Classified Structures at Gettysburg National Military Park*, structures 98–102.

7. Timothy H. Smith, *Farms at Gettysburg: The Fields of Battle* (Gettysburg: Thomas, 2007), 29.

8. Historic American Buildings Survey, Library of Congress, Survey Number HABS PA-358.

9. Damage Claims, Roll 140.

10. Thomas L. Livermore, *Days and Events, 1860–1866* (Boston: independently published, 1920), 243.

11. Elliott's map of the battlefield of Gettysburg, Pennsylvania (Philadelphia: S. G. Elliott, ca. 1864).

12. William J. Wray, *Life of the 23rd Pennsylvania Birney's Zouaves*, original publication 1904 (New York: Bloch, 2000).

13. National Park Service, *List of Classified Structures at Gettysburg National Military Park*, structures 98–102.

14. Historic American Buildings Survey, Library of Congress, Survey Number HABS PA-580.

15. John W. Busey and Travis W. Busey, *Confederate Casualties at Gettysburg: A Comprehensive Record* (Jefferson, NC: McFarland, 2016), 1858.

16. National Park Service, *List of Classified Structures at Gettysburg National Military Park*, structures 46–52A.

17. Busey and Busey, *Confederate Casualties at Gettysburg*, 2015.

18. Gregory A. Coco, *A Strange and Blighted Land* (Thomas Publications, 1995).

19. National Park Service, *List of Classified Structures at Gettysburg National Military Park*, structures 359, 360. This list shows only the kitchen pump and well, and indicates that this is the Basil Biggs farm. Biggs did not purchase the farm until 1865.

20. Francis M. Wafer diary, Douglas Library, Queen's University at Kingston, Kingston, Ontario, Canada, quoted in Gregory Coco, *A Vast Sea of Misery* (Thomas Publications, 1988).

21. Busey and Busey, *Confederate Casualties at Gettysburg*, 1881.

22. Damage Claims, Roll 134.

23. Historic American Buildings Survey, Library of Congress, Survey Number HABS PA-341.

24. 1860 United States Federal Census, Borough of Gettysburg, Adams County, Pennsylvania, p. 58, lines 23–34, dwelling 407, family 458.

25. 1860 United States Federal Census, p. 60, lines 3–6, dwelling 416, family 469.

26. US Department of the Interior, National Park Service, *Impact of War: The Slyder Family Farm*, NPS Teachers' Guide (Gettysburg: US Department of the Interior, National Park Service, n.d.), 26.

27. Edward S. Salomon, "Gettysburg" (paper presented to Military Order of the Loyal Legion of the United States, California Commandery, January 17, 1912).

28. US Department of the Interior, National Park Service, *Impact of War*, 27.

29. US Department of the Interior, National Park Service, 27.

30. Peter Thorn, damage claim, Adams County Historical Society, Gettysburg.

31. Busey and Busey, *Confederate Casualties at Gettysburg*, 272.

32. Damage Claims, Roll 139.

33. Taken from Lightner's personal story, "A Farmer's Experience," *Gettysburg Compiler*, July 6, 1910.

34. William J. Switala, *Underground Railroad in Pennsylvania* (Mechanicsburg, PA: Stackpole Books, August 2008), 26–27.

35. Busey and Busey, *Confederate Casualties at Gettysburg*, 2010.

36. Damage Claims, Roll 133.

37. Elliott's map.

38. Damage Claims, Roll 139.

39. Association of Military Surgeons, *The Military Surgeon*, ed. Samuel Cecil Stanton, 1913 (repr., Whitefish, MT: Kessinger, 2010), 411, 413.

40. Decimus et Ultimus Barziza, *The Adventures of a Prisoner of War*, ed. R. H. Shuffler (Austin: University of Texas Press, 1964), 54–55.

41. John William Crapster O'Neal, "List of Marked Confederates Buried upon the Battlefield of Gettysburg," Gettysburg National Military Park Archives, n.d.

42. Allen Guelzo, "The Confederate Who Came to Dinner: The Story of James Francis Crocker," *Gettysburg Magazine*, Winter 2012.

Chapter 9

1. William J. Switala, *Underground Railroad in Pennsylvania* (Mechanicsburg, PA: Stackpole Books, August 2008).

2. Damage Claims Roll 139.

3. Captain Richard W. Musgrove, personal notes, July 4, 1863, Gregory Coco Papers, Box B-69, Gettysburg National Military Park Archives.

4. Cornelia Hancock, *Letters of a Civil War Nurse*, ed. Henrietta Stratton Jaquette (Lincoln: University of Nebraska Press, 1998), 8.

5. Justin Dwinell, unpublished, undated medical report of the Battle of Gettysburg, n.p., MSC 129, National Library of Medicine, Bethesda, MD.

6. Levi W. Baker, *History of the 9th Massachusetts Battery* (South Framingham, MA: Lakeview Press, 1888).

7. William Watson, *Letters of a Civil War Surgeon*, ed. Paul Fatout (West Lafayette, IN: Purdue Research Foundation, 1961).

8. US Department of the Interior, National Park Service, Nomination Form, National Register of Historic Places—Daniel Sheaffer Farm, Adams County, Pennsylvania.

9. *Daily Evening Bulletin* (Philadelphia), July 16, 1863.

10. John William Crapster O'Neal, "List of Marked Confederates Buried upon the Battlefield of Gettysburg," Gettysburg National Military Park Archives, n.d.

11. US Department of the Interior, National Park Service, Nomination Form, National Register of Historic Places—Rock Creek/White Run Union Hospital Complex, Adams County, Pennsylvania.

12. US Department of the Interior, National Park Service, Nomination Form, National Register of Historic Places—Rodkey-Diener Farm, Adams County, Pennsylvania.

13. Bushman family records, provided by Bushman descendant Susan Chapman.

14. 1860 United States Federal Census, Borough of Gettysburg, Adams County, Pennsylvania, p. 40, lines 4–17, dwelling 270, family 316.

15. File 214-963, Record Group 92, "Records of the Office of the Quartermaster General (OQMD)," Quartermaster General Files, National Archives and Records Administration.

16. O'Neal, "List of Marked Confederates."

17. US Department of the Interior, National Park Service, Nomination Form, National Register of Historic Places—Peter Conover Farm, Adams County, Pennsylvania.

18. US Department of the Interior, National Park Service, Nomination Form, National Register of Historic Places—Henry Beitler Farm, Adams County, Pennsylvania.

19. File 214-832, Record Group 92, "Records of the Office of the Quartermaster General (OQMD)," Quartermaster General Files, National Archives and Records Administration.

20. Obituary of Samuel Durboraw, *Adams Sentinel*, March 15, 1864.

21. John W. Busey and Travis W. Busey, *Confederate Casualties at Gettysburg: A Comprehensive Record* (Jefferson, NC: McFarland, 2016).

22. Busey and Busey.

23. Information on both Pettygrew and Lusk is found in their Find a Grave descriptions: "Andrew J. Pettygrew," Find a Grave, accessed May 4, 2020, https://www.findagrave.com/memorial/19455288/andrew-j_-pettygrew, and "John Lusk," Find a Grave, accessed May 4, 2020, https://www.findagrave.com/memorial/19361978/john-lusk.

24. Michael A. Dreese, *The 151st Pennsylvania Volunteers at Gettysburg: Like Ripe Apples in a Storm* (Jefferson, NC: McFarland, 2009), 102.

Chapter 10

1. Camp Letterman Papers, Lewis Leigh file, Gettysburg National Military Park archives.

2. Gregory A. Coco, *Wasted Valor: The Confederate Dead at Gettysburg* (Gettysburg: Thomas, 1990), 70.

3. Damage Claims, Roll 135.

4. John W. Busey and Travis W. Busey, *Confederate Casualties at Gettysburg: A Comprehensive Record* (Jefferson, NC: McFarland, 2016), 2011.

5. Busey and Busey, 2017.

6. Damage Claims, Roll 136.

7. Damage Claims, Roll 137.

8. "Battle Days in 1863," *Gettysburg Compiler*, July 4, 1906.

9. Damage Claims, Roll 138.

10. William E. Miller, "The Cavalry Battle Near Gettysburg," Gettysburg National Military Park Archives.

11. Miller.

12. William E. Miller, Medal of Honor citation, July 21, 1897, for actions of July 3, 1863, Congressional Medal of Honor Society.

13. Busey and Busey, *Confederate Casualties at Gettysburg*, 2089.

14. 1860 United States Federal Census, Borough of Gettysburg, Adams County, Pennsylvania, p. 3, lines 18–22, dwelling 19, family 22.

15. National Park Service, *List of Classified Structures at Gettysburg National Military Park*, structures 337–340, 343.

16. National Park Service, structure 337.

17. 1860 United States Federal Census, p. 42, lines 26–29, dwelling 288, family 334.

18. John William Crapster O'Neal, "List of Marked Confederates Buried upon the Battlefield of Gettysburg," Gettysburg National Military Park Archives, n.d.

19. Nicholas Paonessa, supervisor, *Case Report: Bloodstains of Gettysburg: The Use of Chemiluminescent Blood Reagents to Visualize Bloodstains of Historical Significance* (Niagara Falls, NY: Forensic Identification/Crime Scene Unit, Niagara Falls Police Department, 2006), accessed August 14, 2019, https://www.bluestar-forensic.com/medias/content/gettysburg_iabpanews.pdf.

20. Damage Claims, Roll 136.

21. 1860 United States Federal Census, p. 52, lines 1–7, dwelling 358, family 408.

22. Timothy H. Smith, Farms at Gettysburg, 48.
23. Report of the Quartermaster General, July 16, 1863, Adams County Historical Society, Gettysburg.
24. O'Neal, "List of Marked Confederates."

Chapter 11

1. 1860 United States Federal Census, Borough of Gettysburg, Adams County, Pennsylvania, p. 39, lines 5–13, dwelling 264, family 308.
2. Annie Young to her cousin Mina, July 17, 1863, Gregory Coco Papers, Box B-72-1, File 186, Gettysburg National Military Park Archives.
3. Samuel Wilkeson, "Details from Our Special Correspondent," *New York Times*, July 6, 1863.
4. John W. Busey and Travis W. Busey, *Confederate Casualties at Gettysburg: A Comprehensive Record* (Jefferson, NC: McFarland, 2016), 2081.
5. Busey and Busey, 2080.
6. Damage Claims, Roll 135.
7. John William Crapster O'Neal, "List of Marked Confederates Buried upon the Battlefield of Gettysburg," Gettysburg National Military Park Archives, n.d.
8. Busey and Busey, *Confederate Casualties at Gettysburg*, 2121.
9. Michael W. Hofe, *Let There Be No Stain upon My Stones* (Gettysburg: Thomas, 1995), 42–44.
10. Damage Claims, Roll 135.
11. Damage Claims, Roll 139.
12. O'Neal, "List of Marked Confederates."

Chapter 12

1. Historic American Buildings Survey, Library of Congress, Survey Number HABS PA-1963.
2. Elliott's map of the battlefield of Gettysburg, Pennsylvania (Philadelphia: S. G. Elliott, ca. 1864).

3. John William Crapster O'Neal, "List of Marked Confederates Buried upon the Battlefield of Gettysburg," Gettysburg National Military Park Archives, n.d.
4. Damage Claims, Roll 132.
5. Damage Claims, Roll 138.
6. Historic American Buildings Survey, Library of Congress, Survey Number HABS PA-1965.
7. O'Neal, "List of Marked Confederates."
8. Damage Claims, Roll 133.
9. "Youth Held Prisoner Two Days to Shoe Horses for Confederates during Battle," *Gettysburg Times*, commemorative ed., June 24, 1988.
10. Damage Claims, Roll 134.
11. Damage Claims, Roll 135.
12. Damage Claims, Roll 138.
13. Clifton Johnson, *Battleground Adventures* (Boston: Houghton Mifflin, 1915), 189.
14. US Sanitary Commission hospital map, 1863, Gettysburg National Military Park Archives.
15. 1860 United States Federal Census, Borough of Gettysburg, Adams County, Pennsylvania, p. 24, lines 23–30, dwelling 160, family 194.
16. National Park Service, *List of Classified Structures at Gettysburg National Military Park*, structures 159, 160.
17. File 214-766, Record Group 92, "Records of the Office of the Quartermaster General (OQMD)," Quartermaster General files, National Archives and Records Administration.
18. Historic American Buildings Survey, Library of Congress, Survey Number HABS PA-1964.
19. Elliott's map.
20. Damage Claims, Roll 134.

Chapter 13

1. William K. Zieber, *Hanover (PA) Herald*, July 15, 1905.
2. "Marion Hall Had Role of School and Hospital," *Evening Sun* (Hanover, PA), June 22, 1963.

3. "The Old Forney Tavern," *Record Herald* (Hanover, PA), November 1, 1915.
4. George Reeser Powell, *History of York County*, vol. 1 (Chicago: J. H. Beers and Company, 1907).

Chapter 14

1. Church history, dedication service program, Great Conewago Presbyterian Church, June 26, 1988.
2. H. C. Bradsby, M.A. Leeson, and S. Aaron, *1886 History of Adams County* (Chicago: Warner Beers, 1886; repr. Knightstown, IN: Bookmark, 1887), 336–337.
3. Obituary of Boreas Deatrick, *New Oxford Item*, June 14, 1917.
4. John W. Busey and Travis W. Busey, *Confederate Casualties at Gettysburg: A Comprehensive Record* (Jefferson, NC: McFarland, 2016), 2129.

Chapter 15

1. George C. Platt, Medal of Honor citation, July 12, 1895, for actions of July 3, 1863, Congressional Medal of Honor Society.
2. Martin Schwenk, Medal of Honor citation, April 23, 1889, for actions of July 3, 1863, Congressional Medal of Honor Society.
3. Timothy H. Smith, special issue on Fairfield, *Adams County History* 19 (2013): 90.
4. Smith, 90–91.
5. Smith, 5.
6. Smith, 102.

7. Smith, 36–37.
8. Robert L. Bloom, *A History of Adams County, Pennsylvania, 1700–1990* (Gettysburg: Adams County Historical Society, 1992), 139.
9. Damage Claims, Roll 137.
10. John W. Busey and Travis W. Busey, *Confederate Casualties at Gettysburg: A Comprehensive Record* (Jefferson, NC: McFarland, 2016), 2055.

Chapter 16

1. "History of Franklin Township," Franklin Township Board of Supervisors, accessed January 11, 2019, http://franklintwp.us/history/.
2. John W. Busey and Travis W. Busey, *Confederate Casualties at Gettysburg: A Comprehensive Record* (Jefferson, NC: McFarland, 2016), 2054.
3. Damage Claims, Roll 136.
4. "Isaac Rife," Find a Grave, accessed March 30, 2020, https://www.findagrave.com/memorial/15944674/isaac-rife.
5. Busey and Busey, *Confederate Casualties at Gettysburg*.
6. Damage Claims, Roll 138.
7. "Elizabeth Rife Mickley/Young," Find a Grave, accessed March 30, 2020, https://www.findagrave.com/memorial/6896829/elizabeth-mickley_young.
8. Damage Claims, Roll 136.
9. Damage Claims, Roll 139.
10. Civil War Trails, historical marker outside inn.
11. Damage Claims, Roll 136.

Index